Atlas of
Descriptive
Histology

Atlas of Descriptive Histology

THIRD EDITION

Edward J. Reith, Ph.D.

Department of Anatomy
College of Medicine, University of Florida

Michael H. Ross, Ph.D.

Department of Anatomy
College of Medicine, University of Florida

HARPER & ROW, PUBLISHERS
New York, Hagerstown, San Francisco, London

Project Editor: Henry Krawitz
Production Supervisor: Will C. Jomarrón
Compositor: Ruttle, Shaw & Wetherill, Inc.
Printer and Binder: The Murray Printing Company

ATLAS OF DESCRIPTIVE HISTOLOGY, *Third Edition*

Library of Congress Cataloging in Publication Data

Reith, Edward J
    Atlas of descriptive histology.

    Includes index.
    1. Histolgy—Atlases. I. Ross, Michael H., joint author. II. Title. [DNLM: 1. Histology—Atlases. QS517 R379a]
QM557.R4   1978   611'.018   77-22970
ISBN 0-06-045368-0

CONTENTS

PREFACE   ix
PREFACE TO THE FIRST EDITION   xi

INTRODUCTION   *1*

Chapter 1. EPITHELIUM   *3*
  PLATE 1-1. Squamous Epithelia   6
  PLATE 1-2. Cuboidal, Columnar, and Pseudostratified
             Columnar Epithelia   8
  PLATE 1-3. Transitional Epithelium, "Nonsurface"
             Epithelium, and Epithelioid Cells   10
  PLATE 1-4. Columnar Epithelium, Electron Microscopy   12
  PLATE 1-5. Striated Border, Terminal Web, Junctional
             Complex, Basement Lamina, Electron
             Microscopy   14

Chapter 2. CONNECTIVE TISSUE   *16*
  PLATE 2-1. Loose Connective Tissue   20
  PLATE 2-2. Connective Tissue, Electron Microscopy   22
  PLATE 2-3. Connective Tissue Cells, Electron
             Microscopy   24
  PLATE 2-4. Dense Connective Tissue   26
  PLATE 2-5. Regular Connective Tissue   28
  PLATE 2-6. Elastic Fibers, Elastic Tissue, and
             Embryonic Connective Tissue   30

Chapter 3. SUPPORTING TISSUE   *32*
  PLATE 3-1. Cartilage   34
  PLATE 3-2. Cartilage I, Electron Microscopy   36
  PLATE 3-3. Cartilage II, Electron Microscopy   38
  PLATE 3-4. Cartilage, Fetal Skeleton   40
  PLATE 3-5. Cartilage and Spongy Bone   42
  PLATE 3-6. Fibrocartilage   44

CONTENTS

PLATE 3-7. Compact Lamellar Bone   46
PLATE 3-8. Cortical Bone, Electron Microscopy   48
PLATE 3-9. Endochondral Bone Formation I   50
PLATE 3-10. Endochondral Bone Formation II   52
PLATE 3-11. Intramembranous Bone Formation   54
PLATE 3-12. Developing Bone I, Electron Microscopy   56
PLATE 3-13. Developing Bone II, Electron Microscopy   58
PLATE 3-14. The Osteoclast, Electron Microscopy   60

Chapter 4. BLOOD   62
PLATE 4-1. Erythrocytes and Agranulocytes   64
PLATE 4-2. Granulocytes   66

Chapter 5. MUSCLE TISSUE   68
PLATE 5-1. Smooth Muscle   70
PLATE 5-2. Smooth Muscle, Longitudinal Section,
            Electron Microscopy   72
PLATE 5-3. Smooth Muscle, Cross Section, Electron
            Microscopy   74
PLATE 5-4. Skeletal Muscle   76
PLATE 5-5. Skeletal Muscle I, Electron Microscopy   78
PLATE 5-6. Skeletal Muscle II, Electron Microscopy   80
PLATE 5-7. Cardiac Muscle   82
PLATE 5-8. Cardiac Muscle, Intercalated Disc,
            Electron Microscopy   84
PLATE 5-9. Cardiac Muscle, Purkinje Fibers   86

Chapter 6. NERVOUS SYSTEM   88
PLATE 6-1. Sympathetic Ganglion   90
PLATE 6-2. Sympathetic Ganglion I, Electron
            Microscopy   92
PLATE 6-3. Sympathetic Ganglion II, Electron
            Microscopy   94
PLATE 6-4. Dorsal Root Ganglion   96
PLATE 6-5. Peripheral Nerve   98
PLATE 6-6. Perineurium, Electron Microscopy   100
PLATE 6-7. Cerebrum   102
PLATE 6-8. Cerebellum   104
PLATE 6-9. Spinal Cord   106

Chapter 7. CARDIOVASCULAR SYSTEM   108
PLATE 7-1. Heart   110
PLATE 7-2. The Aorta   112
PLATE 7-3. Muscular Arteries and Veins   114
PLATE 7-4. Arterioles and Lymphatic Vessels   116
PLATE 7-5. Arteriole, Electron Microscopy   118

Chapter 8. LYMPHATIC TISSUE AND ORGANS   120
PLATE 8-1. Tonsil and Lymph Node I   122
PLATE 8-2. Lymph Node II   124

PLATE 8-3.   Lymph Node III, Electron Microscopy   126
PLATE 8-4.   Lymph Node IV, Electron Microscopy   128
PLATE 8-5.   Spleen I   130
PLATE 8-6.   Spleen II   132
PLATE 8-7.   Thymus   134

Chapter 9. INTEGUMENT   *136*
PLATE 9-1.   Skin I   138
PLATE 9-2.   Skin II   140

Chapter 10. DIGESTIVE SYSTEM   *142*
PLATE 10-1.   Tongue I   144
PLATE 10-2.   Tongue II   146
PLATE 10-3.   Soft Palate   148
PLATE 10-4.   Salivary Glands I   150
PLATE 10-5.   Salivary Glands II   152
PLATE 10-6.   Developing Tooth   154
PLATE 10-7.   Esophagus   156
PLATE 10-8.   Esophagus and Stomach, Cardiac
               Region   158
PLATE 10-9.   Stomach, Fundic Region   160
PLATE 10-10.   Stomach, Pyloric Region   162
PLATE 10-11.   Small Intestine   164
PLATE 10-12.   Duodenum   166
PLATE 10-13.   Villi   168
PLATE 10-14.   Intestinal Glands and Muscularis
               Externa   170
PLATE 10-15.   Appendix and Large Intestine   172
PLATE 10-16.   Mucosa of Large Intestine   174
PLATE 10-17.   Liver I   176
PLATE 10-18.   Liver II   178
PLATE 10-19.   Gall Bladder   180
PLATE 10-20.   Pancreas   182

Chapter 11. RESPIRATORY SYSTEM   *185*
PLATE 11-1.   Olfactory Mucosa   186
PLATE 11-2.   The Larynx   188
PLATE 11-3.   Trachea and Bronchus   190
PLATE 11-4.   Bronchus and Bronchiole   192
PLATE 11-5.   Respiratory Bronchiole, Alveolar
               Duct, Alveolar Sac, and Alveolus   194

Chapter 12. URINARY SYSTEM   *196*
PLATE 12-1.   Kidney I   198
PLATE 12-2.   Kidney II   200
PLATE 12-3.   Kidney III   202
PLATE 12-4.   Ureter   204
PLATE 12-5.   Urinary Bladder   206

CONTENTS

Chapter 13. MALE REPRODUCTIVE SYSTEM   208
    PLATE 13-1. Testis I   210
    PLATE 13-2. Testis II   212
    PLATE 13-3. Efferent Ductules and Epididymis   214
    PLATE 13-4. Ductus Deferens and Seminal Vesicle   216
    PLATE 13-5. Prostate Gland   218

Chapter 14. FEMALE REPRODUCTIVE SYSTEM   221
    PLATE 14-1. Ovary I   222
    PLATE 14-2. Ovary II   224
    PLATE 14-3. Corpus Luteum   226
    PLATE 14-4. Uterine Tube   228
    PLATE 14-5. Uterus   230
    PLATE 14-6. The Cervix   232
    PLATE 14-7. Vagina   234
    PLATE 14-8. Mammary Gland, Inactive   236
    PLATE 14-9. Mammary Gland, Proliferative   238
    PLATE 14-10. Mammary Gland, Lactating   240
    PLATE 14-11. Placenta I   242
    PLATE 14-12. Placenta II   244

Chapter 15. ENDOCRINE SYSTEM   247
    PLATE 15-1. Thyroid Gland   248
    PLATE 15-2. Parathyroid Gland   250
    PLATE 15-3. Pituitary Gland I   252
    PLATE 15-4. Pituitary Gland II   254
    PLATE 15-5. Adrenal Gland I   256
    PLATE 15-6. Adrenal Gland II   258
    PLATE 15-7. Pineal Gland   260

Chapter 16. THE ORGANS OF SPECIAL SENSE   263
    PLATE 16-1. The Eye I   264
    PLATE 16-2. The Eye II   266
    PLATE 16-3. The Eye III   268
    PLATE 16-4. The Eye IV   270
    PLATE 16-5. The Ear   272
    PLATE 16-6. Organ of Corti   274

INDEX   277

PREFACE

THE THIRD EDITION of this book was prepared with the same objectives as those of the original work. It introduces little change with respect to the approach selected in describing to the student the microscopic appearance of the various tissues and organs of the body. The gratifying and wide acceptance of previous editions of the *Atlas* by students and teachers has reinforced our original thinking with regard to its basic philosophy. Indeed, it is this acceptance that has dictated restraint in modifying the format.

The most apparent change in the *Atlas* is the inclusion of a number of electron micrographs dealing chiefly with tissues. The intent of these micrographs is not to expand into the area of cell fine structure, but rather to give the student more confidence in the interpretation of a slide preparation. The electron microscope is able to resolve many structures that are either not visible with the light microscope or not fully apparent. By referring to the electron micrographs and their accompanying text, the student is able to bring to bear information pertinent to the interpretation of the slide preparation. Accordingly, the electron micrographs were selected for their specific value in serving as a source of background information in the interpretation of a tissue section with the light microscope.

The less obvious changes in the third edition include changes in nomenclature that have come about in recent years, as well as the introduction of certain theoretical concepts of histology as they relate to understanding the image seen in the light microscope.

EDWARD J. REITH, Ph.D.
MICHAEL H. ROSS, Ph.D.

Gainesville, Florida

PREFACE TO THE
FIRST EDITION

THIS BOOK IS DESIGNED to assist the student in the laboratory. It was not designed to present the theoretical subject matter of histology as it is found in standard textbooks, but rather to present an account of microscopic appearances in the language of the histologist.

Histology involves not only the analysis of three-dimensional structure by the examination of two-dimensional specimens, but also the application of whatever methods and techniques help the histologist to understand structure, function, and cellular interrelationships in a more dynamic way. Autoradiography, tissue culture, histo- and cytochemistry, electron microscopy, X-ray diffraction, etc., have all been incorporated into the thinking of the histologist, and much of this information has been incorporated into histology textbooks. The student is concerned not only with the necessity of becoming familiar with much of this information, but also with the necessity of learning how to "read" slides. Yet one of the perplexing features of textbook accounts is that very often they do not make a sharp distinction between microanatomy and actual microscopic appearance. Cellular details are often described in textbooks, but the details may not be evident in a routine H & E section. When a student looks through a microscope to examine a slide, he wants to know what is on the slide and what interpretations can be made from it. This book is designed to assist the student in the laboratory when he is confronted with these questions.

A series of extensively labeled photomicrographs have been selected which usually include illustrations at low magnification, thereby providing a panoramic view of the section, and then significant areas were selected for examination at higher magnification. In the descriptive accounts, much emphasis is placed on characteristics of the histologic section and particularly on the reasons why a structure is identified as such.

The interpretation of a histologic slide primarily involves the recognition of forms, general organization, and location of parts. Identification by specific color reaction is less important. This point is emphasized by the use of black and white in the *Atlas*. The histologist can recognize cross striations of muscle regardless of whether they are stained red with eosin, dark blue with iron hematoxylin, or unstained and examined with phase contrast optics; he can recognize nuclei regardless of whether they are stained dark blue by hematoxylin of an H & E stain or red by the acid fuchsin of a trichrome. He does this by considering their form, arrangement, and location. The histology student should attempt to develop this skill, for he will quickly learn that a particular organ or tissue stained at different times, by different people, may not have quite the same color characteristics. This is not to say that the histologist does not make use of staining reactions; he does. However, he depends more on differences rather than specific color reaction. It should be noted that whereas the black-and-white reproductions do show the differences in staining reaction, they emphasize the more important criteria, namely, shape, location, and organization.

The student will find this book useful chiefly in the laboratory. However, he will also find it useful in preparing for examinations at home, especially those that involve a "practical," for in reality the photomicrographs are the closest thing to an actual slide and far closer to the slide than composite illustrations.

EDWARD J. REITH, Ph.D.
MICHAEL H. ROSS, Ph.D.

New York City

Atlas of Descriptive Histology

INTRODUCTION

The illustrations in this book contain light micrographs of routine histological sections, as well as a number of electron micrographs. All except two of the light micrographs are paraffin sections, and most of them have been stained with hematoxylin and eosin (H & E).

In order to adequately interpret a light micrograph (or a specimen on a slide), it is useful to know how specimens are prepared, because during their preparation tissues undergo a number of alterations. Water-soluble materials are lost while the specimen is in aqueous solutions; lipids are lost while in lipid solvents; shrinkage occurs during a number of steps; and, finally, fixation (the first step) has a profound effect on the staining of certain tissue components.

For routine light microscopy, the tissue is first placed in a fixative, which is intended to preserve the structure of the tissue and to prepare it for future treatments. After the tissue has been fixed, it is embedded in a hard substance, such as paraffin, so that adequately thin sections can be cut. This introduces several additional steps because paraffin is not miscible with water. Therefore, the water must be removed from the tissue and replaced by a liquid which is miscible with paraffin. In order to accomplish this, the specimen is dehydrated through a graded series of alcohol solutions and placed in a nonaqueous liquid, e.g., xylene. It is then infiltrated with melted paraffin. The paraffin (containing the tissue) is allowed to cool and harden. It is trimmed to form a block and then sectioned with a microtome. The sections are placed on a slide with a small amount of albumin serving as an adhesive. The specimen, however, is still unsuitable for examination with a microscope, since paraffin is infiltrated throughout the tissue; moreover, the tissue section is colorless and must be stained. Prior to staining, the paraffin is dissolved out and the tissue is rehydrated (by being passed through a graded series of alcohol solutions to water). The tissue is then stained. At this point the slide is still not ready for microscopic examination. In order to obtain a permanent preparation, the stained tissue section must be dehydrated again and, using a nonaqueous mounting medium, covered with a coverslip.

Hematoxylin and eosin are dyes commonly used in preparing routine stained specimens. Hematoxylin stains nuclei, some cytoplasmic components, such as the ergastoplasm (a ribosome-containing component), and some extracellular materials, such as the matrix of cartilage. Eosin stains most cytoplasmic components (e.g., the cytoplasmic filaments of muscle cells) and extracellular fibers. In addition to hematoxylin and eosin, a large number of other stains can be applied to tissue sections. Some of these are employed to illustrate materials which are not adequately visualized by H & E. However, these special methods should be thought of as supplementing, not replacing, the H & E preparations.

Tissues for electron microscopy are prepared using essentially the same principals as for light microscopy. There are, however, certain differences related to the fact that in the electron microscope electrons are used as a "light source." The electrons are made to pass through the specimen and then impinge on photographic film (or on a screen for direct visualization). Image formation in the electron microscope is dependent upon the fact that some electrons do not pass through the specimen to fall on the photographic film; rather, they are deflected by substances of high mass normally within the specimen or added to the specimen during fixation and staining.

Because of the higher resolution of the electron microscope, it is necessary to use fixatives which maximally preserve structure. These fixatives retain many of the substances which are ordinarily lost during the preparation of tissue for the light microscope. Current procedures of fixation involve the use of glutaraldehyde, which is especially useful in retaining protein constituents of the cell, and osmium tetroxide, which retains the lipid components, especially phospholipid. Because it contains a heavy metal, the latter fixative also plays a major role in electron deflection and consequent image formation. Instead of paraffin, the tissues are embedded in a plastic permitting extremely thin sections to be cut. Special microtomes, usually equipped with diamond knives, are utilized for this purpose. After cutting the tissue, the sections are placed on a copper-mesh grid and then stained. The stains employed contain heavy metals, e.g., uranyl acetate and lead nitrate. In contrast to the procedure for light microscopy, where paraffin must be removed before staining, the plastic-embedded preparation does not require removal of the embedding medium prior to staining. The grid containing the stained section is then placed in the electron microscope and the portion of the specimen which spans the openings in the grid may be visualized and photographed.

1 EPITHELIUM

EPITHELIUM consists of cells that are closely applied to each other with no intervening fibrous material. It is found on surfaces and as the functional units (parenchyma) of glands. The outer surface of the body, the body tubes, and the body cavities (except joint cavities and bursae) are lined by epithelium. The tissue under these various surface epithelia is *connective tissue* and separating the epithelium from the underlying connective tissue is a basement membrane. Prior to the era of electron microscopy, unless specifically stained, basement membranes were visible only under certain epithelia such as the tracheal epithelia. When the basement membrane of the trachea was examined with the electron microscope, it was found to consist of a thin amorphous layer, designated the basal lamina, and a thicker layer containing delicate collagen (reticular) fibrils, designated the reticular lamina. The basal lamina is immediately subjacent to the epithelium and the reticular lamina faces the underlying connective tissue. Subsequent studies have shown that almost all epithelia possess a basal lamina but not a reticular layer. This has led to some looseness in the use of the various terms. Although the thin amorphous layer is usually referred to as the basal lamina, it is also called the basement membrane (or basal membrane) even though there is no associated reticular layer.

Blood vessels are present in connective tissue, but they do not penetrate the basement membranes to enter the epithelial layers. Therefore, epithelial surfaces are sometimes described as being avascular.

Typically, glands develop from epithelial surfaces by growing into the underlying connective tissue. In some cases, the connection of the gland to the surface is retained, as in the salivary glands; in other cases the connection is lost, as in the thyroid gland. As already mentioned, the gland cells, being epithelium, are separated from the connective tissue and its blood vessels by a basement membrane. However, in some glands (e.g., liver), the relationship between epithelium and blood vessels becomes extremely intimate and in many species there is no basal lamina.

Some glandular tissue within the body does not develop from surfaces. For example, in the ovary the theca lutein cells of the corpus luteum are derivatives of the connective tissue that surrounds the Graafian follicle. Yet these cells assume most of the characteristics of glandular epithelium. The interstitial cells of Leydig in the testis also develop from connective tissue, and they too assume some of the characteristics of epithelial cells. Still another example can be cited in the development of certain tubules of the kidney. In this process, mesodermal cells of the embryo aggregate and surround themselves by a basal lamina. They then establish a lumen and become tubules. Finally, the mesodermally-derived tubules fuse with other tubules which have grown from an epithelial surface. By all adult criteria, the cells of the renal tubules are epithelium, although they are derived from the mesoderm of the embryo.

Epithelial cells perform a variety of functions. They absorb substances from the lumen of the alimentary canal and the lumen of the kidney tubules, and they secrete other substances into these lumens. Epithelial cells engage in a wide range of synthetic activity throughout the body. They synthesize an intracellular protein, keratin, which covers the surface of the body; they synthesize mucus to lubricate body tubes; they synthesize digestive enzymes and hormones; and in the liver, they subject many materials that are absorbed from the alimentary canal to a host of chemical transformations before these materials pass into the systemic circulation. As a final example, it is pointed out that epithelial cells are the transducer components of the special senses, namely, sight, hearing, smell, position, movement, and taste.

Epithelium is classified according to the arrangement and shape of its cells. Epithelium which is only one cell deep is called *simple;* epithelium which is more than one cell deep is called *stratified.* On the basis of cell shape, epithelium is designated as *squamous, cuboidal,* or *columnar.* Thus by joining these descriptive terms, we may describe an epithelium as simple squamous, as stratified squamous, or stratified cuboidal, etc. In the case of stratified epithelia, only the surface cells are used for the descriptive nomenclature. For example, stratified squamous epithelium is so designated because it consists of more than one cell layer and its surface cells are squamous. In a number of glands the epithelial cells have a pyramidal shape; these may be classified as either cuboidal or columnar, depending upon the height of the cell. In many cases the size and shape of a cell may constitute one of the indices of its function or state of activity. For example, the cells which make up the thyroid follicle are columnar when active, owing to stimulation by thyroid stimulating hormone (TSH). On the other hand, when the cells are not under the influence of TSH they may be cuboidal or squamous.

In two locations, epithelium has special names, *endothelium* and *mesothelium.* Endothelium lines the inner surface of the heart, blood vessels, and lymphatic vessels. Mesothelium lines the serous membranes of the body, namely, the pleura, the pericardium and the peritoneum.

The free surface of epithelial cells may contain cilia, stereocilia, or microvilli according to the function of the cells. Cilia enable the cells to move mucus or other materials along the surface. Stereocilia are special surface modifications that are found in the ductus epididymis and the ductus deferens. Microvilli are found on the surface of cells that engage in absorptive activity. Although they cannot be identified individually with the light microscope, the microvilli in the intestines are arranged as closely packed cylindrical projections which constitute the striated border. In the kidney, microvilli of certain tubule cells are also closely packed, somewhat longer than those in the intestines but not so uniform in height; collectively, they constitute the brush border.

Plate 1-1. Squamous Epithelia

The flat face of *simple squamous epithelium* (mesothelium) of the peritoneum is shown in Figure 1. The specimen was prepared by stripping off the surface of the peritoneum and treating the spread with silver to delineate the cell boundaries. The specimen was also stained to reveal the nuclei (**N**). The silver appears as the black precipitate; it marks the extent of the cytoplasm (**C**). Note that each cell has a polygonal shape and is in immediate apposition with its neighbors. The mesothelial cells are shaped like thin plates. When they are sectioned at right angles to the surface (Fig. 2), the nuclei (**N**) appear as elongated structures which produce a slight bulging of the cell, and the cytoplasm (**C**) appears as a thin band along the surface. Under the epithelium is the supporting connective tissue (**CT**). [Below the connective tissue are smooth muscle (**SM**) cells cut in cross section. The highly irregular contour of the surface mesothelium is due to the contracted state of the smooth muscle.]

The simple squamous epithelium (endothelium) lining a lymphatic vessel is shown in Figure 3. The nuclei (**N**) of the endothelial cells are the dark-staining elongated structures which bulge slightly into the lumen. The cytoplasm (**C**) appears as the linear extension that continues from the extremities of the nuclei. Actually, this thin line represents two plasma membranes and a small amount of intervening cytoplasm. Over the nuclei, the cytoplasm is so attenuated that the nuclei appear to be naked and exposed to the lumen. It is not possible to determine where one endothelial cell ends and the next begins.

Mesothelium, endothelium, and other simple squamous epithelia all have the same general appearance. Any differences in appearance between the epithelia in Figures 2 and 3 are not to be regarded as significant. Histologically, mesothelium and endothelium are distinguished from each other on the basis of their location, not their appearance.

Stratified squamous epithelium of the tongue is shown in Figure 4. The surface cells and their nuclei (**arrows**) are flat; hence, the name "squamous"; the deeper cells are less flat and the deepest cells are columnar, cuboidal, or polyhedral. The boundaries

(**arrowheads**) between the cells can be seen in the middle of the layer. Note that the cells are in intimate contact with each other. The deepest epithelial cells, i.e., those in immediate proximity to the connective tissue, are referred to as the basal layer (**BL**).

Provision must be made for the replacement of surface cells that are lost for one reason or another. In the case of mesothelial cells, these can be replaced by underlying connective tissue cells and presumably from neighboring mesothelial cells. However, the replacement of epithelium by underlying connective tissue cells is unique and is confined to mesothelium. Endothelial cells are replaced by division of neighboring endothelial cells. Other kinds of simple epithelia are likewise replaced by cells within the epithelial layer. For all stratified epithelia, surface cells are replaced by cells which move up from the basal layer where they are produced.

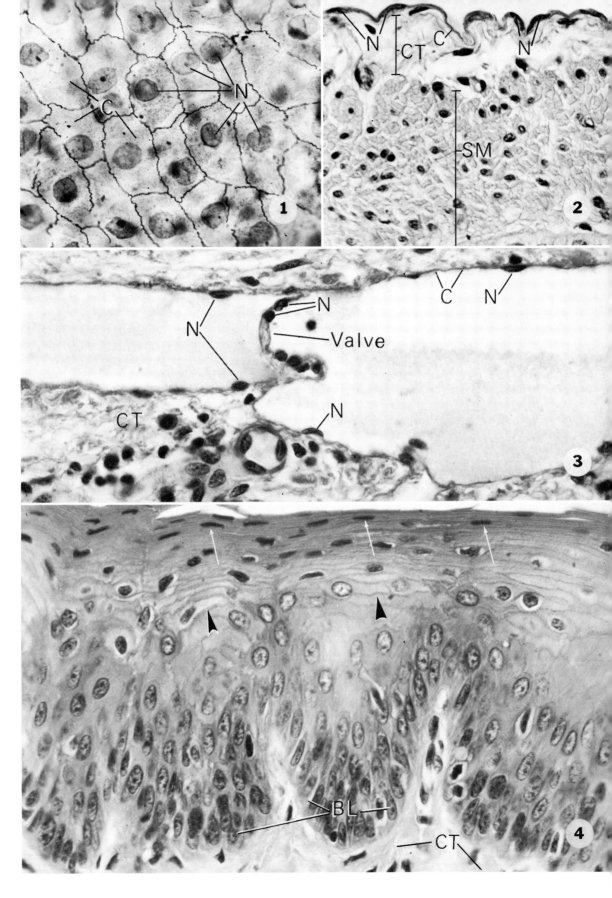

PLATE 1-1

EPITHELIUM

Plate 1-2. Cuboidal, Columnar, and Pseudostratified Columnar Epithelia

The *cuboidal epithelium* (**Ep**) that lines the surface of the ovary is shown in Figure 1. A small amount of cytoplasm surrounds each nucleus. The boundaries between the cells are not distinct and the epithelium appears as a row of nuclei. However, even without being able to see distinct cell boundaries, it is relatively easy to envision that the height and breadth of the individual cells is approximately equal, therefore, this epithelium is designated as cuboidal. Under the epithelium is the supporting connective tissue (**CT**).

The *columnar epithelium* of the gall bladder is shown in Figure 2. The part of the cell which contacts the basement membrane is referred to as basal; it contains the elongated nucleus. The part of the cell near the surface is referred to as apical. The cytoplasm of these cells appears homogeneous and stains with eosin. The cells are closely packed. In some places the lateral cell boundaries are perceptible, helping to define their shape. If the nuclei are examined critically, one gets the impression that the cells are arranged in two layers. This is a reflection of the oblique plane of section. Because of this, the epithelium appears taller than it actually is, and the nuclei tend to appear at more than one level. The columnar epithelium of the small intestines is shown in Figure 3. Here, two kinds of cells are present: columnar absorptive cells and goblet cells (**GC**). The absorptive cells are tall and thin. They possess an elongate nucleus consistent with the shape of the cell. The free surface contains a striated border (**SB**). The round nuclei within the epithelial layer belong to lymphocytes (**Lym**). The goblet cells contain a "cup" of mucus in their apical portions, just above the nucleus. The cytoplasm in the basal portion of these cells is very attenuated, and in one of the cells (**arrow**), it appears as a thin cytoplasmic stalk.

Figure 4 shows the ciliated *pseudostratified columnar epithelium* of a bronchus. Each cilium is connected to a basal body (**BB**), which collectively appear as the dark band at the base of the cilia (**C**). Three cell types are present: columnar cells, goblet cells (**GC**), and basal cells (**BC**). Basal cells are close to the basement membrane. They have a small amount of cytoplasm which does not reach the surface. In this preparation, the nuclei of the

KEY

BB, basal bodies
BC, basal cells
C, cilia
CT, connective tissue
Ep, epithelium
GC, goblet cells
Lym, lymphocytes
S, stereocilia
SB, striated border
TB, terminal bars
arrow, cytoplasmic "stalk" of goblet cell

Figs. 1–4 (monkey), x 640; Fig. 5 (rabbit), x 640.

basal cells are spherical; the nuclei of the columnar cells are slightly larger and ovoid; the nuclei of the goblet cells appear as the dark, elongated, horizontally oriented structures at the base of the mucous cup. This epithelium is designated pseudostratified because all the cells contact the basement membrane.

The pseudostratified columnar epithelium of the ductus epididymis is shown in Figure 5. Most of the cells in this figure are columnar. Some basal cells (**BC**) are also present. The surface projections of the columnar cells are stereocilia (**S**). Electron micrographs show these to be long, branching microvilli. In the light microscope they have a wavy, tapering appearance. The terminal bars (**TB**) appear as small dark bodies near the surface of the epithelium where adjacent cells meet.

Neither stratified columnar epithelium nor stratified cuboidal has wide distribution. Stratified columnar epithelium occurs at certain junctional sites where stratified squamous epithelium meets pseudostratified or simple columnar epithelium. Examples are: soft palate (see Plate 10-3); pharynx (where oropharynx meets nasopharynx); larynx (Plate 11-2); and anal canal. Stratified columnar may also be found lining the large ducts of glands, e.g., the salivary glands and pancreas.

Stratified cuboidal epithelium is found chiefly as the lining of ducts, e.g., in the sweat glands (Plate 9-2, Fig. 2), in smaller ducts of pancreas and salivary glands, and in the mammary gland (Plate 14-8, Fig. 2).

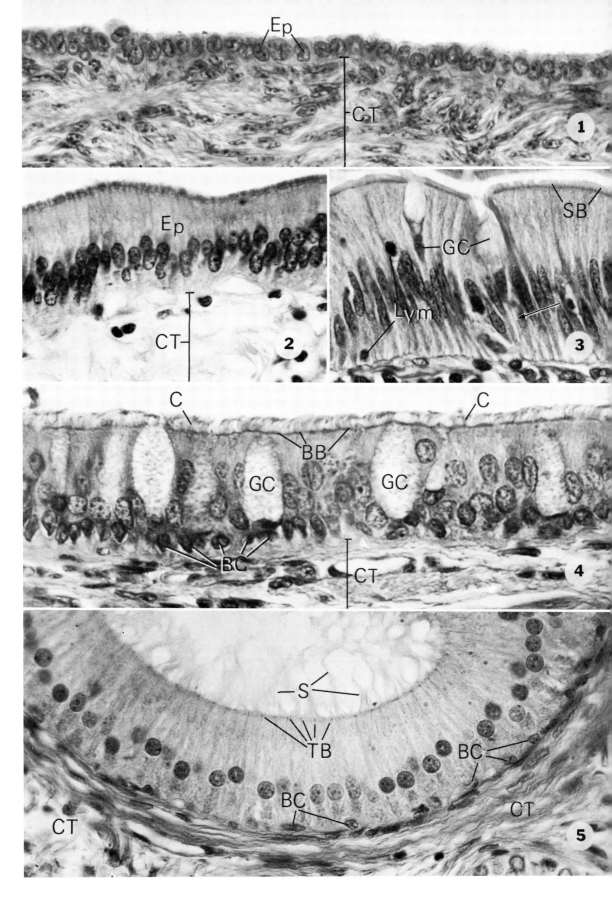

PLATE 1-2

Plate 1-3. TRANSITIONAL EPITHELIUM, "NONSURFACE" EPITHELIUM, AND EPITHELIOID CELLS

Transitional epithelium is present on the inner surface of the renal pelvis, the ureters, the urinary bladder, and part of the urethra. Figure 1 shows the transitional epithelium (**Ep**) from an empty urinary bladder and the underlying connective tissue (**CT**). The epithelium appears to be about four or five cells deep. The cells on the surface are large and dome shaped and occasionally two nuclei (**arrow**) are seen in a single cell. The cells immediately under the surface cells are pear shaped and slightly smaller than the surface cells. The deepest cells are smaller than the surface cells, and as a consequence the nuclei of these cells appear more crowded. When the bladder is distended, the epithelial cells are flattened and the epithelium appears to be only two or three cells deep. It should be noted, however, that a specimen of the bladder wall is usually in a contracted state when it is removed, unless special steps have been taken to preserve it in a distended state.

An example of a *"nonsurface" epithelium* is illustrated in Figure 2. It shows the cuboidal cells of the liver. The cells are arranged as interconnecting sheets, and when sectioned, they appear as cords one or more cells deep according to the plane of section. The nuclei of these cells are spherical; they are surrounded by a granular cytoplasm. The elongated spaces between the cords of cells are vascular channels (sinusoids) (**S**). Although liver cells do not occupy a surface, or constitute a surface in the usual sense, their epithelial nature is indicated by the fact that they contact each other by their lateral borders, a minimum of intercellular "cementing" material is between the cells, and obviously no fibrous material is between the cells. These cells are glandular epithelium (of the liver) which have developed from the endoderm. They retain a connection with the alimentary canal by extremely small canals, the bile canaliculi. These are actually channel-like spaces between adjacent hepatic cells, and they can just barely be seen with the light microscope (see Plate 10-18).

Figure 3 shows interstitial (Leydig) cells of the testis. These cells (**Epd**) possess certain epithelial characteristics. However, they do not develop from a surface; instead they de-

KEY

Ep, epithelium
Epd, epithelioid cells
CT, connective tissue
S, sinusoid
arrow (Fig. 1), binucleate cell
arrows (Fig. 4), nuclei of epithelioid cells of the thymus gland

Figs. 1–4 (monkey), x 640; Fig. 4 (human, 7 mos.), x 640.

velop from connective tissue type cells. They are referred to as *epithelioid cells* because of the following characteristics: the nuclei are spherical and vesiculated, and they are surrounded by a discernible amount of vesiculated cytoplasm. Moreover, the cell borders can be seen and the cells contact similar neighboring cells much the same as epithelial cells contact each other.

Figure 4 shows cells which are also referred to as epithelioid. They develop from the endodermal epithelium; however, they come to assume certain connective tissue characteristics. These are the "reticular" cells or the epithelioid cells of the thymus gland. They possess relatively large, pale-staining nuclei (**arrows**). These stand out among the more numerous, smaller, intensely staining nuclei of the lymphocytes (thymocytes). In some cases, the cytoplasm of the epithelioid cells can be seen; however, the cells are not seen to contact similar neighboring cells in the typical manner of epithelial cells.

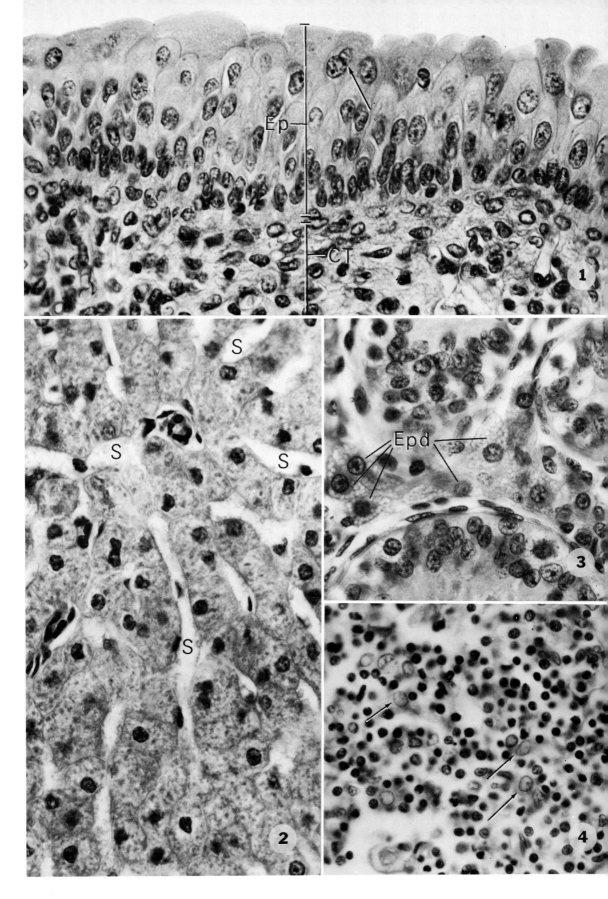

PLATE 1-3

Plate 1-4. Columnar Epithelium, Electron Microscopy

This electron micrograph of the small intestine illustrates some of the salient features of epithelium, particularly as they relate to the light microscopic image. It includes some of the underlying connective tissue, which in this instance is almost entirely occupied by a capillary containing a number of red blood cells (**RBC**).

The epithelium is the same type as that illustrated in Figure 3, Plate 1-2. However, all of the cells are the absorptive type; no goblet cells are included. Also, though distinctly columnar, the cells are not nearly as tall as the absorptive cells in Figure 3. The two round cells at the base of the epithelium are lymphocytes (**Lym**) which migrated from the connective tissue. Similar lymphocyte invasion of the epithelium, a typical occurrence, is also seen in Figure 3, Plate 1-2.

In appraising the electron micrograph, note first the relationship between the cells above the level of the nuclei. The cytoplasm of each cell comes into intimate apposition with its neighbors and consequently the cell boundaries at this magnification are difficult to discern. Below this level prominent intercellular spaces are present (**asterisks**). Here it is easy to define the limits of the individual cells. Next, examine the very basal aspect of the epithelium. Note that each cell extends by means of lateral cytoplasmic processes (**arrows**) to meet with its neighbors, thus again providing intimate cell apposition. [At one site these basal processes are discontinuous (**circles**). This is probably due to the recent migration of the lymphocytes from the connective tissue into the epithelium.] The basal cytoplasmic extensions rest on the basement membrane, or using the more proper electron microscopic term, *basal lamina.* [The basal lamina is actually not recognizeable at this low magnification, but can be seen in the next plate.] The intercellular spaces, in effect, form a continuous compartment between the epithelial cells; the compartment itself being bounded above by the apical cytoplasm, where adjoining cells meet and below by the lateral basal processes which also join with one another. The visualization of this intercellular space is also possible with the light microscope (Plate 1-2, Fig. 3, and Plate 10-13, Fig. 2). The presence of intercellular spaces

KEY

Lym, lymphocyte
RBC, red blood cells
arrows, basal lateral processes
asterisks, intercellular spaces
circles, discontinuity between basal processes
curved arrows, junctional complexes

Fig. x 4,100.

of this type is characteristic of epithelia actively engaged in fluid transport, i.e., the active movement of fluid across an epithelium from lumen to the underlying connective tissue, and thus may be observed not only in the intestine, but in many other epithelia where fluid is actively transported. The essential point, however, is that despite the intercellular spaces, these cells, as an epithelium, do maintain intimate apposition with one another, and in this way provide a selective barrier.

Two other features pertinent to epithelial cells as they relate to light micrography are also evident in this micrograph. One concerns the appositional integrity of the individual cells, namely, the *junctional complexes* (**curved arrows**). Each complex appears as a short, thin, dark line in the electron micrograph. The complex provides strong adhesion between adjoining cells and serves as a permeability barrier. Their unit structure and functional aspects, are dealt with on the next text page. The junctional complexes are comparable to the fine dot-like structures seen in the light microscope where they are referred to as *terminal bars* (see Plate 1-2, Fig. 5).

The other feature worthy of mention here relates to the microvilli which extend from the apical surface of the epithelial cells. In the small intestine the microvilli appear as closely packed finger-like cytoplasmic projections, extremely uniform in size and shape. Because of their uniformity, at the light microscope level, they have a finely striped or striated appearance, hence the term *striated border.* Examination of Plate 1-2, Fig. 3, once again, reveals the striated border as seen at medium power magnification in the light microscope.

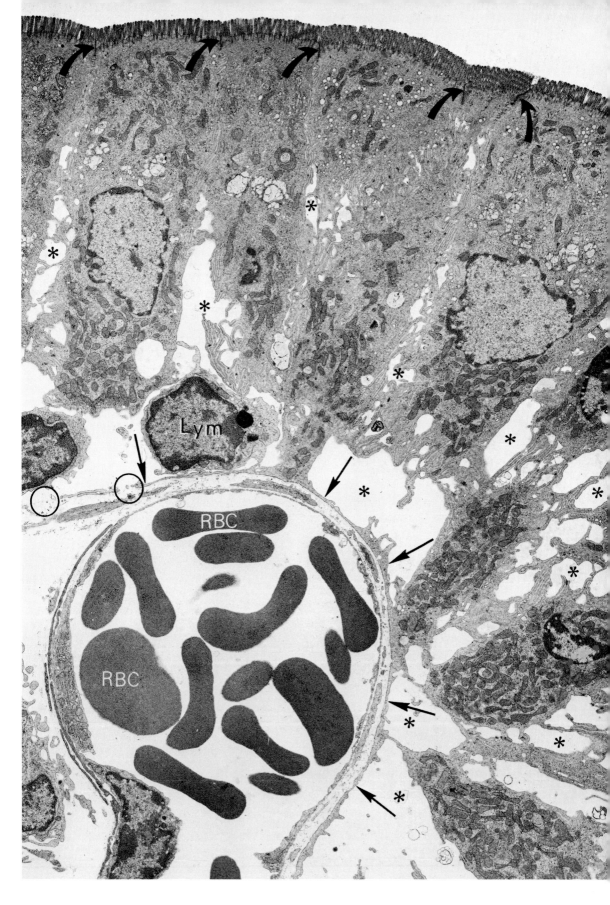

PLATE 1-4

Plate 1-5. STRIATED BORDER, TERMINAL WEB, JUNCTIONAL COMPLEX, BASEMENT LAMINA, ELECTRON MICROSCOPY

Figure 1 shows a portion of the apical cytoplasm of two epithelial cells from the same specimen as in Plate 1-4. The micrograph reveals the microvilli (**M**), the junctional complex (**JC**) and below this, the non-specialized region of cell apposition (**NS**).

Microvilli of the intestinal absorptive cell are uniform in size and shape. They display numerous fine core filaments (**arrows**) which course the length of the microvilli and enter the underlying cytoplasmic region of the cell, as the *terminal web* (**TW**). The latter is a filamentous component which extends across the breadth of the cell as a narrow band in the most apical region of the cell. Other cell organelles are excluded from the terminal web (or may only transiently pass thru, as in the case of pinocytotic vesicles which originate from the plasma membrane at the base of adjacent microvilli). At the light microscope level, the terminal web appears as a slightly darker staining region in contrast to the striated border above and the cytoplasm immediately below. The staining of the terminal web is undoubtedly due to the numbers of filaments (**double arrows**) aggregated in this region of the cell.

Two of the three functionally important components of the complex can be seen in Figure 1. One is the *zonula occludens* (**ZO**), a surface specialization involving the membranes of adjacent cells. The outer leaflets of the opposing cell membranes within this specialization are fused. (The points of fusion are actually in the form of a honeycomb network which can be seen in freeze fracture preparations.) The fusion between the cells results in a narrow zone in which the intercellular space is functionally obliterated. This fused zone forms a band around the cell thus preventing the free passage of substances across the epithelium via the intercellular space.

Immediately below the zonula occludens is the second structural component of the junctional complex, namely, the *zonula adherens* (**ZA**). It, too, is a modification of the cell surface. Here the plasma membranes of the adjacent cells diverge slightly, leaving a uniform intercellular space of 15 to 20 nm.

The fine filaments of the terminal web converge and insert into a dense material bordering the cytoplasmic side of the plasma membrane of the zonula adherens. It is probable that the zonula adherens is the main element that contributes to the visualization of the terminal bar seen in the light microscope. Although the zonula adherens appears relatively electron lucent, with no apparent structural content, as the name implies, it is thought to serve as a zone of strong adhesion between adjacent cells. Core filaments of the microvilli and filaments of the terminal web are regarded to be actin. There is evidence indicating that these two groups of filaments are functionally joined by myosin as shown in Figure 2 to constitute a contractile apparatus. The circles in the figure represent myosin. (Myosin is usually lost during the routine preparation of the tissue.) Note the attachment of terminal web filaments to the density of the zonula adherens.

The *macula adherens* also serves as a strong attachment site, but occurs as focal or spotlike (macula) attachments between adjacent cells in contrast to the bandlike zonula adherens which rings the cell. The macula adherens is not present in Figure 1, nor in Figure 2. (An example of this type of junctional specialization can be seen in the cardiac muscle, Plate 5-8, upper inset.) The macula adherens corresponds to the desmosome of the light microscopist. When discernible in the light microscope, it appears as a fine dot or fusiform thickening.

Figure 3 shows the basal portion of the epithelium. The epithelial compartment extends as far as the basement lamina (**arrows**). The lamina has been cut on edge and it appears as a delicate linear structure, so thin, that it cannot be resolved with the light microscope. Note that the basal processes of adjacent epithelial cells meet and in effect, they "close off" the intercellular epithelial space. The "basal closure" is simply a close approximation of the basal processes of adjacent cells without the presence of a junctional complex.

The figure also shows a small part of a red blood cell (**RBC**), a capillary lumen (**CL**), and the capillary endothelium (**arrow heads**).

KEY

CL, capillary lumen
F, fibroblast process
JC, junctional complex
M, microvilli
NS, non-specialized region of cell apposition
RBC, red blood cell
TW, terminal web
ZA, zonula adherens
ZO, zonula occludens
arrows, core filaments of microvilli (Fig. 1)
arrows, (Fig. 3) basal lamina
arrowheads, capillary endothelium
double arrows, filaments of terminal web

(Fig. 2 from Rodewald et al., J. Cell Biol. *70:* 541, 1976)

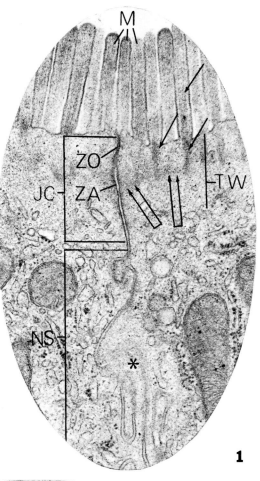

1

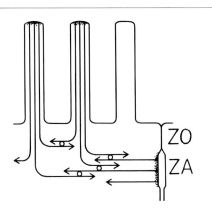

2

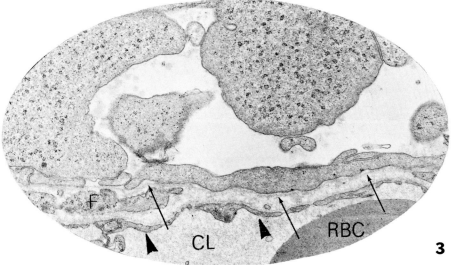

3

PLATE 1-5

2 CONNECTIVE TISSUE

CONNECTIVE TISSUE consists of cells and extracellular material, namely, fibers and ground substance. The various combinations of cells and extracellular material account for the different kinds of connective tissue. For purposes of convenience, connective tissues can be classified as follows:

A. Connective Tissue Proper*
    General
    1. loose
    2. dense
    Special
    3. regular
    4. elastic
    5. adipose
    6. reticular
    Embryonic
    7. mesenchyme
    8. mucous
B. Supporting Tissue (see Chapter 3)
    1. cartilage
    2. bone

1,2. Both *loose* and *dense connective tissue* contain fundamentally the same components. The difference between them is in the ratio of cells to extracellular fibers. Loose connective tissue contains relatively more cells and fewer fibers; dense connective tissue contains fewer cells and more fibers. Moreover, the fibers in loose connective tissue are thinner and more delicate.

Ground substance occupies the space between the cells and fibers of connective tissue. It is not a conspicuous feature of routine H & E sections because it is easily lost during tissue preparation. Ground substance contains mucopolysaccharides (glycosaminoglycans) of different types. Some of these

---

* Unless otherwise indicated, the term "connective tissue" hereafter refers to general connective tissue.

mucopolysaccharides may contain "acid" groups, such as sulfate, which stain with basic dyes. Special preparations are usually employed to demonstrate ground substance.

Three kinds of fibers are present in connective tissue: collagenous fibers, elastic fibers, and reticular fibers. *Collagenous fibers* form interlacing bundles and are sometimes also referred to as white fibers. In connective tissue these fibers are produced by cells called fibroblasts*. Collagenous fibers and fibroblasts are the most characteristic components of connective tissue. In routine H and E preparations, the collagenous fibers stain with eosin. Collagenous fibers are also produced by other cell types, namely, bone cells, cartilage cells, odontoblasts, cementoblasts and smooth muscle cells. *Elastic fibers,* as the name suggests, impart elastic properties to a tissue. In connective tissue, elastic fibers are less numerous than collagenous fibers; they are also produced by fibroblasts. Although elastic fibers may stain lightly with eosin, special stains which contain orcein or resorcin fuchsin are usually employed for their demonstration. Chondrocytes of elastic cartilage and smooth muscle cells also produce elastic fibers. *Reticular fibers* are related to collagenous fibers in that the collagen fibril is the basic subunit of structure in both. Reticular fibers are associated with a larger amount of protein-polysaccharide matrix which binds the fibrils together, and typically, reticular fibers are much thinner than collagenous fibers. Reticular fibers are present in large numbers in connective tissue (mesenchyme) of embryonic tissues. However, with development, collagenous fibers come to replace most of the reticular fibers, except those which are present where epithelium adjoins connective tissue, and around muscle cells, fat cells, and small blood vessels and nerves. Because of their small size, reticular fibers are inconspicuous in routine H & E preparations although they do stain with eosin. They are demonstrated with special silver staining procedures which cause the reticular fibers to appear black. Reticular fibers can also be demonstrated with the periodic acid Schiff (PAS) reaction because of the carbohydrate associated with the collagen fibrils.

Several cell types are present in connective tissue: fibroblasts, mast cells, macrophages, fat cells, and white blood cells which have migrated from the nearby blood vessels. Connective tissue is also described as containing undifferentiated cells which retain the ability to develop into other cell types.

As mentioned above, *fibroblasts* are the most characteristic cells of connective tissue. They are associated with the production of collagenous, elastic, and reticular fibers, and also with the production of ground substance. Macrophages are also called *histiocytes.* They may be fixed or wandering. *Mast cells* are found throughout connective tissue. However, they are especially numerous around small blood vessels. The cytoplasm of these cells is filled with granules which stain metachromatically with certain basic dyes. Mast cell granules contain heparin and histamine. *Fat cells* have the ability to store large amounts of lipid.

It is not practical to try to identify each of the various connective tissue cell types in H & E preparations. However, the following points may be helpful. One can often distinguish a fixed cell from a wandering cell (see

---

* The term fibrocyte is sometimes employed to designate a relatively quiescent fibroblast in adult tissue.

Plate 2-2). Fat cells can be identified because of their large size and empty appearance. Fibroblasts, fixed macrophages, and mast cells are difficult to distinguish from one another. The cytoplasm of these cells is generally difficult to delineate from the extracellular fibrous material, and the cells frequently appear as naked nuclei. The question of identifying cell types, however, is not simply a matter of considering the cells as if they were isolated units. In a histology slide, cells are seen in relation to other structures, and the position of connective tissue cells with respect to these other structures, e.g., blood vessels, surfaces, and fibers, may serve as an aid to their identification. For example, in very fibrous tissue, the fibroblast is the predominant cell type, and this fact in itself serves as a major factor in its identification. On the other hand, fibroblasts are also present in extremely cellular tissues, such as one often sees under epithelial surfaces, where other cell types may be equally or more numerous. In these situations, the identification of fibroblasts may be more difficult. Mast cells are relatively numerous in the vicinity of small blood vessels. Despite this, mast cells can be positively identified only by taking special precautions to preserve the granules (e.g., fixation with lead subacetate) and subsequent staining with a basic dye. In special circumstances, the cell type can be identified with more assurance owing to a manifestation of its functional role. Thus, macrophages can be identified if they contain phagocytized material within their cytoplasm. The fibroblast usually possesses a small, flattened nucleus. However, when it is actively engaged in the production of collagen, the nucleus of the cell becomes enlarged and pale staining. Moreover, the cytoplasm becomes conspicuous, and parts of it stain with hematoxylin or basic dyes.

The term *lamina propria* is applied to the connective tissue which serves as a supporting framework for the epithelium of mucous membranes. This connective tissue is usually very cellular. In some places it contains large numbers of lymphocytes, and in these cases it is referred to as diffuse lymphoid tissue. *Plasma cells* are frequently found in the lamina propria. These cells are related to B-lymphocytes and are involved in antibody production. They have a spherical nucleus which is eccentrically located and traditionally described as being "cartwheel." The cytoplasm of plasma cells is more extensive than the cytoplasm of lymphocytes, and it stains with hematoxylin, except for the region which contains the Golgi apparatus.

3. *Regular connective tissue* consists of bundles of parallel collagenous fibers. This kind of tissue constitutes capsules of organs, tendons and ligaments.

4. *Elastic tissue* contains a predominance of elastic material. This need not be in the form of fibers; rather, it may be in the form of broad and interconnecting bands, or else as fenestrated membranes. The two locations in which large amounts of elastic material are found are the walls of the elastic arteries and the elastic ligaments of the spinal column (ligamenta flava and ligamentum nuchae).

5. In certain locations, the connective tissue of the body contains large numbers of fat cells. This tissue no longer retains the characteristics of general connective tissue, but has a distinctive histological appearance, and is called *adipose tissue.*

6. The designation *reticular tissue* is applied to the reticular fibers and

special cells (reticular cells) which form the framework of lymphoid organs and bone marrow. *Blood* is a derivative of connective tissue (bone marrow and lymphoid organs) in which the intercellular material is liquid.

7, 8. *Mesenchyme* is embryonic connective tissue; *mucous connective tissue* is embryonic connective tissue with a large amount of ground substance which gives it a jelly-like quality.

CONNECTIVE TISSUE

Plate 2-1. LOOSE CONNECTIVE TISSUE

The tissue which surrounds the epithelial elements of an inactive mammary gland lobule serves as an example of loose connective tissue (**LCT**) (Fig. 1). In an H & E preparation, the nuclei of the connective tissue cells appear as the dark-staining bodies (**arrows**). The cytoplasm, however, cannot be distinguished from the thin, irregularly arranged collagenous fibers that are between the cells. The small, walled, ring-like structures within the connective tissue are blood vessels (**BV**). Surrounding the inactive lobule and its loose connective tissue is dense connective tissue (**DCT**). As stated in the introduction, both contain fundamentally the same elements; however, loose connective tissue is more cellular and less fibrous, whereas dense connective tissue is relatively less cellular and more fibrous. In the loose connective tissues, the fibers are extremely thin; in the dense connective tissue the fibers are thick. This is readily apparent in Figure 1.

It should be emphasized that the classification of loose and dense connective tissue is based on relative factors and intermediate forms do exist. An example of an intermediate form is shown in Figure 2, the connective tissue of the rete testis. This moderately dense connective tissue (**CT**) contains a variety of connective tissue cells and interlacing bundles of collagenous fibers which separate the cells. Compared to the loose connective tissue seen in Figure 1, the fibrous material here is clearly abundant, and at the same time it is almost if not equally as cellular. For most of the cells, only the nuclei are evident; the cytoplasm is difficult to delineate from the extracellular fibrous material. On the basis of the nuclear shapes, staining, and arrangement, it is evident that the cells are not grouped or organized in any special pattern.

To summarize, the light microscopic appearance of loose connective tissue includes the presence of several cell types not organized in any special pattern, and, between the cells, interlacing bundles of fibers. The presence of epithelium (**Ep**) in Figure 2 permits one to compare epithelium and connective tissue. The epithelial cells are arranged to form a surface. They are closely applied and are not separated by fibers.

It is not possible to identify the ground

KEY

BV, blood vessels
CT, connective tissue
DCT, dense connective tissue
Ep, epithelium
LCT, loose connective tissue
arrows, nuclei of connective tissue cells

Fig. 1 (human), x 160; Fig. 2 (human), x 480.

substance in routine H & E preparations. Also, it is extremely difficult and usually impractical to try to identify elastic fibers without employing specific stains. It is safe to say, however, that most of the fibers are collagenous.

The relationship between the cells and fibers, and the character of each of these elements, is best appreciated when visualized at the ultrastructural level. Plate 2-2 is an electron micrograph which reveals the salient features of a connective tissue comparable to that seen in Figure 2.

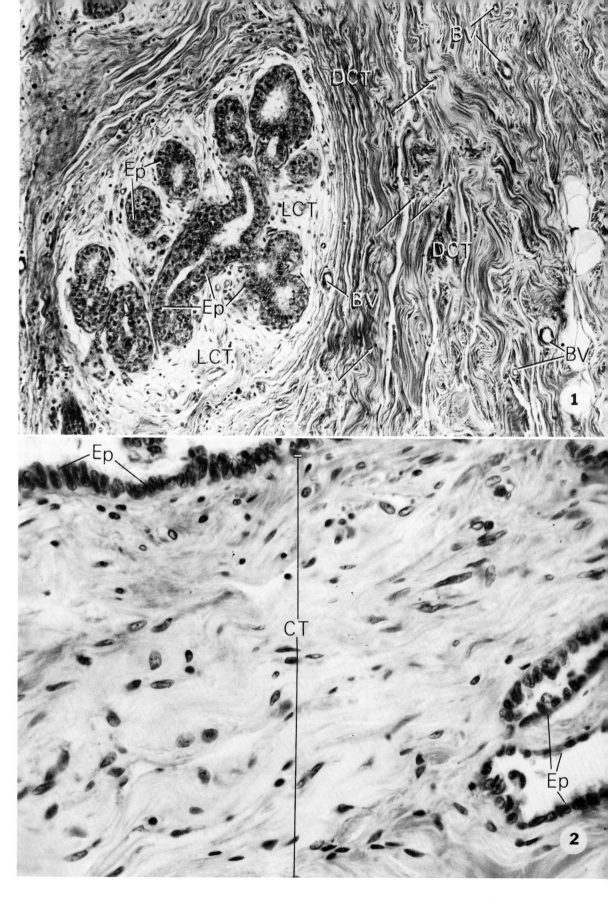

PLATE 2-1

CONNECTIVE TISSUE

Plate 2-2. CONNECTIVE TISSUE, ELECTRON MICROSCOPY

The formed elements which constitute a connective tissue, namely the fibers and cells, are readily characterized at the ultrastructural level. The specimen shown here is from a section through the wall of an oviduct. The tissue is rather cellular, but it also contains a considerable amount of fibrous material. In terms of its constituent elements, it is comparable to the connective tissue shown in Figure 2 of the preceding plate. With the electron microscope, the morphological character of the tissue constituents become immediately apparent. The fibroblasts (**F**), which constitute the bulk of the connective tissue cell population, usually exhibit long cytoplasmic processes which pass between the collagen bundles. The processes extend for indeterminant distances and may become so attenuated (arrowheads) that their thinness precludes the possibility of being visualized with the light microscope.

In addition to the fibroblast population, there are at least two other connective tissue cell types present in this specimen (see rectangles). One is a cell with both myoid and fibroblast-like features. This, we refer to as a myofibrocyte (**My**). The other is a cell which has certain features that suggest it is a monocyte (**M**), or a closely related cell type. These two cell types, along with a fibroblast, are illustrated at higher magnification in the following plate.

The collagen fibers (**CF**), between which the fibroblasts processes pass, have a stippled appearance at this relatively low magnification. This is due to the cut, end-on profiles of the individual collagen fibrils. It is these threadlike units, the fibrils, which when aggregated in bundles form the fiber that is visualized at the light microscope level.

In the specimen shown here, almost all of the collagen fibers (**CF**) have been cross sectioned and consequently it is possible to discern their variable size and shape. In the routinely prepared light microscopic specimen, during the fixation and dehydration stages of its preparation, there may be considerable initial hydration, and then with subsequent dehydration, shrinkage of the tissue occurs. One consequence of this is the artificial separation of the collagen fibers. The fibers are then discerned in the light

microscope as wispy, isolated, thread-like elements, rather than the more even distribution seen in the electron micrographs.

Typically one finds small blood vessels passing through the substance of the connective tissue and in this instance there is a capillary (**Cap**) present as well as a longitudinally sectioned venule (**V**). The latter contains a number of red blood cells (**RBC**).

22

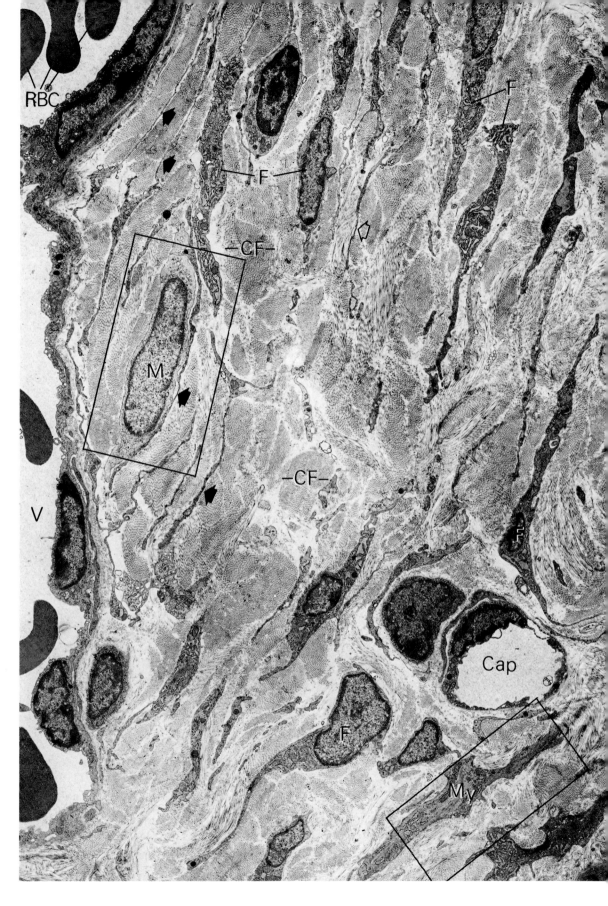

PLATE 2-2

Plate 2-3. CONNECTIVE TISSUE CELLS, ELECTRON MICROSCOPY

As noted on the previous page, the cytological features displayed by the various connective tissue cell types at the ultrastructural level serve as an accurate "fingerprint marking" which allows one, with few exceptions, to readily identify the cell type in question. For example, Figure 1 reveals portions of two adjacent fibroblasts. Despite the fact that only a small portion of each cell is evident, they can be immediately identified as fibroblasts on the basis of the presence of a moderate amount of granular endoplasmic reticulum (**GER**) and by the elongate processes which both cells exhibit.

The cisternae of the endoplasmic reticulum are notably dilated, as seen in the lower cell, and contain a homogeneous substance of moderate density. This substance is a product of the synthetic activity of the ribosomes on the surface of the reticulum and, having been released into the cisternae, represents a precursor of the collagen seen in the extracellular space. In this same cell, the section reveals a portion of the Golgi apparatus (**G**). The latter consists of a multitude of small vesicles and flattened sac-like profiles.

The portion of the cell shown in Figure 2 is in many respects similar to the fibroblasts just described, and at the light microscopic level it would probably be indistinguishable from them. Note that in one area, profiles of granular endoplasmic reticulum are evident (**GER**) and their contents exhibit the same texture and density as that of the fibroblast. However, the cell differs from the fibroblast in that the cytoplasm reveals a fine filamentous component, just barely visible at this magnification. Associated with these areas are "cytoplasmic densities" (**arrows**); the combination of these dense areas and the cytoplasmic filaments is a feature characteristic of smooth muscle cells. It is evident that this cell type designated as a myofibrocyte, functions both as a fibroblast and a contractile, or muscle cell. Other examples of this kind of cell can be found in the testis, ovary, spleen, and nerve (perineurium).

The last cell type on this plate, Figure 3, is one which would probably also be recognized as a fibroblast if viewed in the light microscope. As seen here, the cell exhibits a flattened nucleus and a little cytoplasm about

KEY

CF, collagen fiber
GER, granular endoplasmic reticulum
G, Golgi apparatus
SER, smooth endoplasmic reticulum
arrows, cytoplasmic densities
arrowheads, longitudinally sectioned collagen fibrils.

it. The cytoplasm is somewhat nondescript, the most notable feature being the small vesicular profiles of smooth endoplasmic reticulum (**SER**). Presumably this cell is a monocyte which may be in transition to a tissue macrophage. Again, the essential point here is that we are viewing a cell type which is cytologically different from a fibroblast, though with the light microscope, in a routinely stained H & E section, the distinction between these two cells is not possible.

In all three figures, the collagen fibrils can be clearly identified as the subunits of the collagen fibers (**CF**). In most locations the fibrils have been cross sectioned and here they appear as closely packed circular profiles; in other locations the fibrils have been sectioned more longitudinally (**arrowheads**) and here the typical cross banded pattern is evident. Again, it is indicated that individual fibrils cannot be identified with the light microscope, rather, one sees a bundle of fibrils and this bundle is then referred to as a collagen fiber. One can also ascertain from these illustrations that the diameter of the collagen fiber depends on how many fibrils are within the bundle.

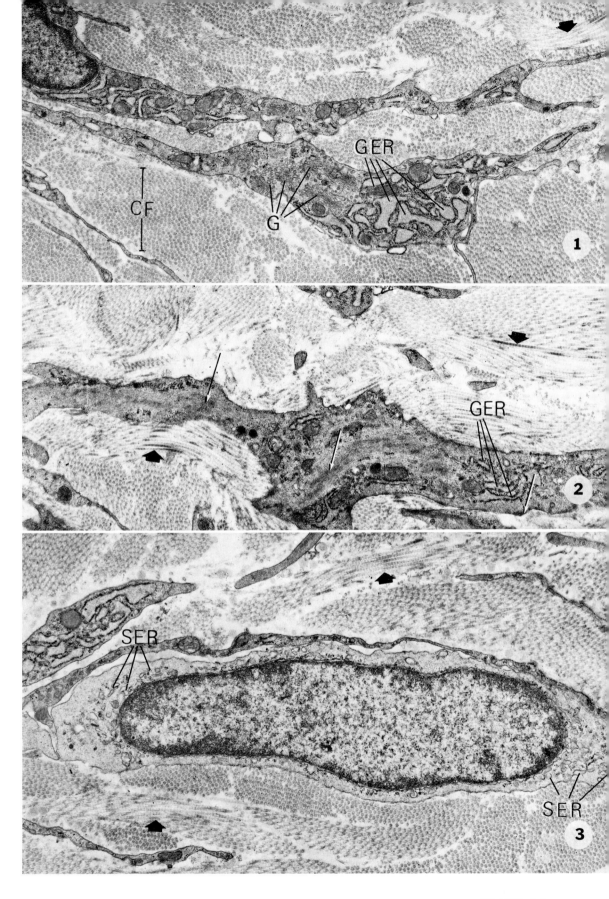

PLATE 2-3

CONNECTIVE TISSUE

Plate 2-4. DENSE CONNECTIVE TISSUE

A section of dense connective tissue is shown in Figure 1. It consists of thick interlacing bundles of collagenous fibers and connective tissue cells interspersed throughout. The collagenous fibers are by far the most prominent component of the specimen. Although elastic fibers are also present, special methods are required for their demonstration. Reticular fibers are located around the small blood vessels; however, they also require special methods for their demonstration. At this relatively low magnification (Fig. 1), the connective tissue cells can be identified chiefly on the basis of their nuclear staining. The nuclei appear as small dark bodies throughout the field.

Figure 2 shows a field of dense connective tissue at higher magnification. The thick bundles that are seen at low magnification are comprised of large numbers of collagenous fibers (**CF**). Reference to Plate 2-3 will reveal that each fiber that can be seen with the light microscope actually consists of numerous fibrils which can be resolved only with the electron microscope.

Although it is not practical to try to identify the various kinds of connective tissue cells, some generalizations can be made. A cell in which the nucleus is surrounded by a definable amount of cytoplasm can generally be regarded as a wandering cell rather than one that is fixed. Two such cells (**arrowheads**) are shown in Figure 2. The nucleus of each is surrounded by a clearly defined amount of cytoplasm. A wandering macrophage has this appearance, and these are probably macrophages. However, such an identification is somewhat tenuous unless phagocytized material can be identified within the cytoplasm. The nuclei of several other connective tissue cells are also evident. The cytoplasm, however, is not evident. While most of these cells are likely to be fibroblasts, one cannot precisely identify the individual cells as such (see preceding plate).

The **inset** shows a lymphocyte next to the cell which has been identified as a macrophage. The lymphocyte has a small, spherical, intensely staining nucleus. A small amount of cytoplasm is discernible around the nucleus. However, it should be noted that one does not always see cytoplasm around a lymphocyte in a histological section.

KEY

arrow, blood vessel
arrowheads, nonfixed (wandering) cells

Fig. 1 (human), x 160; Fig. 2 and inset (human), x 640.

26

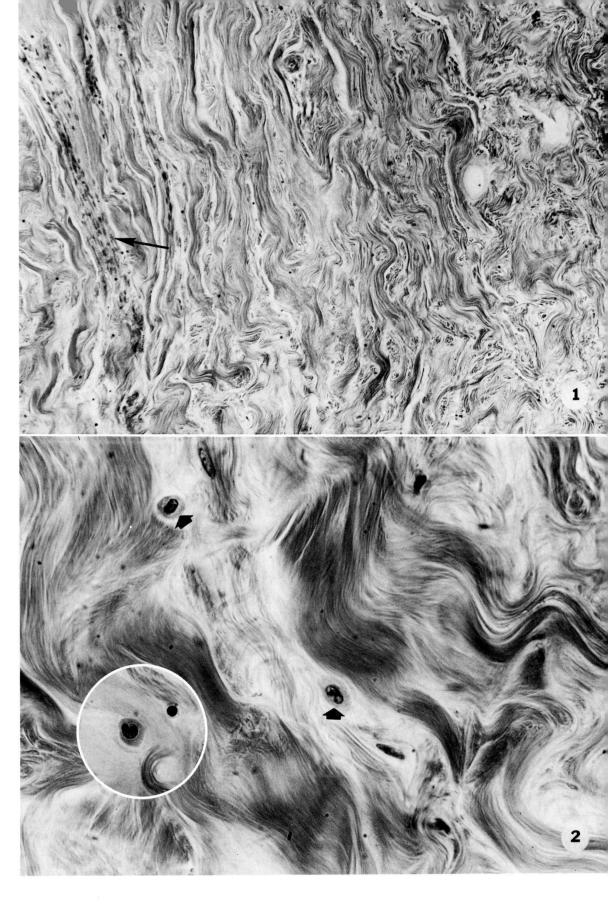

PLATE 2-4

Plate 2-5. REGULAR CONNECTIVE TISSUE

Regular connective tissue consists of connective tissue in which the fibrous elements are organized in a parallel array. This is epitomized in ligaments and tendons.

Figure 1 is a longitudinal section of a ligament. It shows rows of collagenous fibers separated by rows of cells practically all of which are fibroblasts. The nucleus of each is conspicuous but the cytoplasm of these cells is difficult to discern. The lateral extent of the collagenous bundles is not always clear; however, it is suggested by the location of the cells. The nuclei stand out; however, the cytoplasm of the cells is not evident. One regularly sees folds and even cracks in routine H & E preparations of ligaments (and also tendons). These folds are frequently at right angles to the long axis of the collagenous bundles. They are considered to be the result of the vibrational impact of the cutting knife. Indeed, even smaller cross-directional markings may be present, and these should not be confused with the cross striations of striated muscle.

Examination of Figure 2, a higher magnification of a ligament, indicates that the cells between the collagenous bundles are of one type; they are fibroblasts. The nuclei of these cells are shaped like oval plates. Therefore, when the broad face of the nucleus is viewed, it appears oval, and when the nucleus is viewed on edge, it appears flat. Ligaments are described as being less regularly organized than tendons.

A tendon is illustrated in Figure 3. It also consists of parallel bundles of collagenous fibers which are separated by rows of fibroblasts. The nuclei of these cells are viewed on edge and they appear as the thin, dark-staining profiles. A small amount of striated muscle (**StM**) is shown where it connects to the tendon. Although both tendon and muscle appear as oriented fibers and nuclei, the muscle contains cross striations, but the tendon does not.

The capsules of organs also contain rather organized bundles of collagenous fibers. These are more likely to be disposed in sheets than in cords. Therefore, the term "lamellated" is sometimes applied to this form of regular connective tissue.

KEY

StM, striated muscle

Fig. 1 (cat), x 160; Fig. 2 (cat), x 440; Fig. 3 (human), x 440.

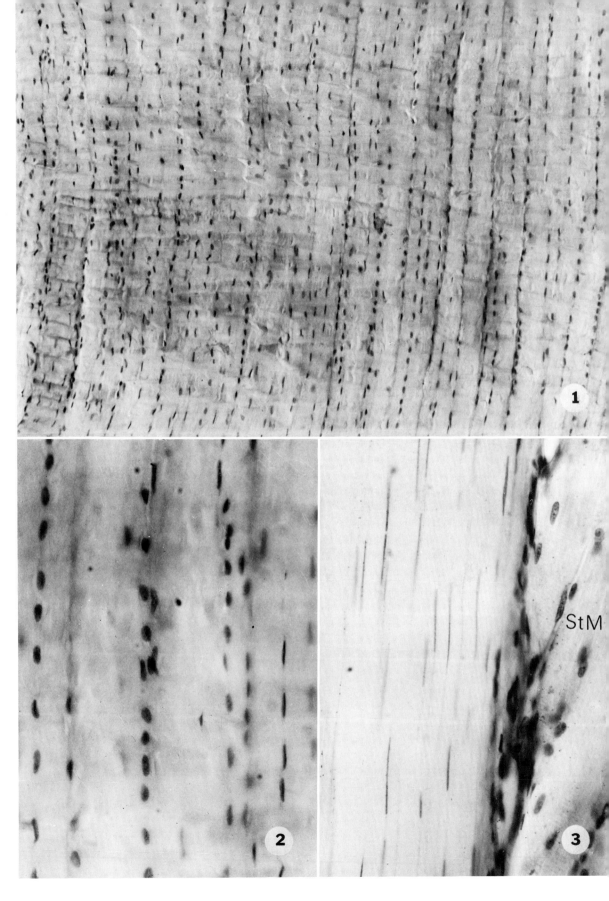

StM

PLATE 2-5

Plate 2-6. ELASTIC FIBERS, ELASTIC TISSUE, AND EMBRYONIC CONNECTIVE TISSUE

Elastic fibers are present in loose and dense connective tissue throughout the body, but in lesser amounts than collagenous fibers. Moreover, as noted previously, elastic fibers are not conspicuous in routine H & E sections and thus there is no reminder of their presence. However, with special stains, designed to display elastic fibers, they are readily seen. Certain of these stains can then be followed by the usual H & E procedure in which case, not only the elastic fibers but the other tissue components are revealed. Figure 1 is a section of the connective tissue of skin. This specimen was prepared to show elastic fibers; it was then stained with H & E. The connective tissue at the top of the figure is loose (papillary layer of dermis) and contains delicate elastic fibers (**arrows**). (These should not be confused with the nuclei of the connective tissue cells which also appear dark). The connective tissue in the bottom part of the figure is dense (reticular layer of dermis), and the elastic fibers (**arrowheads**) are thicker and coarser. This connective tissue, however, is not classified as elastic, because the preponderance of fibrous material is collagenous.

Figure 2 shows the wall of an elastic artery (pulmonary artery) which has been stained to demonstrate the elastic material. The specimen was not subsequently stained with H & E. The elastic material appears black and is a conspicuous component of the arterial wall. It is organized in the form of fenestrated membranes, or sheets, rather than as fibers. The plane of section is such that the membranes are seen "on edge." Tissues of the body containing large amounts of elastic material are limited in distribution to the walls of elastic arteries and some ligaments that are associated with the spinal column.

Mesenchyme is embryonic connective tissue. It is highly cellular and contains a minimum of fibers, none of which are organized into thick bundles. (This is in contrast to adult connective tissue wherein the cells may be few and the collagenous bundles thick). Figure 3 shows the mesenchyme from the cheeks of a fetal head. The nuclei of the mesenchymal cells stain with hematoxylin and are readily evident. The cytoplasm, however, is difficult to distinguish from the extracellular

KEY

BV, blood vessel
Ep, epithelium
StM, developing striated muscle
arrowheads, coarse elastic fibers
arrows, delicate elastic fibers

Fig. 1 (human), x 160; Fig. 2 (human), x 150; Fig. 3 (fetal pig), x 400; Fig. 4 (human), x 400.

material. Extremely delicate strands of collagenous fibers are present between the cells. The specimen also shows some developing striated muscle cells (**StM**), blood vessels (**BV**), and the epithelial surface (**Ep**).

Mucous connective tissue is embryonic connective tissue that is characterized by the presence of large amounts of ground substance which gives it a jelly-like quality. It is present in many parts of the embryo, for example, under the skin and in the umbilical cord. A section of the umbilical cord is shown in Figure 4. The cells are widely scattered. The cytoplasm of the cells cannot always be distinguished from the intercellular fibrous material and precipitated mucoid material.

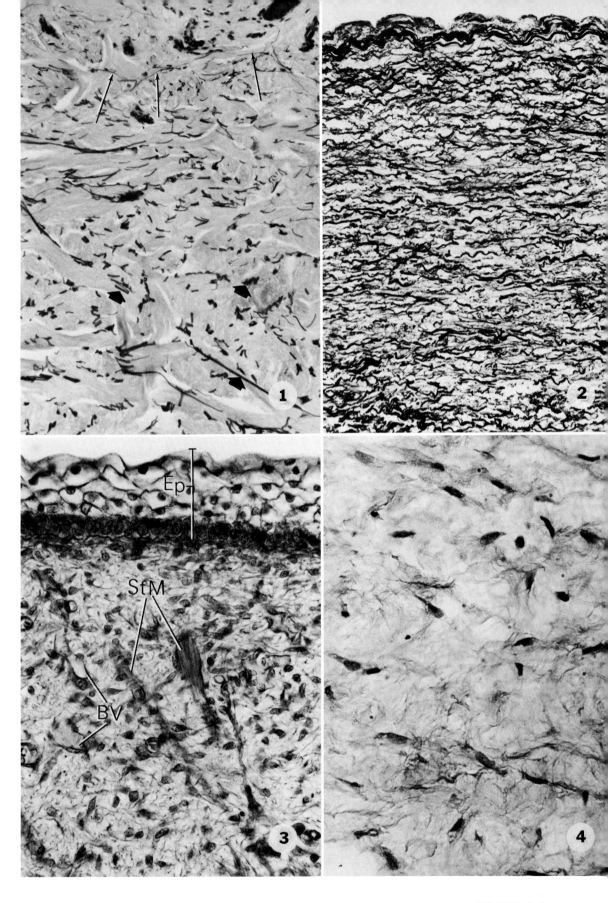

PLATE 2-6

3 SUPPORTING TISSUE

CARTILAGE AND BONE are the essential weight bearing components of the skeleton and for this reason they are also referred to as supporting tissues. Cartilage, in common with other connective tissue, consists of cells and intercellular material, except that in cartilage the intercellular material is solidified and the cells are of one type, called chondrocytes. Cartilage cells elaborate a gel-like matrix which contains small diameter collagen fibrils imbedded in ground substance. The ground substance consists of protein-polysaccharide compounds some of which are sulfated. Generically, the protein-polysaccharide compounds are designated glycosaminoglycans or proteoglycans. (An older designation for these compounds, still in use, is mucopolysaccharides.) The chondrocytes surround themselves with this matrix and occupy spaces called lacunae. Elastic fibers are also present in the matrix of elastic cartilage. Cartilage is unique among the various members or relatives of the connective tissue family in that it is not vascularized. Three chief kinds of cartilage can be distinguished: *hyaline cartilage, elastic cartilage,* and *fibrocartilage.*

Bone is a modified form of connective tissue in which the intercellular matrix becomes calcified. The intercellular matrix of bone also contains ground substance (glycosaminoglycans) and collagenous fibers. Two types of bone can be distinguished: dense or compact, and spongy or cancellous. The essential features in both *spongy* and *compact bone* are the presence of a mineralized matrix, small canals (canaliculi) which contain slender processes of bone cells, and spaces (lacunae) which contain bone cells (osteocytes). In cancellous bone the matrix, lacunae, and osteocytes are organized to form spicules or trabeculae and a cut surface of cancellous bone has a spongy appearance. The cut surface of dense bone has a more solid appearance. An additional feature of dense bone is that much dense bone (especially in the adult) consists of special arrangements of blood vessels and bone elements to form structural units called Haversian systems.

At the microscopic level, bone can also be designated as lamellar and non-lamellar. Spongy bone is non-lamellar, dense bone may be lamellar or non-lamellar. Haversian systems consist of lamellar bone.

The special feature of the Haversian system is the presence of blood

32

vessels in a central canal (the Haversian canal) which in a long bone is typically oriented parallel to the long axis of the bone. The mineralized tissue of the Haversian system is disposed in layers around the Haversian canal. In any given layer, the collagen fibers are oriented in essentially the same direction, but the direction differs in different layers much as the direction of wood grain differs in different layers of plywood (lamellated wood). It is the orientation of collagen, differing in each layer, which gives lamellar bone its layered appearance. Lamellar bone is not confined to Haversian systems and it occurs in several other arrangements (see Plate 3-7).

In non-lamellar bone, the collagen is not disposed in a layered manner. The collagen of non-lamellar bone is disposed in bundles of varying thickness, however, the orientation of the bundles is not regular. The collagen bundles may be interwoven (woven bone) or they may be disposed in a more parallel pattern (parallel fibered bone).

The initially developed bone in a specific location is always in the form of spicules (primary spongiosa, or primary spongy bone). If this is destined to become dense bone, the compaction of the primary spongy bone involves a filling in of the connective tissue spaces between the initially deposited bone spicules with additional bone. This may result in the development of dense non-lamellar bone or in some locations, in primary osteons. (Osteons may also be classified as primary and secondary. Primary osteons are first generation bone which develop in some locations where primary spongy bone is made compact. Secondary osteons are the result of internal remodeling of previously present dense bone. The term Haversian system refers to secondary osteons, moreover, when the term osteon is used without the qualifying term "primary" it should be construed to mean secondary osteon.)

Special preparations are needed to examine bone because of its mineral content. Two of the most common are ground sections and decalcified sections. Ground sections are prepared by removing as much soft tissue and organic matter from the bone as possible and allowing the bone to dry. Thin slices are then cut with a saw, and these are ground to adequate thinness with fine grinding stones. The specimen may be treated with India ink to highlight the spaces that were formerly occupied by organic matter, e.g., cells and other soft tissue components. In such preparations, the canaliculi, lacunae, and Haversian canals appear black (except where the India ink is lost). Ground sections display the architecture of dense bone and especially the organization of Haversian systems by revealing the mineralized material. Unfortunately, the relationship of bone to soft tissue is destroyed in routine ground preparations. In decalcified sections, the cellular and organic components are retained, and the mineral is removed by treating the tissue with demineralizing solutions such as acids or chelating agents. After the bone has been demineralized it is processed in the same manner as other tissues. These preparations usually retain the relationships between the bone and related soft tissue. It may also be necessary to decalcify cartilage of aged tissue.

Plate 3-1. CARTILAGE

Hyaline cartilage is found in the adult as the structural framework for a number of parts of the respiratory system. Figure 1 is a portion of the trachea; Figure 2, a portion of a bronchiole. In both of these cases, the cartilage (**Cart**) appears as an avascular expanse of tissue surrounded by a *perichondrium* (**P**). The latter is the fibrous capsule-like cover of hyaline cartilage. The perichondrium is shown to completely surround the hyaline cartilage of the bronchiole. It also surrounds the hyaline cartilage of the trachea. Perichondrium is more than a simple capsule in that it serves as a source of new chondrocytes during growth of cartilage. The outer part of the perichondrium is more fibrous; the inner part is more cellular. It is this more cellular inner part that is chondrogenic.

A more detailed examination of hyaline cartilage reveals the following features (Fig. 3): Cartilage consists of a homogeneous appearing matrix (**M**) in which are small spaces, called lacunae (**L**), that contain chondrocytes (**Ch**). The matrix contains collagenous fibers which are masked by the solidified ground substance and are not evident in routine H & E sections. The ground substance contains, among other components, sulfate containing compounds (e.g., sulfated glycosaminoglycans). Because of this, the matrix of cartilage stains with hematoxylin or basic dyes, and is said to be basophilic. However, if the sulfated material is not adequately retained during the preparative processes, the matrix may stain with eosin. The matrix immediately surrounding a lacuna stains more intensely and is referred to as the capsule (**Cap**). In a number of instances the capsule and cartilage cell can be clearly distinguished (**arrowhead**, Fig. 3). Frequently, two or more chondrocytes are extremely close, separated only by a thin partition of matrix. These are said to be isogenous clusters of cells because they are considered to be derived from a single predecessor cell. The matrix that surrounds such a group of related lacunae (territorial matrix) (**TM**) stains somewhat less than the capsule, but more intensely than the more removed matrix (extraterritorial matrix). Cartilage cells are often distorted during tissue preparation and in some cases fall out of their space so that occasional empty lacunae

KEY

Cap, capsule
Cart, cartilage
Ch, chondrocytes
Ep, epithelium
L, lacuna
M, matrix
P, perichondrium
TM, territorial matrix
broad arrow, lacuna showing capsule and chondrocyte
thin arrows, empty lacunae

Fig. 1 (dog), x 160; Fig. 2 (monkey), x 160; Fig. 3 (monkey), x 640.

(**arrows**) are seen. Cartilage cells characteristically contain glycogen and lipid but special methods are required for their demonstration.

Cartilage is capable of both appositional growth, i.e., growth at the surface, and interstitial growth, i.e., growth within the substance of the cartilage. During appositional growth and development of cartilage, fibroblasts in the chondrogenic layer of the perichondrium begin to elaborate matrix which ultimately surrounds the cell. It follows, then, that the cells which have just become chondrocytes are close to the perichondrium. They are also flatter and smaller, and in smaller lacunae than the more deeply located cells. In the process of interstitial growth, cells which have recently divided are close to each other forming isogenous clusters and sometimes two cells may be seen in the same lacuna.

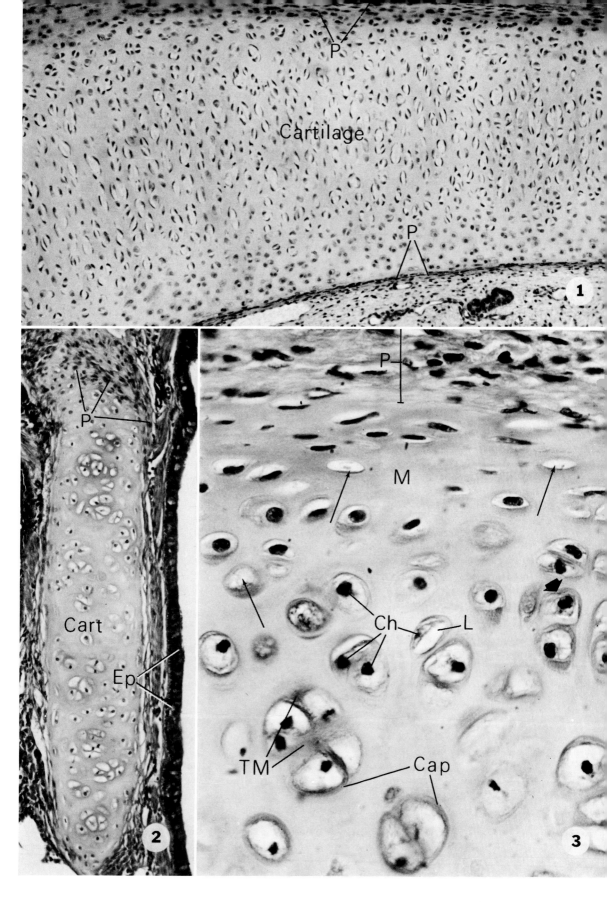

PLATE 3-1

Plate 3-2. Cartilage I, Electron Microscopy

This electron micrograph shows at relatively low magnification a small area of cartilage (**Cart**) and its perichondrium (**P**). The perichondrial cells exhibit long flat cytoplasmic processes which extend between the collagen bundles. Their nuclei are flattened and possess scant surrounding cytoplasm. While these cells constitute the cellular component of the perichondrium, and thus are referred to as perichondrial cells, they are typical fibroblasts in all respects. As fibroblasts, they are responsible for the production of the collagen and elastic material as well as the ground substance of the perichondrium. In contrast, the fully differentiated, mature condrocytes exhibit round to ovoid nuclei with a moderate amount of cytoplasm. Not being subject to the shrinkage encountered in routine light microscopic preparations, the chondrocyte in the EM preparation does not separate from its surrounding cartilage matrix; consequently, one does not see an empty or partially empty lacuna.

The cartilage shown here is in a growing state. Therefore, it is possible to point to the changes which occur during the process of appositional growth. The cells labelled A, B, and C represent transitional stages in the differentiation of a fibroblast to a chondrocyte. Cell A can still be regarded as belonging to the perichondrium, though it probably does not retain the characteristic thin processes of the fibroblast. It is still a flat cell and has a relatively smooth surface contour, i.e., it lacks the scalloped or microvillous surface characteristic of the chondrocyte. Cell B is similar to A in shape but it exhibits a slightly scalloped surface on its left side (this is just barely discernible at the low magnification of the micrograph). In addition, the matrix along this surface shows a greater density than that seen on the opposing side of the cell. The more dense material represents cartilage matrix. Cell C represents a further transition and can be regarded as a young chondrocyte. The entire surface of the cell has a scalloped appearance and it is completely surrounded by cartilage matrix. Also, the nucleus of the cell has now become ovoid, and the cell has altered its shape toward a more polygonal form. With time it will assume the more rounded shape of the older cartilage cells.

KEY

A, B, C, progression in chondrocyte differentiation
Ca, calcium
Cart, cartilage
G, glycogen
L, lipid
P, perichondrium

Fig. (mouse), x 6,000.

Glycogen (**G**), which normally accumulates in cartilage cells and appears as aggregates of electron dense particles, is already present in relatively small amounts in the cartilage cells shown here. However, in routine H & E preparations the glycogen is not retained. Similarly, lipid (**L**) which also accumulates in the chondrocyte is retained in the EM preparations, but is lost in the routine light microscopic preparations. The loss of glycogen and lipid, which are both plentiful in the older chondrocyte, results in the typical washed out appearance and poor cytological detail when viewed in the light microscope. The extremely electron dense material seen in the cartilage matrix represents calcium salts (**Ca**) which may be found in increasing amounts as the individual ages.

The cytological features of the perichondrial cell and chondrocyte, and their surrounding matrices are shown at higher magnification in the next plate. The rectangles delineate the areas illustrated at higher magnification.

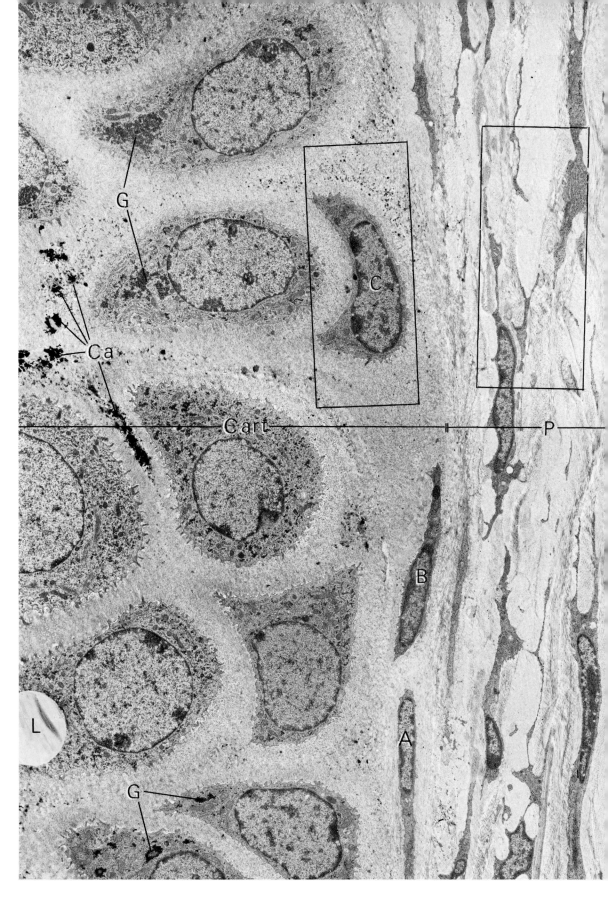

PLATE 3-2

Plate 3-3. Cartilage II, Electron Microscopy

Figures 1 and 2 are higher powers of the cells and extracellular matrices seen in the preceding plate. They allow for a more detailed comparison of the perichondrium and cartilage. The perichondrium in Figure 1 reveals portions of two fibroblasts or perichondrial cells. One of the cells reveals multiple arrays of rough surfaced or granular endoplasmic reticulum (**GER**), a feature characteristic of the fibroblast. The surface of the cell is relatively smooth. Also characteristic of the fibroblast are the long tenuous cytoplasmic processes (**F**) which extend between the bundles of collagen fibrils, i.e., the collagen fibers (**CF**). During the process of its differentiation and maturation, the fibroblast undergoes alteration in shape, changing from a flat elongate cell to one that is ovoid to round. The surface of the differentiated chondrocyte (Fig. 2) exhibits small irregular projections which give the cell a ruffled or scalloped appearance (**arrowheads**). These projections first appear at the time that cartilage matrix formation is initiated. Other than the accumulation of lipid and glycogen, the cytoplasm of the cartilage cell does not appear appreciably different than the cytoplasm of the fibroblast. The chondrocyte in Figure 2, because of the particular site through which the cell was sectioned, does not reveal its granular endoplasmic reticulum. This organelle is particularly well developed in the active chondrocyte. However, the cell does display a fairly prominent portion of its Golgi apparatus (**GA**). Also, note that the glycogen (**G**) within the cell can be just resolved as a particulate component at this magnification. The other very electron dense, extracellular material represents calcium deposits (**Ca**).

The extracellular formed elements of the perichondrial matrix consist mostly of collagen fibrils which are aggregated into bundles, i.e., collagen fibers (**CF**), oriented in varying directions. The upper inset shows bundles of cross and obliquely sectioned collagen fibrils from the area included within the circle of Figure 1. Note the very tight packing of the fibrils. Elastic fibers (**E**) are also evident in the perichondrium. They are comprised of an electron lucent core material and numerous surrounding, very electron dense, microfibrils. The microfibrils (**arrows**)

KEY

Ca, calcium
CF, collagen fibers
E, elastic fibers
F, fibroblast process
G, glycogen
GA, Golgi apparatus
GER, granular endoplasmic reticulum
arrowheads, scalloped surface
arrows, microfibrils of elastic fibers

Figs. 1 and 2 (mouse), x 16,000; insets x 31,000.

are just perceptible at this magnification. In contrast to the perichondrial connective tissue matrix, the cartilage matrix (Fig. 2), exclusive of the calcium deposits, appears almost homogeneous, particularly when observed at lower magnifications. It contains extremely fine (5 to 20 nm) matrix fibrils. Typical collagen fibrils are absent from the matrix, though the larger population of matrix fibrils are regarded to be a form of collagen. In contrast to the collagen fibril, the fibrils of the cartilage matrix lack a periodic banding. The lower inset shows the cartilage matrix from the area included in the circle of Figure 2. Note the fineness of the fibrils and the absence of typical collagen fibrils. The relative homogeneity of the cartilage matrix, as seen here, accounts for its amorphous appearance when observed in the light microscope.

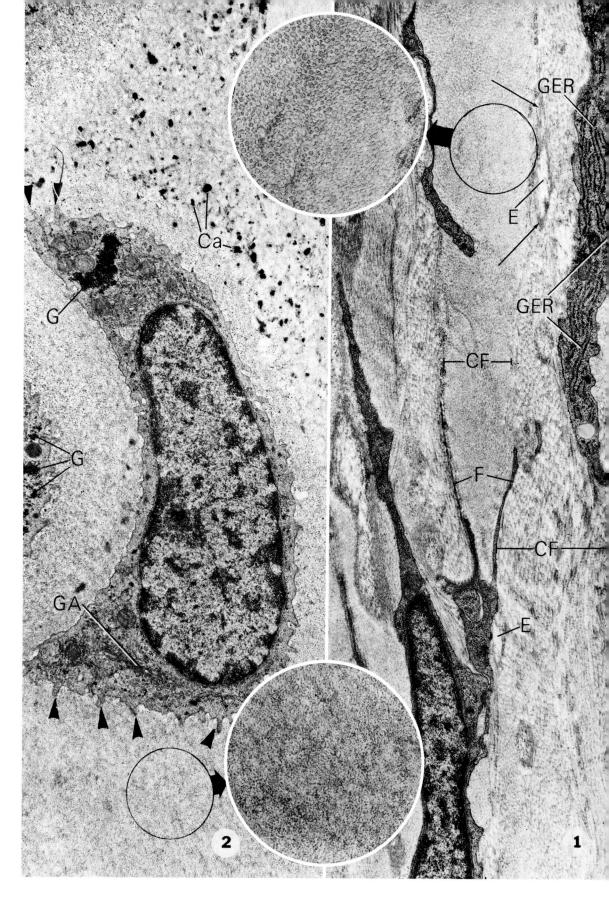

GER

E

GER

CF

F

CF

E

1

Ca

G

G

GA

2

PLATE 3-3

Plate 3-4. Cartilage, Fetal Skeleton

Hyaline cartilage is present as a precursor to bones in the fetus. Most of this cartilage will be replaced by bone tissue, except where one bone rubs against another bone, as in a joint. In these locations, cartilage persists as an articular structure. Evidently bone is not able to rub against bone and form a freely movable joint, whereas cartilage is able to do this. In addition, cartilage, being capable of interstitial growth, persists in weight-supporting bones as a "growth plate" as long as growth in length occurs. The role of cartilage on articular surfaces and in bone growth is considered in the following plate.

Figure 1 is a section through a fetal foot. The cartilage matrix appears extremely dark because it is stained intensely with hematoxylin. The intensity of staining is due to either of two factors, sulfated glycosaminoglycans or calcium, or to a combination of the two. The matrix of cartilage that is about to be replaced by bone becomes impregnated with calcium salts and the calcium stains intensely with hematoxylin. It should be noted that the multitude of light spaces within the matrix are due to the lacunae.

The cartilage is surrounded by perichondrium, except where it faces a joint cavity (**JC**). Here the naked cartilage forms a surface. In a number of places, developing ligaments (**L**) can be seen where they join the cartilage. The nuclei of the fibroblasts are conspicuous. They are aligned in rows and are separated from other rows of nuclei by collagenous material. Some blood vessels (**BV**) can be seen in various parts of the section, but not in the cartilage; this is avascular.

Figure 2 is a more magnified view of the rectangle in Figure 1. In reference to the joint, note the following: the joint cavity (**JC**) is a space between the cartilage whose boundaries are completed by a wall of connective tissue (**CT**). This connective tissue surface will constitute the synovial membrane in the adult and contribute to the formation of a lubricating fluid (synovial fluid) that is present in the joint cavity. Therefore, all the surfaces which will enclose the adult joint cavity derive orginally from mesenchyme. This is at least one major exception to the general principle that epithelium is found on surfaces, and should be kept in mind.

KEY

BV, blood vessels
CT, connective tissue
JC, joint cavity
L, ligament

Fig. 1 (rat), x 65; Fig. 2 (rat), x 160; Fig. 3 (rat), x 640.

Synovial fluid is a viscous fluid and contains among other things, glycosaminoglycans that are related to other connective tissue glycosaminoglycans.

Figure 3 provides a closer view of the cartilagenous surface and shows closely situated lacunae with their chondrocytes. The nuclei of the chondrocytes appear spherical and are clearly distinguishable. However, the cytoplasm is not always evident so that in some cases it appears that only a nucleus is present in the lacuna. The capsules of lacunae near the surface are discernable. In a number of cases, it is evident that cell division has recently occurred because two cells occupy the same lacuna. In other cases, two lacunae are extremely close with only a thin plate of matrix separating them. This is also an indication of recent cell division.

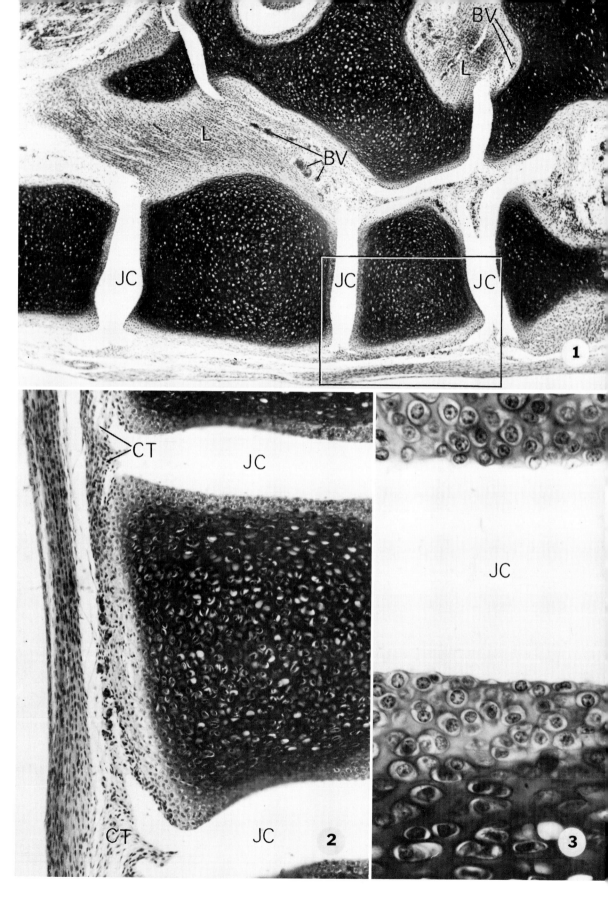

PLATE 3-4

Plate 3-5. CARTILAGE AND SPONGY BONE

Cartilage is retained on the articular surface of bones as a friction plate in a synovial joint (Fig. 1). This is hyaline cartilage (**HC**), but it is not surrounded by a perichondrium. One surface of the cartilage is free and serves for articulation; the other surface is in contact with bone of the spongy or cancellous type. The general features of cartilage are evident in Figure 1, namely, a more or less homogeneous-appearing matrix which contains lacunae and their cells. However, certain features relating to the histological appearance of cartilage and its comparison to bone are brought out in this specimen, and for this reason a brief consideration of spongy bone will be given below.

Spongy bone (**SB**) consists of trabeculae and spicules of mineralized matrix in which are small spaces, the lacunae. Each lacuna contains a bone cell (osteocyte). The nuclei of the bone cells stain with hematoxylin and stand out against the eosinophilic staining of the matrix. Between the trabeculae and spicules are the numerous round cells of the red bone marrow (**RBM**).

When comparing cartilage and bone, note the following: in articular cartilage the lacunae and cells near the surface are smaller and flatter in comparison to the more deeply located lacunae and cells. However, there are intermediate sizes between these two extremes. In bone, on the other hand, the lacunae are essentially the same size and are spaced in a characteristic manner. Moreover, in the bone, if the spicules exceed a certain size, they contain blood vessels (**BV**), whereas cartilage is avascular. A somewhat less regular feature of bone is the wavy nature of its matrix. These wave patterns (**arrows**) are characteristic of spongy bone and woven compact bone. (In contrast, as shown in Plate 3-7, the matrix of lamellar compact bone is more highly organized). The boundaries between bone and the articular cartilage are marked by **arrowheads.**

Hyaline cartilage (**HC**) is also present in developing long bones as a growth unit called the *epiphyseal disc.* Because of its capacity for interstitial growth, which is not shared by bone tissue, the epiphyseal disc (Fig. 2) is an essential feature of bone that is growing in length. In this specimen bone is in contact

KEY

BV, blood vessels
HC, hyaline cartilage
L, lacunae
P, perichondrium
RBM, red bone marrow
SB, spongy bone
broad arrows, boundary between bone and hyaline cartilage
thin arrows, bone lines

Figs. 1 and 2 (dog), x 160; Fig. 3 (dog, Weigert stain), x 160.

with the top of the cartilaginous growth plate and this is an indication that the resorption of cartilage from this surface by invading pericapillary cells has come to an end.

Elastic cartilage differs from hyaline cartilage inasmuch as the matrix contains elastic fibers (Fig. 3). These impart unique properties of elasticity to elastic cartilage that are not shared by hyaline cartilage. Elastic cartilage is found in the auricle of the external ear, in the auditory tube, and in part of the larynx.

Figure 3 shows the perichondrium (**P**), lacunae (**L**), cartilage cells, and matrix of elastic cartilage. The cells have shrunk and separated from the walls of the lacunae, and in many instances, the nuclei and cytoplasm of the chondrocytes are clearly evident. The elastic fibers appear as the black fibers within the matrix. Note again that the cells and lacuna nearer the perichondrium are smaller than those more centrally situated, and that intermediate sizes are present.

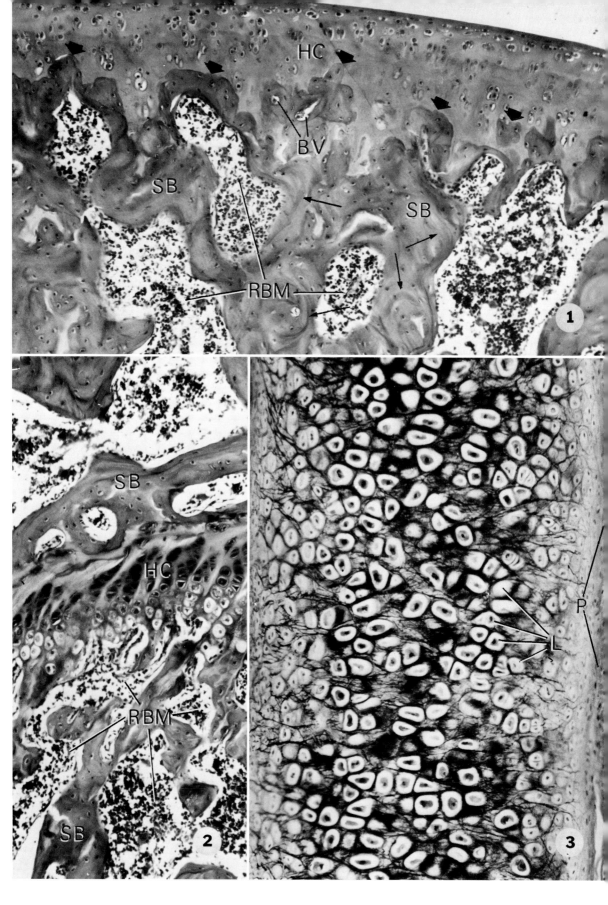

PLATE 3-5

Plate 3-6. FIBROCARTILAGE

Fibrocartilage is an intermediate between fibrous (collagenous) tissue and hyaline cartilage. It is regularly present where fibrous tissue is subjected to pressure, namely, at the intervertebral discs and the symphysis pubis. It is also present at a number of other places. For example, it is present at the knee joint, mandibular joint, sternoclavicular joint, shoulder joint, and it may be present along the grooves or insertions for tendons or ligaments.

Histologically, fibrocartilage appears as fields of cartilage imperceptibly blending with regions of fibrous tissue or, sometimes, hyaline cartilage. No perichondrium is present. A low-magnification view of fibrocartilage is shown in Figure 1. Much of the field has a fibrous appearance, and nuclei of fibroblasts are to be seen scattered about. However, even at this low magnification, at least one field appears to show characteristics of cartilage (**rectangle**). This is examined at higher magnification in Figure 2. Examination of this figure shows a region where the intercellular material is homogenous (**HM**) and typical of cartilage. Lacunae (**L**) with distinct capsules can be identified. However, even in places where the intercellular material is fibrous (**FM**), some distinct lacunae, chondrocytes, and capsules can be seen (**arrows**). The presence of a capsule around a cell is indicative of a cartilage cell, and when fibrous material shares the field with these cells and their capsules, one can identify the tissue as fibrocartilage. The nuclei of other cells which are not apparently contained in a lacuna and surrounded by a capsule are also seen. These are nuclei (**F**) which belong to fibroblasts.

KEY

F, fibroblast nuclei
FM, fibrous matrix
HM, homogenous matrix
L, lacunae
arrows, lacunae and chondrocytes in fibrous matrix

Fig. 1 (dog), x 160; Fig. 2 (dog), x 640.

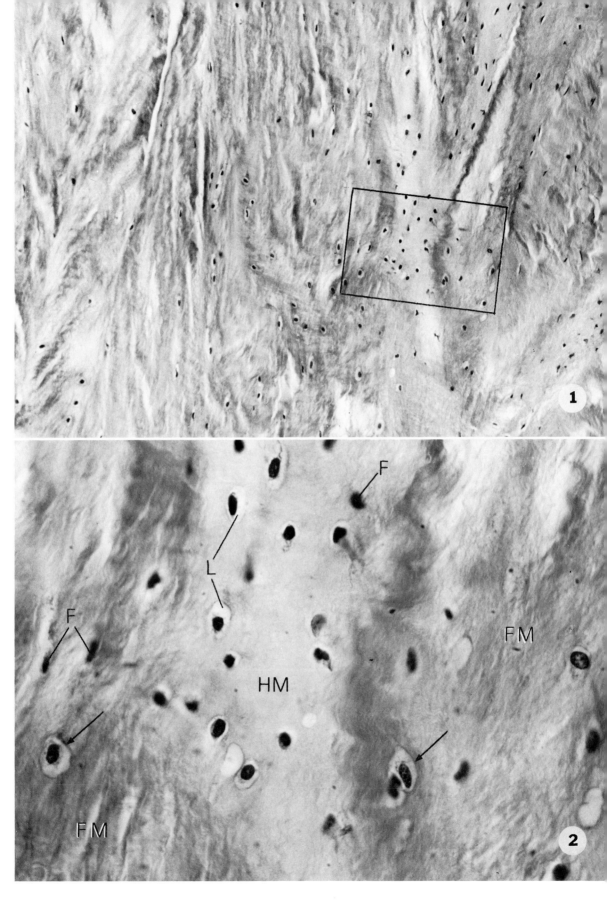

PLATE 3-6

Plate 3-7. COMPACT LAMELLAR BONE

Haversian systems, or osteons, are roughly cylinderical structures which may branch. In the shaft of a long bone, the long axes of the osteons are generally oriented parallel to the long axis of the bone, so that a cross section through the shaft of a long bone would also cut the osteons in cross section.

Figure 1 is a ground section of dense lamellar bone which was treated with India ink. The center of each Haversian system contains a canal, called the *Haversian canal* (**HC**), which travels through its long axis. This is surrounded by concentric layers of mineralized material which, in cross section, appear as rings much the same as growth rings of a tree. The Haversian canal is also surrounded by concentric arrangements of lacunae. These appear as the small dark oval structures with their long axis oriented circumferentially. Although the Haversian canals may vary somewhat in size, the lacunae are much smaller, far more numerous, and relatively uniform in size. Small canals (canaliculi) radiate outward from the Haversian canals to the lacunae. These appear as the delicate black radiations from the Haversian canal that pass through the lamellae to the lacunae (see **inset,** Fig. 1). The canaliculi also connect neighboring lateral lacunae, but these connections are less conspicuous. As already mentioned, the lacunae contain bone cells and the canaliculi contain the slender processes of bone cells. However, neither of these are evident in ground sections.

In Figure 1, a number of Haversian systems appear complete; these have been most recently formed. Other Haversian systems show incomplete outer lamellae (**arrows**); these belong to older Haversian systems which have been partly resorbed. In some cases only small parts of older Haversian systems remain between the complete newer ones. These remains are called *interstitial lamellae* (**IL**).

The Haversian canal contains small blood vessels and delicate connective tissue. The blood vessels reach the Haversian canals from either the periosteum or bone marrow through other tunnels called *Volkmann's canals* (**VC**) (Fig. 1). These can be distinguished from the Haversian canals in that they cut through

KEY

CL, circumferential lamellae
HC, Haversian canal
IL, interstitial lamellae
VC, Volkmann's canal
arrows (Fig. 1), incomplete lamellae
arrows (Fig. 3), canaliculi

Fig. 1 (dog), x 65, (inset), x 260; Figs. 2 and 3 (dog), x 160.

lamellae, whereas the Haversian canals are surrounded by concentric rings of lamellae.

The general features of dense lamellar bone are shown in Figure 2, a decalcified section. In the center of each osteon is a Haversian canal (**HC**) and, in some cases, the blood vessels can be seen. The matrix stains pink with eosin; the nuclei of osteoblasts stain with hematoxylin and stand out sharply against the pink background of the matrix.

The ringlike arrangement of the lamellae is not conspicuous in Figure 2, but is particularly striking in Figure 3. Figures 2 and 3 are photographs of the same slide (and same field), except that phase contrast optics were employed for Figure 3. The canaliculi are also evident in Figure 3 (**arrows**). Collagenous fibers travel spirally in the lamellae, but while those in a particular lamella travel in the same direction, those in neighboring lamellae travel in a different direction. This accounts for the striking appearance of the lamellae when viewed with phase contrast optics.

In addition to interstitial lamellae and concentric lamellae of osteons, there is yet a third group of lamellae called circumferential lamellae. These extend around much of the shaft of a long bone on both its outer and inner surface. The upper portion of Figure 3 shows some circumferential lamellae (**CL**). They extend uninterruptedly from one side of the illustration to the other and they appear as long parallel layers. Elongate lacunae among these lamellae have their long axis disposed in the same direction as the lamellae.

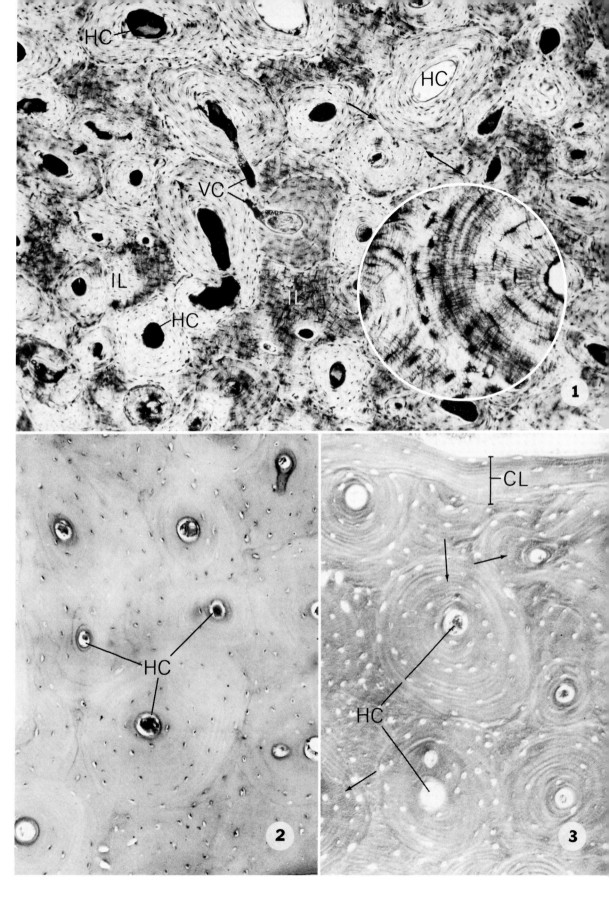

PLATE 3-7

Plate 3-8. Cortical Bone, Electron Microscopy

This electron micrograph shows at low magnification an osteon from the femur of a young rabbit. The bone was decalcified leaving the cells and extracellular soft tissue components (collagen) essentially intact. The particular osteon illustrated here consists of three complete lamellae, numbered 1 to 3 and, immediately surrounding the Haversian canal (**HC**), a fourth lamella which is incomplete (**asterisks**). The outer limit of the osteon is marked by a cement line (**CL**) and beyond this is an interstitial lamella (**IL**).

In examining the Haversian canal the most apparent structures are the blood vessels. Both are capillaries (**Cap**). The smaller vessel is surrounded by pericytes, whereas the larger one does not possess this additional cellular investment. It should be noted that the closely packed preosteoblasts around the capillaries can easily be mistaken for smooth muscle cells of larger blood vessels with the light microscope. However, the electron microscope shows that veins and arteries are not present in Haversian canals, rather, as already indicated there are two types of capillaries. The cells within the Haversian canal (other than those associated with the capillaries) are either osteoblasts or preosteoblasts. The osteoblasts (**Ob**) line the Haversian canal. The remainder of the cells are regarded as preosteoblasts (**POb**). They are less differentiated cells, but have the capacity to transform into osteoblasts as the lining osteoblasts become incorporated into the bone matrix which they produce. In examining the osteoblasts it should be noted that one of them exhibits a process extending into a canaliculus (**double arrow**) of the incomplete lamella. Similarly, the osteocyte in the lower portion of the figure also shows cytoplasmic processes entering canaliculi (**arrows**).

The canaliculi (**C**) within the lamellae, and those extending across the lamellae appear less numerous than the number in a light micrograph (see **inset,** Plate 3-5). The difference is a reflection of the thickness of the section, more canaliculi being included in the relatively thick light microscope section than the number included in the thin section utilized in electron microscopy.

KEY

Cap, capillary
C, canaliculus
CL, cement line (of Ebner)
IL, interstitial lamellae
HC, Haversian canal
L, lacuna
Ob, osteoblast
Oc, osteocyte
POb, preosteoblast
double arrow, osteoblast process in canaliculus
single arrow, osteocyte processes in canaliculus
#1,2,3, lamellae

Fig., x 3,000. Electron micrograph, courtesy of S. C. Luk, C. Nopajaroonsri, and G. T. Simon. J.U.R. *46:*184, 1974.

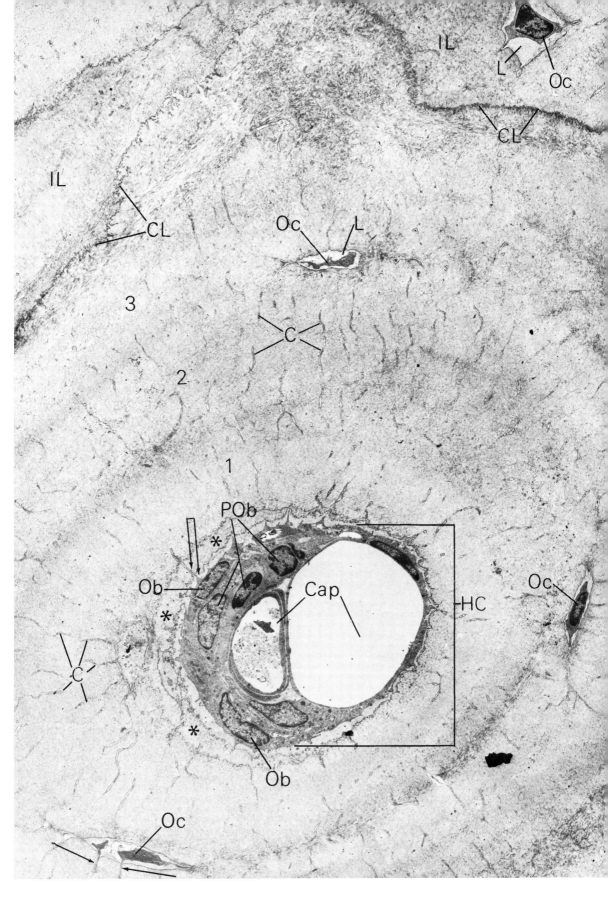

PLATE 3-8

Plate 3-9. ENDOCHONDRAL BONE FORMATION I

Endochondral bone formation involves the simultaneous removal of cartilage and the formation of bone. Moreover, as a bone grows, it undergoes changes in shape, i.e., external remodeling. These changes include the formation of a large medullary cavity. Two specialized cell types have been identified with the process of bone growth and remodeling, osteoblasts and osteoclasts. Osteoblasts are the cells that are engaged in the formation of bone. Although the removal of bone is not as well understood, it has been established that multinucleated cells, called osteoclasts, are engaged in the removal of bone in some situations. (Osteocytes can alter and resorb the bone in their immediate vicinity. The process is called osteocytic osteolysis; its role in bone remodeling, if any, is not clear.)

The early steps of endochondral bone formation are illustrated in the cartilage model on the left side of Figure 1. These steps are: (1) The cartilage cells in the center become enlarged, i.e., hypertrophic (**HC**). (2) The matrix of the cartilage becomes calcified (**CM**). The calcified matrix stains intensely with hematoxylin and appears as the black material between the white spaces occupied by the enlarged cartilage cells. (3) A collar of bone forms around the circumference of the center of the cartilage bar. This bone is called *periosteal bone* (**PB**) because the osteoblasts develop from the periosteum (at this very early stage it might be called perichondral bone). It should be noted that the periosteal bone (or perichondral bone) is in fact intramembranous bone since it develops within the membrane that surrounds the bone (or cartilage).

The cartilage model on the right side of Figure 1 shows the next events and a continuation of the earlier ones. A vascular bud (not shown) and accompanying perivascular cells from the periosteum invade the calcified cartilage and bring about its dissolution, thereby forming a cavity (**Cav**). Careful examination at higher power would reveal that the cells in the center of this cavity are not all cartilage cells; some of them are connective tissue cells. While this new step occurs, the earlier steps continue: (1) the cartilage cells proliferate, thereby providing for an increase in the length of the develop-

KEY

AC, articular cartilage
Cav, cavity
CM, calcified matrix
EB, endochondral bone
EpC, epiphyseal plate
HC, hypertrophic cartilage cells
PB, periosteal (perichondral) bone
P Bud, periosteal bud

Fig. 1 (monkey), x 40; Fig. 2 (human), x 40; Fig. 3 (monkey), x 16.

ing bone; (2) the periosteal bone (**PB**) continues to form; (3) the cartilage cells facing the cavity become hypertrophic (**HC**); (4) the matrix becomes calcified (**CM**) and erosion of cartilage occurs at the two extremities of the expanding cavity; and (5) bone forms on the spicules of cartilage at the erosion front. This is *endochondral bone*.

All of these processes are seen at a more advanced stage in Figure 2. Note the thicker and more extensive periosteal bone (**PB**) which stains with eosin, the enlarged cavity (**Cav**), the edge of the eroded cartilage, and the endochondral bone (**EB**) which has formed around the cartilagenous spicules at the erosion front. This bone also stains with eosin, whereas the calcified cartilage stains intensely with hematoxylin. Some intensely staining calcified cartilage is still present in the spicules of endochondral bone.

At some point, as the continuous processes described above proceed, one end of the cartilage model (the epiphysis) is invaded by blood vessels and connective tissue from the periostium (periosteal bud) (**P Bud**) and it undergoes the same changes that occurred in the shaft (Fig. 3) except that no periosteal (or perichondrial) bone forms. This same process then occurs at the other end of the long bone. Consequently, at each end of a developing long bone a cartilaginous plate (epiphyseal plate) (**EpC**) is between two sites of bone formation. The rectangle in Figure 3 is shown at higher magnification in Plate 3-10.

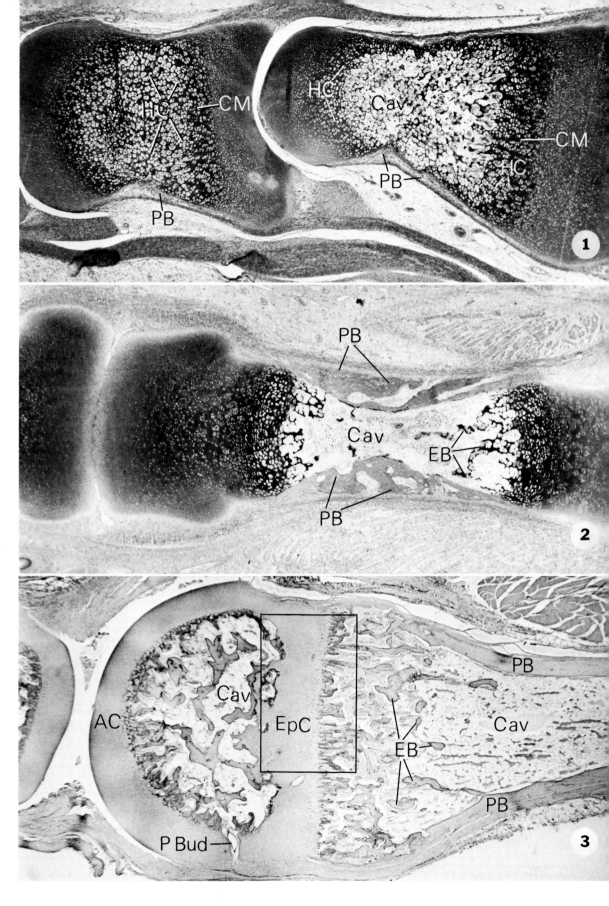

PLATE 3-9

Plate 3-10. ENDOCHONDRAL BONE FORMATION II

A higher magnification of the rectangle in Plate 3-9 is shown as Figure 1. The cartilage of the epiphyseal plate can be divided into different zones which reflect the progressive changes that occur in active endochondral bone formation. These zones are not sharply delineated and the boundary between them is somewhat arbitrary. They lead toward the marrow cavity, so that the first zone is furthest from the cavity. The zones are:

1) The zone of reserve cartilage (**RC**). The cells of this zone have not yet begun to participate in the growth of the bone; they are reserve cells. These cells are small, usually only one to a lacuna, and not grouped. At some time, some of these cells will proliferate and undergo the changes outlined in the next zone. 2) Zone of proliferating cartilage (**PC**). The cells of this zone are increasing in number; they are slightly larger than the reserve cells, close to their neighbors, and they begin to form rows. 3) Zone of hypertrophic cartilage (**HC**). The cells of this zone are aligned in rows and are significantly larger than the cells in the preceding zone. 4) Zone of calcified matrix (**CM**). In this zone the matrix becomes impregnated with calcium salts and, because of this, it stains intensely with hematoxylin. 5) Zone of resorption (**arrows**, Fig. 2). This zone is where an edge of eroded cartilage is in direct contact with the connective tissue. Spicules of cartilage are formed because the pericapillary cells invade and resorb in spearheads rather than along a straight front. Specifically, the pericapillary cells break into the rows of hypertrophied chondrocytes. Endochondral bone (**EB**) formation occurs on the surfaces of these spicules of calcified cartilage.

Osteoblasts (**Ob**) are aligned on the surface of the spicule where bone formation is actively in progress. In most cases, a thin band of material, called osteoid, can be seen on the surface of the spicule in direct contact with the osteoblasts. The osteoid is the recent product of the osteoblasts; it stains with eosin, and is paler or lighter staining than the bone matrix. It is more evident in the illustrations on the following plate. Cartilage cells (**CC**) are still present in the center of some spicules, especially near the epiphyseal cartilage (Fig. 2). The smaller cells in the spicules, more

KEY

B, bone
C, cartilage
Cav, marrow cavity
CC, cartilage cells
CM, calcified matrix
CT, connective tissue
EB, endochondral bone
EBF, endochondral bone formation
HC, hypertrophic cartilage
M, marrow cells
Ob, osteoblasts
Oc, osteocytes
PC, proliferating cartilage
RC, reserve cartilage
arrows, resorption of cartilage

Fig. 1 (monkey), x 40; Fig. 2 (monkey), x 160; Fig. 3 (dog), x 160.

isolated and surrounded by eosinophilic matrix, are osteocytes (**Oc**). Between the spicules in Figures 1 and 2 is loose connective tissue (**CT**).

Figure 3 shows the epiphyseal plate where bone formation is going on at a reduced rate and only on one side of the epiphyseal plate. The functional zones are similar to those described above, but they are reduced in extent, along with the reduction of the thickness of the epiphyseal plate (Figs. 2 and 3 are the same magnification.) The histological signs of endochondral bone formation (**EBF**) are present on the diaphyseal side of the epiphyseal plate, but not on the epiphyseal side. This is indicated because bone (**B**) contacts the cartilage (**C**) on the epiphyseal side, whereas connective tissue (**CT**) is in contact with the cartilage on the diphyseal side. The connective tissue between the spicules contains large numbers of round cells. These are marrow cells (**M**).

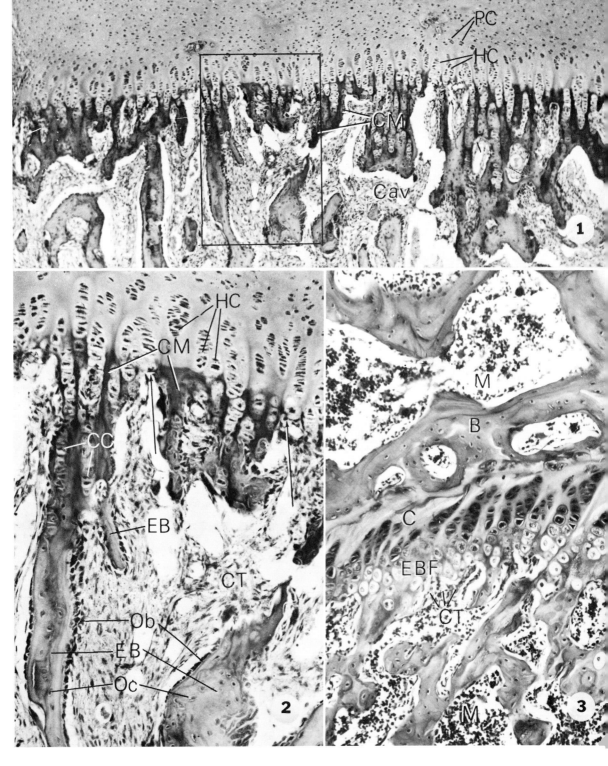

Epiphyseal Plate

PLATE 3-10

Plate 3-11. Intramembranous Bone Formation

The flat bones of the skull, the mandible, and the clavicle ossify, at least in part, via an intramembranous route. The bones which form via an intramembranous route do not provide structural support compared to the support that is required of bones that ossify via an endochondral route.

The formation of intramembranous bone in the mandible is shown in Figure 1. This is a low-power panoramic view which shows some developing spicules of bone and their relationship to the surface of the face. The bone spicules (**BS**) appear as the elongated irregular dark profiles in the connective tissue. The oval structure is Meckel's cartilage (**MC**).

The sequence of events in intramembranous bone formation can be studied by examining a spicule (**rectangle**) at higher magnification (Fig. 1, **inset**). The earliest steps are illustrated at the top and later events at the bottom. During intramembranous bone formation, cells of the connective tissue differentiate into osteoblasts (**Ob**) and aggregate at the site where the bone is laid down. The osteoblasts engage in the production of osteoid (**Os**) which consists of collagenous fibers and a homogenous matrix. Osteoid can be recognized because it is situated on the surface of bone spicules, osteoblasts are usually seen in contact with it, and it stains less intensely with eosin than does the "matrix" of the bone. Osteoid becomes calcified and is then bone. When osteoblasts have surrounded themselves with their product and come to lie in lacunae, they are called osteocytes.

Intramembranous bone formation and the remodeling of the skull are illustrated in Figure 2. Note that osteoblasts and osteoid are present along almost the entire surface of bone on the skin side. Lines can be seen in the spicules (**BS**) which reflect the general contours and pattern of bone deposition. These lines are intact on the side of the spicule upon which bone is being deposited, but they are interrupted where bone is being resorbed (**arrow**).

Figure 3 shows developing intramembranous bone at higher magnification. The nuclei of the osteocytes (**Oc**) stain with hematoxylin and stand out against the pink-staining matrix. The osteoblasts (**Ob**) are located on the surface of the bone spicule, immediately

KEY

BS, bone spicules
BV, blood vessels
MC, Meckel's cartilage
Ob, osteoblasts
Oc, osteocyte
Ocl, osteoclast
Os, osteoid
arrow, edge where bone was resorbed

Fig. 1 (pig), x 65; Fig. 2 (human), x 65; Fig. 3 (human), x 160; Fig. 4 (rabbit), x 640.

adjacent to the lightly staining osteoid (**Os**) which they have just formed. Two osteoclasts (**Ocl**) can be seen on the under surface of one of the spicules. Loose connective tissue is between the bone spicules, the blood vessels (**BV**) are located within this connective tissue at approximately equal distance from the neighboring bone spicules.

Osteoclasts are multinucleated cells which engage in the removal of bone. They are immediately adjacent to the bone which is actually being removed (Fig. 4). A ruffled border is present at the cell-bone junction, but this can only be seen in the most favorable preparations. After osteoclasts have been at work for some time, they form a slight concavity on the surface of the bone. This concavity is called Howship's lacuna.

Notice in these figures, the blood vessels are located at approximately an equidistant point from the advancing fronts of bone formation. The bone at this point of development resembles spongy bone and it is designated primary spongiosa. Most of this bone will continue to develop into compact bone. With continued bone formation, the bone trabeculae will become thicker and ultimately bone comes to replace most of the connective tissue surrounding the blood vessels. This will then be compact woven bone.

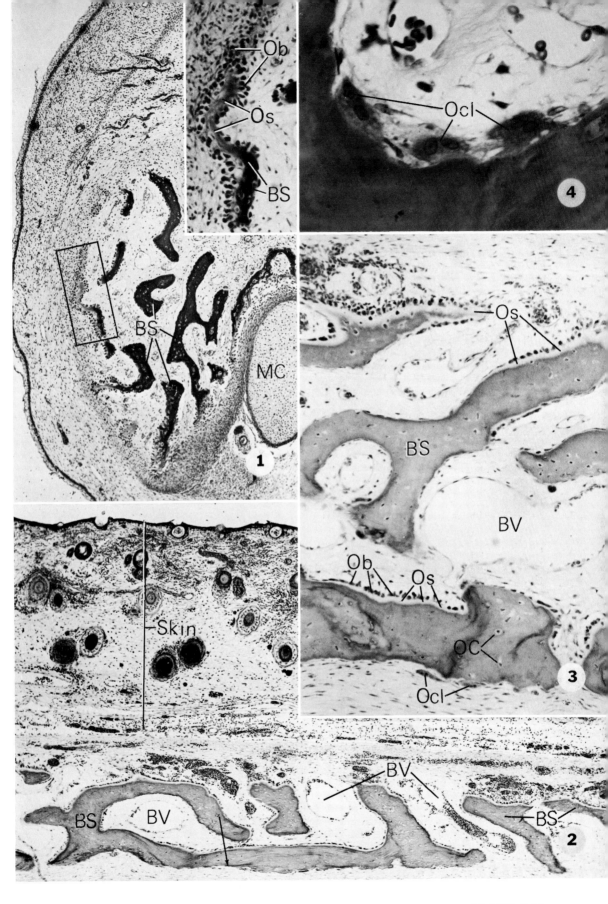

PLATE 3-11

Plate 3-12. DEVELOPING BONE I, ELECTRON MICROSCOPY

This electron micrograph reveals the periosteal surface of a growing long bone. It is from the mid-portion of the shaft, a region of the bone which develops by intramembranous ossification. Accordingly no cartilage is present. The upper part of the illustration reveals typical fibroblasts (**Fib**) and bundles of collagenous fibers (**CF**). This constitutes the layer which, with the light microscope, is referred to as the fibrous portion of the periosteum (**FP**). Below is the cellular layer of the periostium which contains the preosteoblasts (**POb**) and osteoblasts (**Ob**).

The osteoblasts are aligned on the surface of the developing bone. They appear more or less cuboidal in shape. The lateral boundaries of adjacent osteoblasts are not very conspicuous, but the distinction between adjacent cells is somewhat enhanced by differences in electron density of the cytoplasmic matrix. The osteoblasts contain large amounts of rough surfaced endoplasmic reticulum (**RER**) and an extensive Golgi apparatus (see Plate 3-13), features indicative of cells highly active in protein synthesis. Note that the preosteoblasts possess more cytoplasm than the fibroblasts, but on the other hand, its rough surfaced endoplasmic reticulum (**RER**) is not yet as extensive as the reticulum in the osteoblasts.

Below the osteoblasts is the osteoid (**Os**), the material which in the light microscope simply appears as the poorly staining homogenous band between the osteoblasts and the bone. The osteoid consists principally of collagen, ground substance and some processes from the osteoblasts that extend between the collagen fibrils. These are shown at higher magnification in Plate 3-13.

In order to fully understand the biology of bone growth it is necessary to realize that the osteoblasts move away from the bone as they secrete their product, the osteoid. Shortly after the osteoid is produced, it becomes calcified, by a wave of mineralization which follows the movement of the osteoblasts, with the osteoid always intervening. The calcium is in the form of hydroxyapatite crystals. In this specimen most of the calcium salts have been lost from the bone (**B**); consequently it has a relatively electron lucid appearance. However, calcium salts remain

KEY

B, bone
C, canaliculi
CF, collagen fibers
Fib, fibroblasts
FP, fibrous periosteum
Ob, osteoblasts
Oc, osteocyte
Os, osteoid
POb, preosteoblast
RER, rough surfaced endoplasmic reticulum
asterisks, mineralization front

Fig., x 5000

at the mineralization front where it appears as the black electron opaque material (**asterisks**).

At intervals, certain osteoblasts no longer continue to move away from the bone and as a consequence the cell is surrounded by the osteoid it has produced. As the mineralization front progresses, the cell becomes surrounded by bone. It is then contained within a lacuna, and referred to as an osteocyte. A recently formed osteocyte (**Oc**) can be seen in the micrograph. Note that the bone matrix which borders the lacuna has retained its calcium salts. The processes of the osteocyte are contained in canaliculi (**C**).

Other osteocytes also arise in the same manner as just described. Thus, as the bone thickens, the osteoblast layer tends to become depleted as the osteoblasts become transformed into osteocytes. However, the depletion is balanced by the proliferation of connective tissue cells which differentiate first into preosteoblast and then to osteoblasts.

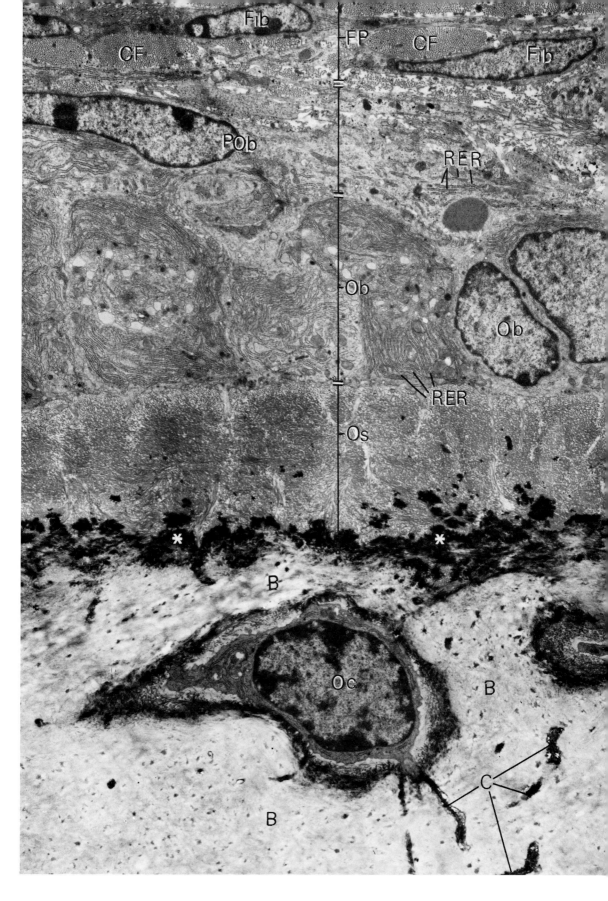

PLATE 3-12

Plate 3-13. DEVELOPING BONE II, ELECTRON MICROSCOPY

The osteoblasts shown in Figure 1 are comparable to those seen in the preceding plate. The higher magnification shows to advantage the cytological detail of the cells.

In characterizing the osteoblast as well as understanding the nature of its product, it is important to realize that osteoblasts are derived from connective tissue cells which are indistinguishable from fibroblasts. They retain much of the cytologic morphology of the fibroblasts and this is evident in the accompanying electron micrograph. In active fibroblasts, there is a large amount of rough surfaced endoplasmic reticulum and an extensive Golgi apparatus. The osteoblasts pictured here also contain a large amount of rough surfaced endoplasmic reticulum (**RER**) and a prominent Golgi apparatus (**GA**), indicative of their role in the production of osteoid. The Golgi apparatus shown in the osteoblast contains typical flattened sacs and transport vesicles. It also shows enlarged vesicles which contain material of various density. Two of the large elongated Golgi vesicles (**arrows**), contain a filamentous component. On the basis of special staining techniques for electron microscopy, such filaments are considered to be collagen precursor.

The osteoblasts in Figure 1 (and those in the preceding plate) have a cuboidal shape and because of their close apposition they bear a resemblance to cuboidal cells in an epithelial sheet. While the osteoblasts are indeed arranged on the surface of the developing bone in a sheet-like manner, they nevertheless exhibit properties of connective tissue cells, not epithelial cells. It should be noted that no basement lamina surrounds the osteoblasts, moreover, although none are pictured in Figure 1, collagen fibrils are occasionally observed between osteoblasts. The osteoblast differs from the typical fibroblast in that the former cell type is highly polar, secreting onto the bone surface. The surface of the osteoblast which faces the osteoid can be regarded to be the secretory face, or secretory pole of the cell.

The secretory face of the osteoblast is shown adjacent to the osteoid at higher magnification in Figure 2. Both the round and the somewhat larger irregularly shaped profiles of the osteoid are collagen fibrils (**C**). Ground

KEY

C, collagen fibrils
GA, Golgi apparatus
N, nucleus of osteoblast
Os, osteoid
POb, preosteoblast
RER, rough surfaced endoplasmic reticulum
arrows, (Fig. 1) elongate Golgi vesicles with collagen precursor
arrow, (Fig. 2) process of osteoblast
arrowheads, large collagen fibrils

Fig. 1, x 14,000; Fig. 2, x 30,000.

substance occupies the space between the collagen fibrils. It should be recalled that the osteoblast is moving away from the bone leaving its product behind. The collagen fibrils closest to the cell are of small diameter and represent the most recently formed fibrils. With time, as the cell recedes and as the mineralization front approaches, the collagen fibrils increase in diameter. This is thought to occur by the accretion of additional collagen onto the fibrils already present. It is not unlikely that some of the large irregularly shaped fibrils (**arrowheads**) arise by a combination of accretion and the fusion of smaller fibrils. By the time the mineralization front reaches the fibrils, they have achieved their greatest diameter. Mineralization results in an impregnation of both the collagen fibrils as well as the ground substance with calcium hydroxyapatite.

The illustration also shows processes of the bone forming cells (**arrow**). These processes will be contained in canaliculi after the osteoblast is transformed into an osteocyte.

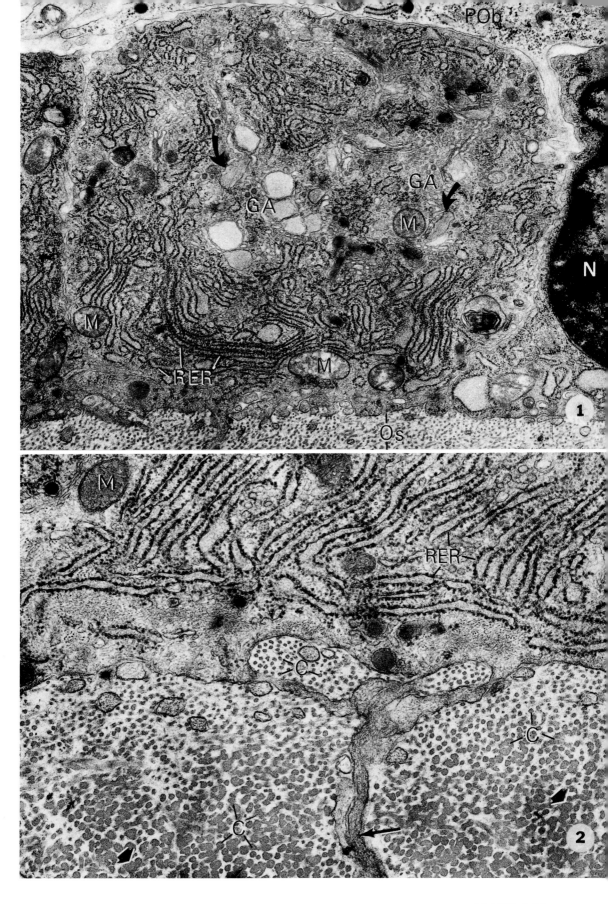

PLATE 3-13

Plate 3-14. The Osteoclast, Electron Microscopy

This illustration shows a segment of bone surface (**B**) and adjacent to the bone, portions of two cells, an osteoblast (**Ob**) and an osteoclast (**Oc**). The difference between these two cell types is reflected not only in their cytological appearance, but also in the character of the underlying extracellular matrix. As already noted, the osteoblast is typically separated from the mineralization front of the bone by osteoid (**Os**). The portion of the cell seen in relation to the osteoid is readily identified as an osteoblast by its extensive rough surfaced endoplasmic reticulum. Similarly the osteoid is recognized by the presence of the numerous collagen fibrils.

In contrast, the osteoclast is adjacent to a mixture of collagen fibrils and hydroxyapatite crystals. In effect, at this site, bone is being broken down. The portion of the osteoclast which is in apposition with this partially digested bone possesses numerous infoldings of the plasma membrane (**inset**). When viewed with the light microscope, the infoldings are evident as the ruffled border. When the plane of section is at right angles to the infoldings, they resemble microvilli. They are however folds, not fingerlike microvillous projections, and when sectioned in a plane paralleling a fold (**asterisks**), a broad nonspecialized expanse of cytoplasm is seen. This is the cytoplasm within the fold of the ruffled border; it is free of organelles except for fine filaments. Apatite crystals (**arrows**) can often be seen in the extracellular space of the infoldings.

The cytoplasm of the osteoclast contains numerous mitochondria (**M**), lysosomes, and Golgi complexes all of which are functionally linked with the resorption and degradation of the bone substance. Electron micrographs show that the apatite crystals are ingested by the cell. After the apatite crystals are ingested, the calcium is mobilized for passage into the blood stream in a manner not yet fully understood. The organic matrix (i.e., collagen and ground substance) is also resorbed by the osteoclast, but again the exact mechanisms are not clear. However, there is evidence that the osteoclast secretes hydrolytic enzymes into the area of bone where actual resorption is in progress.

As in Figure 3-12, the bone, except at the mineralization front (**MF**) and the resorption

front (**RF**), appears unusually light because the mineral component has been lost during the preparation of the specimen. In the lower part of the illustration, some collagen fibrils are evident, the arrows indicate where cross banding is visible.

The proximity of osteoblasts and osteoclasts on the bone surface is not atypical. It highlights the fact that the bone surface is subject to continuous change, especially in growing individuals.

KEY

B, bone
Ob, osteoblast
Oc, osteoclast
M, mitochondria
MF, mineralization front
RB, ruffled border
RF, resorption front
arrowheads, apatite crystals
asterisks, cytoplasm within folds of ruffled border

Fig., x 10,000, (inset) x 25,000.

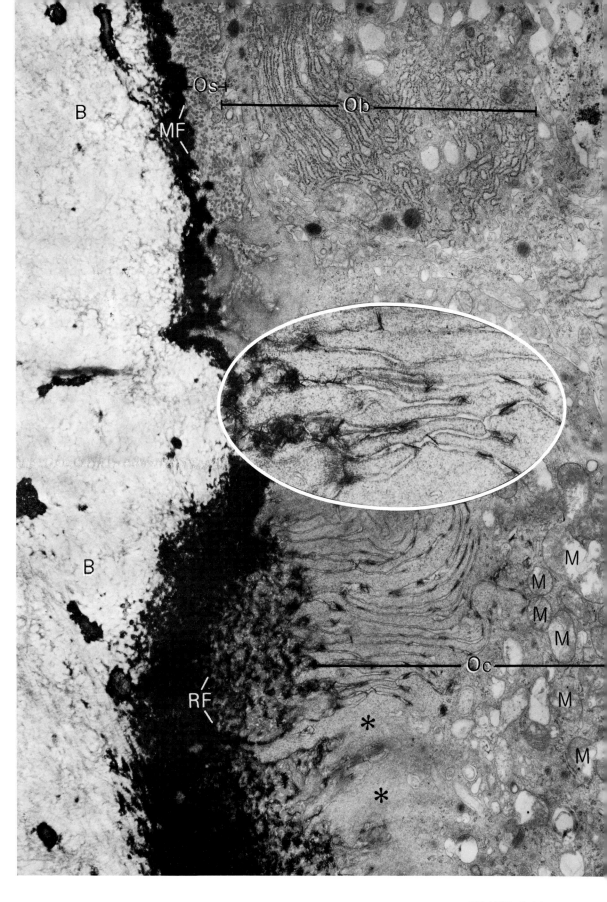

PLATE 3-14

4 BLOOD

BLOOD CAN BE REGARDED as the fluid tissue which circulates through the cardiovascular system. It is a derivative of connective tissue and consequently it is frequently classified under this category. Blood consists of cells and a liquid intercellular material, *plasma*. Approximately 45 per cent of the volume of a normal blood sample consists of cells; the remainder is plasma. The cellular components of blood and their relative numbers are given below.

A. Red Blood Cells (Erythrocytes), 4–5 million per cu. mm.
B. White Blood Cells (Leucocytes), 6–9 thousand per cu. mm.
    1. agranulocytes   (*approx. percentage of white cells*)
       lymphocytes   30–35
       monocytes   3– 7
    2. granulocytes
       neutrophils   55–60
       eosinophils   2– 5
       basophils   0– 1
C. Platelets (Thrombocytes) 200,000–400,000 per cu. mm.

Each blood cell has a life cycle of limited duration, and during only part of this cycle is the cell a component of the peripheral blood. It follows that the production and destruction of blood cells goes on constantly. *Red blood cells, granulocytes, monocytes,* and *platelets* are formed within the red bone marrow; lymphocytes are formed within the bone marrow and lymphoid tissues (see also Chapter 8). During fetal development both red and white cells are also formed in other areas, e.g., in the spleen and liver.

Platelets are cytoplasmic fragments derived from multinucleated giant cells (megakaryocytes) of the bone marrow. In peripheral blood they appear as small blue-stained bodies, frequently in clusters.

Red blood cells and platelets perform their functions while they are within the blood stream. However, the white blood cells regularly leave the blood through the walls of capillaries and venules to enter the connective tissues, lymphoid tissues and bone marrow where they perform specific functions. Thus white blood cells must be regarded as transients within the blood which use the blood stream as a vehicle for being transported to specific sites within the body.

The method which displays the cell types of peripheral blood to greatest advantage is the blood smear. This differs from the usual preparation seen in the histology laboratory in that the specimen is not imbedded in paraffin and sectioned. Rather, a drop of blood is placed directly on a slide. The drop is spread thin with another slide, allowed to dry and then stained. Another point of difference in the preparation of a blood smear is that instead of hematoxylin and eosin, special mixtures of dyes are used for staining of blood cells. The resulting preparation may be examined with or without a cover slip.

Dyes used to stain blood smears are usually based on modifications of the Romanowsky type stain. This consists of a mixture of methylene blue (a basic dye), related azures (also basic dyes), and eosin (an acid dye). In principal, the basic dyes stain nuclei, basophil granules, and RNA of the cytoplasm, whereas the acid dye stains the red blood cells and the granules of eosinophils. It was originally thought that the neutrophil granules were stained by a "neutral dye" that formed when methylene blue and its related azures were combined with eosin. However, the mechanism whereby neutrophil granules are stained is not clear. To complicate matters further, some of the basic dyes (the azures) are metachromatic and impart a violet-to-red color to the material they stain.

Plate 4-1. ERYTHROCYTES AND AGRANULOCYTES

In examining a blood smear, it is useful to survey the smear with a low-power objective in order to ascertain which parts of the preparation show an even distribution of blood cells. In general, the periphery of a blood smear should be avoided, the cells being either distorted, too close to each other (at the end where the drop of blood was placed), or too widely dispersed (at the opposite end, where the smear ended). Furthermore, the edges of a blood smear do not show a true per cent distribution of white cells.

Figure 1 shows a low-power view of a smear with the blood cells well distributed. Most of the cells are *erythrocytes.* They are readily identified because of their number and lack of a nucleus. Scattered among the red cells are a number of white blood cells which, collectively can be distinguished from the erythrocytes without difficulty because of their larger size and/or their staining characteristics.

Erythrocytes have a biconcave shape. In the circulating blood they measure about 8.5 microns in diameter. In blood smears, they measure about 7.5 microns, and in sectioned material about 7 microns. [The latter figure (7μ) is useful to remember since it enables one to ascertain, by comparison, the approximate size of other structures in tissue sections without resorting to a micrometer.] Erythrocytes stain uniformly with eosin, a component of the usual dye mixture (e.g., Wright's) used to stain blood smears. However, because of the biconcave form of the erythrocyte, its center is thinner and appears lighter than the periphery.

In order to distinguish the different kinds of leucocytes in a blood smear, it is advantageous to use the highest available magnification, usually an oil immersion lens. This enables one to ascertain the morphological features of the cytoplasm and use this information in addition to nuclear morphology and cytoplasmic staining in identifying the cell type.

Lymphocytes and monocytes are classified as *agranulocytes,* that is, they are usually free of conspicuous cytoplasmic granules. Moreover, their nuclei are described as nonlobulated. Thus, they are distinguished from granulocytes which possess distinct cyto-

KEY

arrow, Golgi area

Fig. 1 (human), x 400; Figs. 2–6 (human), x 1800.

plasmic granules as well as lobulated or segmented nuclei.

Figures 2 and 3 serve to illustrate characteristic features of *lymphocytes.* Their nuclei stain intensely; they generally have a rounded shape and, as illustrated in Figure 2, the nucleus may possess a slight indentation. These cells measure 8 and 10 microns in diameter, respectively (lymphocytes range from 6 to 12 microns in diameter). Frequently, only a small amount of cytoplasm is present (Fig. 2) and one gets the impression that the nucleus constitutes most of the cellular volume. In other cells (e.g., Fig. 3) a distinct rim of cytoplasm surrounds the nucleus and a lightly stained Golgi area (**arrow**) may be evident. The cytoplasm stains pale blue and occasional azurophilic granules may be observed.

Figures 4 and 5 show characteristic features of *monocytes.* These cells measure about 15 microns in diameter (monocytes range from 9 to 18 microns in diameter). Each cell possesses an indented nucleus, and in both cases, the indentation typically faces the larger cytoplasmic area of the cell. The nuclei are somewhat less "compact" than the nuclei of lymphocytes. The cytoplasm, like that of the lymphocyte stains lightly, but tends to have a grayer or duller blue tint as compared to the lymphocytes. Azurophilic granules are also present and may be more conspicuous, but less numerous, than those of the lymphocyte.

Figure 6 illustrates a cell which is difficult to identify with certainty. The lack of distinctive granules suggests that it is either a monocyte or a large lymphocyte. On the other hand, the nuclear contour and faint cytoplasmic granulation suggest that the cell might be related to the neutrophils. A more frequent difficulty in the identification of monocytes is encountered in deciding between small monocytes versus large lymphocytes, inasmuch as it is possible in most blood smears to find cells with characteristics intermediate between those of lymphocytes and monocytes.

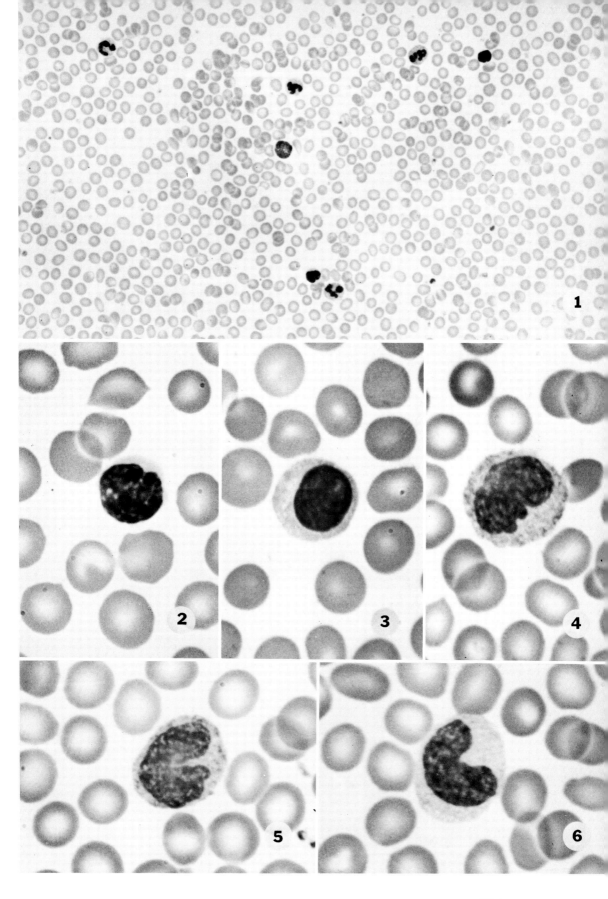

PLATE 4-1

Plate 4-2. GRANULOCYTES

Granulocytes are characterized by the presence of a lobed nucleus and distinctive granules within the cytoplasm. Three kinds of granulocytes are present in a peripheral blood smear: neutrophils, basophils, and eosinophils.

Neutrophils develop in the red bone marrow from cells which have a rounded nucleus. During their maturation, the nucleus changes from a rounded to a segmented, or lobed, form. A fully developed neutrophil nucleus may have as many as five lobes. The configuration and number of lobes varies from one cell to another (Figs. 1–3) and on the basis of the variable nuclear morphology, these cells are sometimes named polymorphonuclear neutrophils. It should be understood, however, that each cell has only one nucleus, each lobe being joined to its neighbor by a strand of nuclear material. Figure 1 shows two neutrophils whose nuclei are incompletely segmented. The nucleus of these cells is C shaped. Such cells are referred to as band cells; a number of other terms have also been coined to describe these cells, however, their use is being discouraged. These cells are regarded as being younger than those cells whose nuclei are lobulated as in Figures 2 and 3.

Neutrophils usually measure from 9 to 14 microns in diameter. The cytoplasm of these cells contain granules which range from 0.1 to about 0.4 micron in diameter and stain variably, either azure, light blue, or violet. Although neutrophils contain characteristic granules, the identification of these cells can usually be accomplished on the basis of the distinctive lobulation and staining of their nuclei. Moreover the fact that these cells are the most numerous of the leucocytes, in a smear of normal blood, in itself constitutes a basis for their identification.

Eosinophils are shown at high magnification in Figures 4 and 5. These measure 12 and 13 microns, respectively (eosinophils range from 10 to 14 microns in diameter). The most conspicuous feature of eosinophils is the presence of numerous cytoplasmic granules which stain with eosin. The granules dominate the cell and frequently obscure the edges of the nucleus. In some cases, the granules may overlie the nucleus. The eosinophilic gran-

KEY

Figs. 1–6 (human), x 1800.

ules have specific morphological characteristics which can be used in the identification of the cells. The granules are relatively uniform in size within a particular cell. They are about 1 micron in diameter, significantly larger than granules of neutrophils, and are typically closely packed. In going "through focus," eosinophilic granules often display a marked refractility.

A *basophil* is shown in Figure 6. It measures 11 microns in diameter (the range being from 9 to 14 microns). These cells contain cytoplasmic granules which stain intensely with methylene blue. The granules are randomly distributed throughout the cell and usually obscure the nucleus to such a degree that it can barely be distinguished. Some of the granules shown in Figure 6 are larger than the eosinophilic granules, others are smaller, and some are as small as those found in the neutrophils. The basophil is the rarest of the leucocytes. It may be necessary to examine a significant part of the blood smear before one can be found.

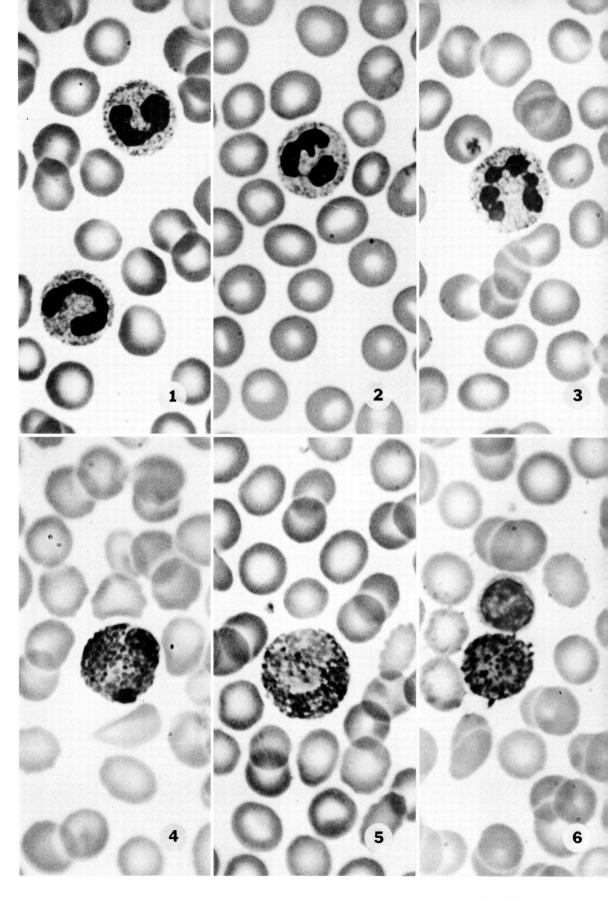

PLATE 4-2

5 MUSCLE TISSUE

MUSCLE consists of long protoplasmic fibers which are specialized to contract. The muscle fibers are cellular elements and should not be confused with connective tissue fibers, which are extracellular and nonprotoplasmic. There are two distinctive types of muscle: smooth and striated. Striated muscle is further subdivided as being skeletal, cardiac, or visceral.

Smooth muscle consists of cells that are almost invariably spindle shaped. They possess a single, elongated nucleus. The cytoplasm of smooth muscle cells contains a variety of organelles; however, in routine H & E preparations, the cytoplasm stains rather evenly with eosin, and the organelles are not visualized. Examination of the cytoplasm with the electron microscope shows longitudinally oriented threadlike structures called myofilaments. These are the contractile elements within the cytoplasm.

Smooth muscle is found in many locations within the body. It is found in large amounts in the walls of the viscera (and for this reason it is also called visceral muscle); it is present in the walls of blood vessels; it is present in small bundles or as single cells in the skin, endocardium, intestinal villi, etc.; and it is associated with many glands and their ducts. If the muscle cells that are associated with the glands (or their ducts) are on the epithelial side of the basement membrane they are called myoepithelial cells. (It should be noted that the myoepithelial cells develop from the same source as the epithelium itself.)

Muscle cells within a bundle or layer are usually oriented in the same direction, but neighboring bundles or layers may be oriented in different directions. For example, in the intestines, two of the muscle layers are oriented at right angles to each other.

Although smooth muscle cells are primarily associated with contraction, they are also able to produce connective tissue fibers. Moreover, a cell type, intermediate between a smooth muscle cell and a fibroblast, occurs in connective tissue. This is the myofibrocyte, shown in Plates 2-2 and 2-3.

Skeletal muscle consists of extremely long multinucleated fibers. When viewed with the light microscope, the cytoplasm is seen to be bounded by a thick "membrane." This membrane was called the sarcolemma by classical histologists and was regarded as being the cell membrane. However, ultrastructural studies reveal that it consists not only of a cell membrane, but of basement membrane material and delicate collagenous fibers. In current usage, the term sarcolemma is restricted to the cell (plasma) membrane as seen with the electron microscope. The nuclei of skeletal muscle fibers are located immediately under the sarcolemma. Skeletal muscle fibers possess cross striations. The striations are the most characteristic histological features of this kind of muscle, and are the basis for the designation "striated muscle." The cytoplasm of skeletal muscle cells contains longitudinal subunits called myofibrils. These can be seen in favorable histological preparations; they are especially evident in cross sections of the muscle fibers, where they give the cut edge of the fiber a stippled appearance.

The cross striations that are seen in routine preparations are a property of the myofibrils. Banded portions of neighboring myofibrils are in register and give the entire muscle fiber its cross striated appearance. Examination of the myofibrils with the electron microscope reveals that they are comprised of myofilaments. There are two types of myofilaments: thin (actin) filaments and thick (myosin) filaments. It is the arrangement of thick and thin filaments which give the myofibril its cross banded appearance.

In addition to its location in the muscles which move the skeleton, multinucleated striated muscle is also found in the muscles of the face, in the muscles that move the eyeballs, in the tongue, in the pharynx, and in the upper part of the esophagus. In the latter two locations, the striated muscle is obviously in a visceral location, and consequently can be classified as visceral striated muscle.

Cardiac muscle is the muscle that is found in the wall of the heart and base of the large veins which empty into the heart. It consists of long fibers which branch and meet neighboring fibers. Cardiac muscle fibers are also cross striated. As in skeletal muscle, the cross striations are ultimately due to the arrangement of thick and thin myofilaments. With the light microscope cardiac muscle fibers also exhibit specialized cross bands called intercalated discs. Examination of these discs with the electron microscope reveals that they are opposing cell membranes with extensive junctional complexes. The fibers of cardiac muscle, then, are distinctly different from the fibers of striated muscle. In cardiac muscle, the cells are aligned end to end to form the functional "fibers" which are seen with the light microscope. On the other hand, a fiber of skeletal or visceral striated muscle is a single protoplasmic unit. The nuclei of cardiac muscle fibers are located at regular intervals in the center of the fibre. (Some of the cardiac muscle fibers are specialized to conduct impulses; these are called Purkinje fibers.)

Plate 5-1. SMOOTH MUSCLE

In longitudinal section, smooth muscle cells appear as elongated fibers, all of which are oriented in the same direction (Fig. 1). Their nuclei (**N**) are also elongated and conform to the general shape of the cell. In this preparation the nuclei appear slightly twisted, like a corkscrew; this is characteristic of nuclei in contracted cells. The cells are slightly separated from each other and this allows one to delineate the cell boundaries. However, the boundaries cannot always be seen in H & E sections (see Fig. 4).

A cross section through smooth muscle cells from the same specimen is shown in Figure 2. The nuclei (**N**) are included in some cells. These appear as dark spherical structures. In most of the cells, however, the nuclei have been missed, and only the eosinophilic cytoplasm appears. Because the cells are staggered, some are cut through the thick central portion, others are cut through the tapering ends. The difference in diameter between neighboring cells is one of the most characteristic features of smooth muscle that is cut in cross section. This also applies to the nuclei, but to a much lesser degree. The two elongated nuclei (**arrows**) belong to connective tissue cells.

Interlacing bundles of smooth muscle cells are shown in Figure 3. One bundle has been cut longitudinally (**L**). This can be recognized by the elongated shape of the nuclei. Other bundles of smooth muscle cells have been cut in cross section or obliquely (**X**). Because the muscle cells within a bundle are oriented in the same direction, they have essentially the same appearance regardless of the plane of section. Therefore, when the bundle is cut longitudinally, the cells and their nuclei all appear elongated; when the bundle is cut in cross section, they appear polygonal. This point is more evident in Figure 4, which is a higher magnification of the same specimen shown in Figure 3. Note where the smooth muscle cells are cut longitudinally (**L**), the nuclei (**N**) are elongated; where they are cut in cross section or obliquely (**X**), the nuclei are spherical or oval.

Connective tissue (**CT**) is between the bundles of smooth muscle cells. Connective tissue can be distinguished from the muscle in several ways: (1) Smooth muscle cells are

KEY

CT, connective tissue
L, smooth muscle, longitudinal section
N, nuclei of smooth muscle cells
X, smooth muscle, cross or oblique section
arrows, connective tissue cell nuclei

Fig. 1 (intestine, monkey), x 640; Fig. 2 (intestine, monkey), x 640; Fig. 3 (uterus, human), x 160; Fig. 4 (uterus, human), x 640.

regularly oriented, but the connective tissue fibers are arranged in a somewhat irregular and wavy pattern; 2) the nuclei of the smooth muscle cells have essentially the same shape in a particular bundle; the nuclei of the connective tissue cells, on the other hand, present a variety of shapes; (3) the muscle cytoplasm stains more intensely than the connective tissue fibers; and (4) when examining smooth muscle, one sees a characteristic number of nuclei per unit area of tissue.

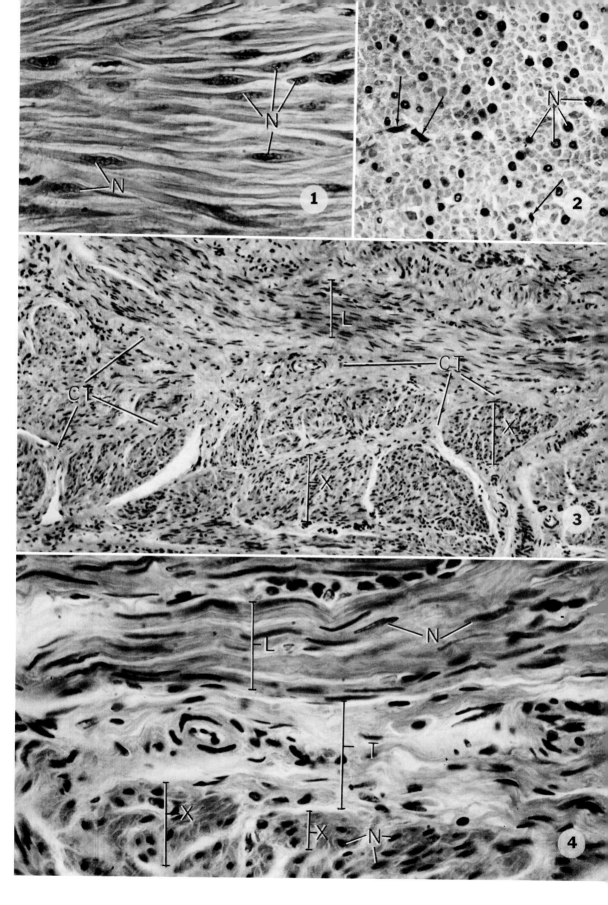

PLATE 5-1

Plate 5-2. SMOOTH MUSCLE, LONGITUDINAL SECTION, ELECTRON MICROSCOPY

The electron micrograph illustrated here shows smooth muscle comparable to that shown in the light micrograph of Figure 1 in the preceding plate. The muscle cells are longitudinally oriented and are seen in relatively relaxed state as evidenced by the smooth contour of their nuclei. The intercellular space is occupied by abundant collagen fibrils (**C**) which course in varying planes between the cells.

At the low magnification utilized here much of the cytoplasmic mass of the muscle cells has a homogeneous appearance. This homogeneous appearance is due to the contractile components of the cell, namely the thin (5nm) actin filaments which are oriented in parallel array in the direction of the long axis of the cell. (The thicker myosin filaments of mammalian smooth muscle cells are extremely labile and tend to be lost during tissue preparation). The non-homogeneous appearing portions of the cytoplasm contain mitochondria and other cell organelles. To illustrate these differences, the area within the small circle in the lower right of the micrograph is shown at higher magnification in the inset nearest the right hand margin of the micrograph. The particular site selected for the inset reveals a filamentous area (**F**) as well as a region containing mitochondria (**M**), a few profiles of rough endoplasmic reticulum (**arrows**), and numerous dense particles, most of which are glycogen. While the distinction between the filamentous containing regions of cytoplasm and those areas containing the remaining organelles are clearly evident in the electron microscope, the routine H & E preparation of light microscopy reveals only a homogeneous eosinophilic staining cytoplasm.

Fibroblasts and other connective tissue cells, when present, are also readily discernible in electron micrographs among the smooth muscle cells of various organs. In this micrograph several fibroblasts (**Fib**) are evident. In contrast to the smooth muscle cell, their cytoplasm exhibits numerous profiles of rough endoplasmic reticulum, as well as other organelles throughout all but the very attenuated cytoplasmic processes. For purposes of comparison, the small circled area of the

KEY

C, collagen
F, filamentous area of cytoplasm
Fib, fibroblast
M, mitochondria
N, nucleus, smooth muscle cell
arrows, endoplasmic reticulum

Fig., x 5,500, insets, x 20,000.

fibroblast on the left side of the micrograph is shown at higher power in the adjacent inset. Note the more numerous dilated profiles of endoplasmic reticulum (**arrows**) and the multitude of small particles (**ribosomes**), most of which are associated with the membranes of the reticulum. The ribosomes are slightly smaller and stain less intensely than the glycogen particles of the smooth muscle cells. The presence of rough endoplasmic reticulum in both the fibroblast and the smooth muscle cell is consistent with the finding that smooth muscle cells, in addition to their contractile role, have the ability to produce and maintain collagen and elastic fibers.

The tissue utilized in this micrograph is from a young animal and it contains fibroblasts which are in a relatively active state; hence the well developed endoplasmic reticulum and abundant cytoplasm. With the light microscope it is not likely that one would be able to readily distinguish between the fibroblasts shown here and the smooth muscle cells. However, if the fibroblasts are less active as in a more mature tissue or in an older individual, its cytoplasm would be less extensive and accordingly, it would be more easily distinguished from the smooth muscle cells.

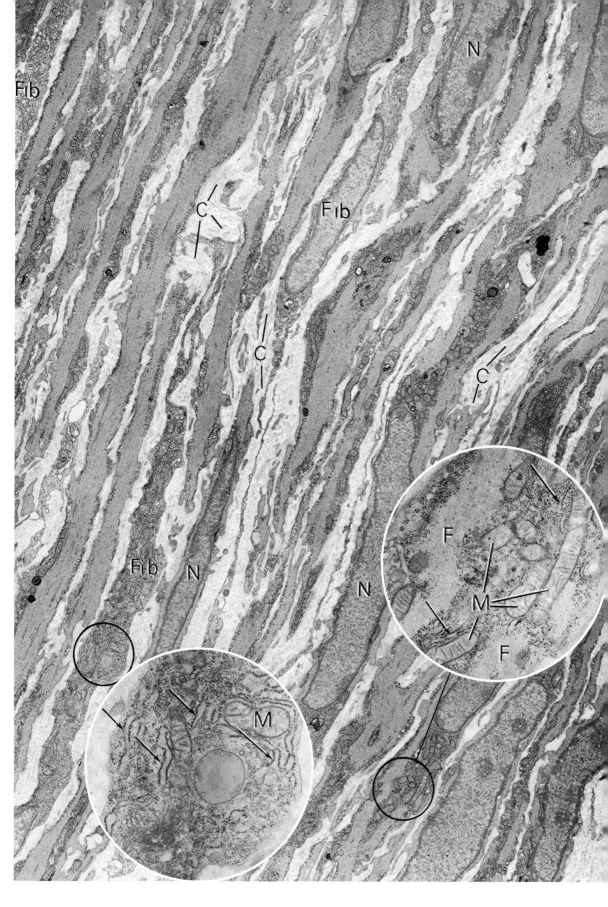

PLATE 5-2

Plate 5-3. SMOOTH MUSCLE, CROSS SECTION, ELECTRON MICROSCOPY

The specimen from which this micrograph was obtained is the same, namely the oviduct, as that shown in the previous plate. It is an electron micrograph of cross sectioned smooth muscle cells and shows, at higher resolution, many of the features of smooth muscle cells seen already with the light microscope. For example, it can be seen that the muscle cells are arranged in bundles comparable to those seen with the light microscope in Figures 3 and 4 of Plate 5-1. On the other hand the bundle arrangement is not readily apparent, even in electron micrographs, when the muscle cells are longitudinally sectioned as in the preceding plate. The cross sectioned profiles of the greatest diameter depict the mid-portion of the muscle cell and these show nuclei, whereas the profiles of lesser diameter depict the tapered ends of the cell and show cytoplasm only. As already indicated in the preceding plate, the smooth muscle cells display cytoplasmic areas which appear homogeneous due to the presence of myofilaments. The homogeneous areas are evident, but the individual myofilaments are not. Also seen within the cytoplasm of the smooth muscle cells are mitochondria. Other cytoplasmic constituents are not resolved at this relatively low magnification.

Generally the cross sectioned smooth muscle cells (**SM**) show an irregular contour when seen at the electron microscopic level. This is due in part to the better resolution obtained with the electron microscope but, even more so, it is a reflection of the extreme thinness of the section. In examining the individual cells at this low magnification, numerous sites are seen where a cell appears to contact its neighbor. Most of these sites do not reflect true cell to cell contacts, however, there are places where the smooth muscle cells do make contact by means of a nexus or gap junction (**inset**). These junctions are similar to gap junctions in other cells. They are considered to be the structural sites of easy ion movement from cell to cell, and also in muscle cells, for the spread of excitation from one cell to another. At the gap junction, the neighboring cells leave a gap of only 20Å between the adjacent plasma membranes. Usually special staining procedures are employed to demonstrate the gap. When seen in face view, the special stains reveal hexagonal patterns on the opposing plasma membranes. In routinely prepared electron micrographs of a gap junction (**arrow, inset**), it appears as though the adjacent plasma membranes make contact (See also Plate 5-8).

The electron micrograph shows connective tissue cells associated with the bundles of smooth muscle cells. The processes of the connective tissue cells tend to delineate and define the limits of the bundles. Fibroblasts (**Fib**) are the most numerous of the connective tissue cells. Their processes are long and in some areas profiles of fibroblast processes virtually ensheath the smooth muscle cell bundle. Although the nuclei of the fibroblasts would be evident with the light microscope, the cellular processes would not. In addition to fibroblasts, another cell type is also seen about or between the bundles of smooth muscle cells. These are the macrophages (**M**) readily identified with the electron microscope by the presence of lyosomal bodies within the cytoplasm. With the light microscope, these cells would be difficult to identify since the lysosomes are not evident without the use of special histochemical staining procedures. However, if the macrophages contained phagocytosed particles of large size, or of distinctive coloration (e.g., hemosiderin) their identification with the light microscope becomes easier.

In the electron micrograph shown here the macrophages appear to have taken up a preferential position, lying in immediate apposition with the fibroblasts. The relationship is so close, that at this magnification the intercellular space is difficult to discern. The dotted line indicates the boundary between the two cell types.

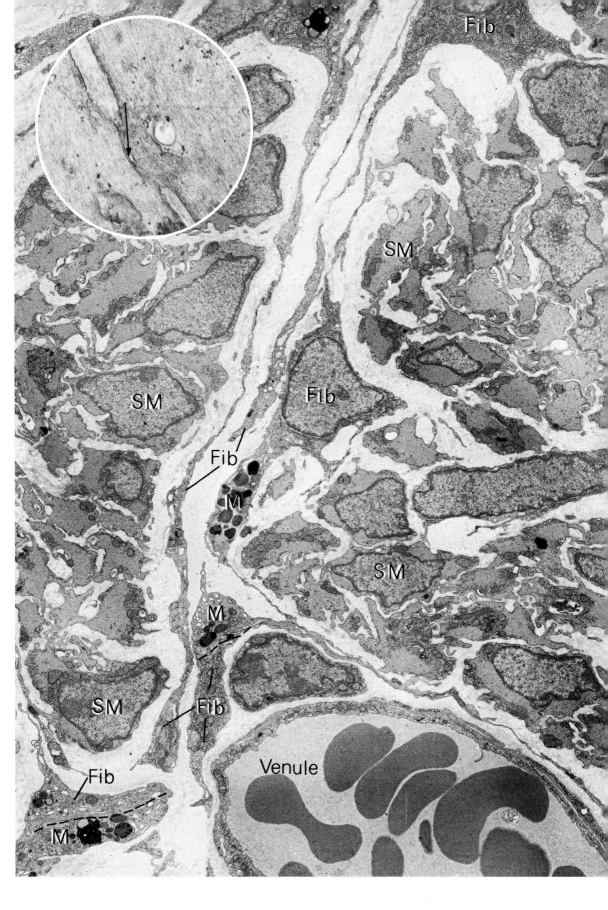

PLATE 5-3

Plate 5-4. SKELETAL MUSCLE

Longitudinally sectioned skeletal muscle is shown in Figure 1. The fibers are oriented vertically in the illustration. The cross striations are the bands which appear at right angles to the long axis of the fibers. They are the most striking feature of skeletal muscle when viewed through the microscope. (The visualization of cross striations may be enhanced by reducing the diameter of the condenser diaphragm.) Although the individual myofibrils are not conspicuous, the suggestion that longitudinal subunits exist is obtained in many places where the myofibrils are slightly out of register. Between the muscle fibers is a small amount of delicate connective tissue, called *endomysium.* This contains an extensive capillary network which travels lengthwise between the muscle fibers. During maximal muscular activity, the capillaries are all patent; in a less active state, only some are patent at a particular time. The capillary walls are not evident, but the closely packed red blood cells are evident (**arrows**). In fact, the arrangement of blood cells in this slide serves as an indication as to the location of the capillaries.

Skeletal muscle cells are multinucleated. The nuclei (**N**) of the skeletal muscle cells are seen advantageously in Figure 2. The nuclei appear as the elongated structures at the edge of the fiber. In some cases, when they are viewed face down, the nuclei appear to be in the center of the cell. Although the cross striations are conspicuous, the longitudinal myofibrils are not clearly delineated, and only in some places are there suggestions of longitudinal subunits. Delicate connective tissue, endomysium (**CT**), is between the fibers; the blood vessels are not evident in this illustration.

A cross section of striated muscle is shown in Figure 3. The fibers appear as polygonal profiles of eosinophilic areas. The cut ends of the myofibrils (also called sarcostyles) give the cut surface a stippled appearance. In many fibers, clefts separate groups of myofibrils into distinct areas called *Cohnheim's fields.* The clefts are now regarded as artifacts and little significance is attached to the Cohnheim's fields. The peripheral location of the nuclei (**N**) is well displayed in cross sections. The thin line (**arrowheads**) which surrounds

KEY

CT, connective tissue (endomysium)
N, nuclei
arrowheads (Fig. 3), See text
arrows, red blood cells in capillaries

Fig. 1, x 400; Fig. 2, x 640; Fig. 3, x 640.

the muscle fibers was formerly considered to be the cytoplasmic boundary of the cell and it was called the sarcolemma. However, as already mentioned it is now known that this thin line includes the plasma membrane of the muscle cell, an amorphous layer of basal lamina material and possibly some collagen fibrils. The term sarcolemma is now used to refer only to the plasma membrane. Separation has occurred between some of the muscle fibers. This reveals the delicate connective tissue (**CT**) which constitutes the endomysium.

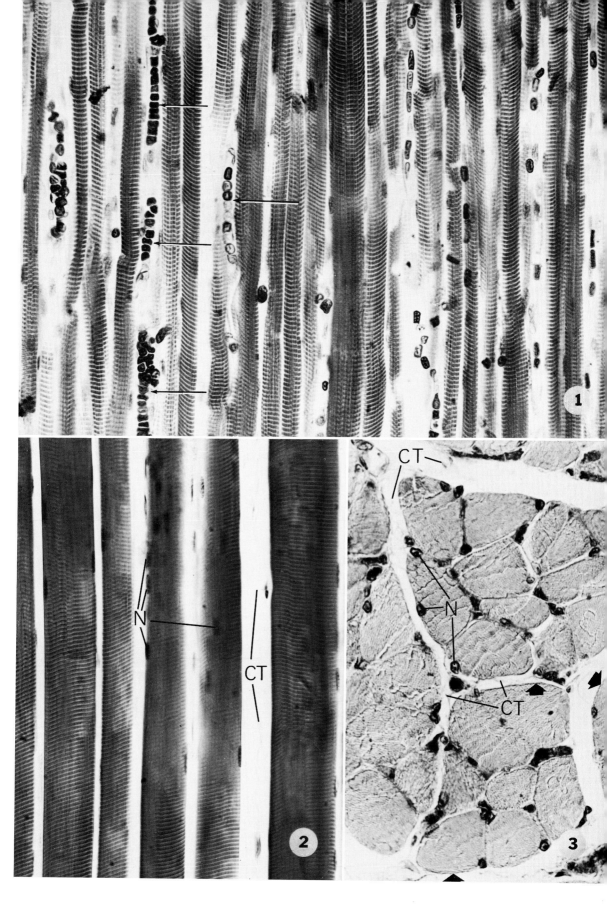

PLATE 5-4

Plate 5-5. Skeletal Muscle I, Electron Microscopy

The cytological organization and functional units of the skeletal muscle cell are revealed in this low power electron micrograph. For purposes of orientation it should be noted that only a small portion of two muscle cells (fibers) are included in the micrograph. Both are seen in longitudinal profile. One of the sectioned muscle cells occupies the upper two thirds of the figure and reveals a nucleus (**N**) at its periphery. Below, and largely covered by the inset is part of the second muscle cell. The connective tissue in the extracellular space between the two cells, i.e. the collagen fibrils (**Col**) and fibroblast (**Fib**) constitutes the endomysium of the muscle.

The individual myofibrils (**Myf**), which were barely perceptible in the light micrograph are clearly seen here in longitudinal profile. The myofibrils, which are more or less cylindrical structures, extend across the micrograph. Each is separated from neighboring myofibrils by a thin sheath of surrounding sarcoplasm (**Sp**).

As mentioned in dealing with the light microscopic image, each repeating set of bands in a striated muscle fiber represents a sarcomere. In the electron micrograph shown here two sarcomeres (**S**), one following the other, but in adjacent myofibrils, have been marked. Each sarcomere extends from one Z line, the thin dark line, to the next Z line. The essential features of a sarcomere are shown at higher magnification in the inset. Here the filamentous nature of the myofibrils are evident. For example, the I band which is bisected by the Z line is seen to consist of thin (5 nm), barely visible filaments. The thin filaments which are composed of actin, are joined to the Z line, and extend across the I band into the A band. The thick filaments, composed of myosin, account for the full width of the A band. In the A band there are additional bands or lines. One of these, the M line, is seen at the middle of the A band. This line appears to be due to the presence of a substance which binds the thick filaments to one another. A second sub-band within the A band is the H band. This band appears as the less dense segment within the A band and it consists of only myosin filaments. The lateral segments (**double ended arrows**) of the A band are rather dense. This more dense ap-

KEY

A (anisotropic), A band
I (isotropic), I band
H (*Ger.* helle = light), H band
M (*Ger.* mitte = middle), M band
Z (*Ger.* zwichenscheibe = intercalated line), Z line

} bands and lines within a sarcomere

CM, cell membrane (sarcolemma)
Col, collagen
Fib, fibroblast
Myf, myofibril
N, nucleus
S, sarcomere
Sp, sarcoplasm between adjacent myofibrils
arrowheads, glycogen
double ended arrows, overlap in A band of thick and thin filaments

Fig., x 6,500; inset, x 30,000.

pearing area is a reflection of the extent to which the actin filaments have extended into the A band and interdigitated with the thick filaments. Since contraction involves the interdigitation of the thick and thin filaments, increasing degrees of contraction result in continued narrowing of the I and H bands. Inasmuch as the individual thick filaments do not change in length, the width of the A band is always the same.

The cross banded pattern which characterizes the striated muscle fiber is a reflection of the arrangement, in register, of the individual myofibrils. Additionally, the cross banded pattern of the myofibril is a reflection of the arrangement, in register, of the myofilaments (**inset**). The "in register" arrangement of myofibrils is an important feature relating to impulse propagation within the cell; this is considered in Plate 5-6.

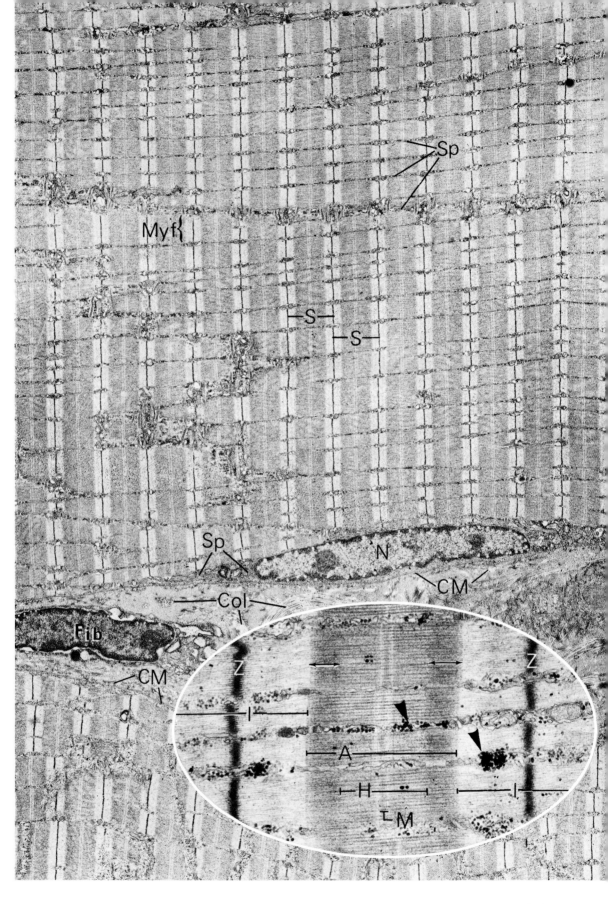

Sp

Myf{

S
S

Sp

N

CM

Col

Fib

CM

Z   Z

I

A

H

M

I

PLATE 5-5

Plate 5-6. Skeletal Muscle II, Electron Microscopy

The electron micrograph shown here illustrates to advantage the nature of the sarcoplasm, especially the membrane system which pervades it. It also again demonstrates the filamentous components which make up the myofibril.

For purposes of orientation, it is pointed out that the muscle fiber is longitudinally sectioned, but it has been turned so that the direction of the fiber now has a vertical orientation. The various bands and lines of a single sarcomere are labeled in the myofibril on the left of the illustration. The thin actin filaments are especially well resolved in the I band in the lower left corner and can be easily compared with the thicker myosin filaments of the A band. The point of juncture or insertion of the actin filaments into the Z line is also readily apparent.

In contrast to the relatively nondescript character of the sarcoplasm as seen in the light microscope, the electron microscope reveals a well developed membrane system called the sarcoplasmic reticulum (**SR**). The reticulum consists of segments of anastomosing tubules which form a network around each myofibril. The electron micrograph here fortuitously depicts a relatively wide area of sarcoplasm in a plane between two myofibrils. Prominent in this area are numerous glycogen particles (**G**). Somewhat less apparent, but nevertheless evident, are the anastomosing tubules of the sarcoplasmic reticulum (**SR**). Near the junction of the A and I bands the tubules of the reticulum become confluent, forming flattened sac-like structures, the terminal cisternae. These cisternae come in proximity to another membrane system, the T (transverse) system.

The T-system consists of tubular structures (**T**), each tubule originating as an invagination of the sarcolemma. The tubules course transversely through the muscle fiber. Because of the uniform register of the myofibrils, each T-tubule comes to surround the myofibrils in proximity to the juncture of the A and I bands. In effect the T-system is not simply a straight tubule, but rather, it forms a grid-like system that surrounds each myofibril at the level of the A-I junction. Thus, in a section passing tangentially to a myofibril, as is seen in the center of the micrograph and in the upper

KEY

A, A band
G, glycogen
I, I band
M, M band
Mi, mitochondria
SR, sarcoplasmic reticulum
T, T-tubule
Z, Z line
arrowhead, junction between tubular component of sarcoplasmic reticulum and terminal cistern.
arrows, longitudinal profile of T-tubule

Fig., x 45,000; insets, x 52,000.

inset, the lumen of the T-tubules may appear as elongate channels (**arrows**) bound by a pair of membranes. The inner, facing pair of membranes belong to the T-tubule. The outer membranes, on either side, belong to the terminal cisternae of the sarcoplasmic reticulum. The communication between a terminal cisternae and the tubular portion of the sarcoplasmic reticulum is marked by an arrowhead in the upper inset. In contrast, a longitudinal section passing through two adjacent myofibrils (see lower **inset**) will reveal the T-tubule to be flattened with the terminal elements of the sarcoplasmic reticulum (**SR**) on either side. The combination of the T-tubule and the adjoining dilated terminal cisternae of the sarcoplasmic reticulum on either side is referred to as a triad.

The nature and geometric configuration of the triad helps explain the rapid and uniform contraction of a muscle fiber. It is postulated that, the depolarization of the sarcolemma continues along the membranes of the T-tubules and thereby results in an inward spread of excitation to reach each myofibril at the A-I junction. This is thought to effect the first stage in the contraction process, that of causing the release of calcium ions from the immediately adjacent terminal cisternae. Relaxation occurs through the recapture of calcium ions by the sarcoplasmic reticulum. In terms of energetics it is also of interest that the mitochondria (**Mi**) occupy a preferential site in the sarcoplasm, being oriented in a circular fashion around the myofibrils in the region of the I band.

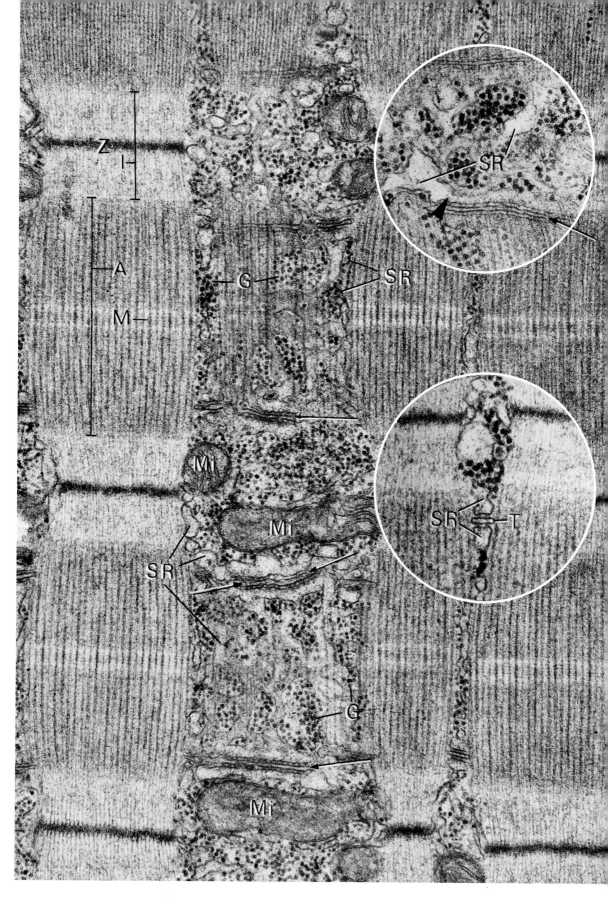

PLATE 5-6

Plate 5-7. Cardiac Muscle

A section of cardiac muscle is shown in Figure 1. Most of the fibers are cut longitudinally (**L**), though some are cut obliquely (**X**). The branching nature of cardiac muscle is readily evident in this figure (**arrows**). The nuclei are located in the center of the fibers. This is evident not only where the fibers have been cut longitudinally but also where they are cut obliquely or in cross section. Between the fibers are many small nuclei which belong to connective tissue cells (**CT**), or cells which make up the blood vessels (**BV**).

The cross striations and intercalated discs can be seen if longitudinal sections of cardiac muscle are examined at higher magnification (Fig. 2). The myofibrils appear as the longitudinal subunits. The intercalated discs (**ID**) appear as the dense cross bands. Intercalated discs are not always evident in H & E preparations. They are frequently difficult to see in human specimens. The discs represent thickened opposing cell membranes. In this respect, cardiac muscle fibers differ significantly from skeletal muscle fibers. The cardiac muscle fibers are end-to-end alignments of cells; each skeletal muscle fiber, on the other hand, is a single protoplasmic unit.

Figure 3 shows cardiac muscle cut in cross section. The field shows the cross-sectioned muscle fibers and connective tissue between the fibers. The muscle fibers have irregular profiles because of the branching that is characteristic of this muscle. A small blood vessel (**BV**) crosses the upper half of the field.

The myofibrils can be seen in cross sections if the magnification is sufficiently high as in Figure 4. They appear as the small eosinophilic bodies which give the cut edge of the muscle fiber a stippled appearance.

KEY

BV, blood vessel
CT, connective tissue
ID, intercalated discs
L, longitudinally sectioned fibers
X, obliquely sectioned fibers
arrows, branching of cardiac muscle fibers

Fig. 1 (human), x 160; Fig. 2 (dog), x 640; Fig. 3 (human), x 160; Fig. 4 (human), x 640.

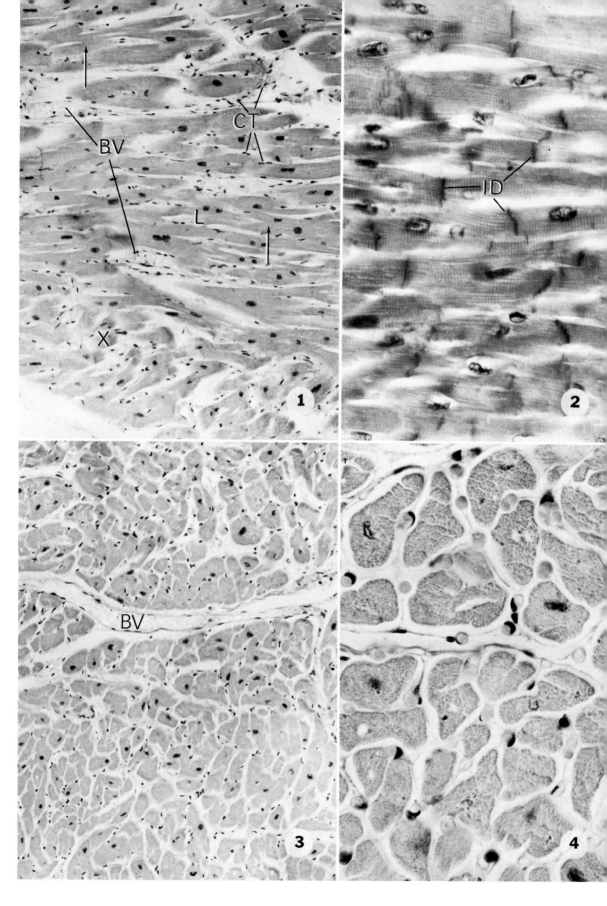

PLATE 5-7

Plate 5-8. CARDIAC MUSCLE, INTERCALATED DISC, ELECTRON MICROSCOPY

The electron micrograph illustrated here reveals portions of two cardiac muscle cells including the site where they join in end to end apposition. The junction between the two cells can be followed in its entirety across the micrograph. It takes an irregular, step-like course making a number of near right angle turns so that part of the junction is disposed crosswise, part is disposed longitudinally and part is disposed obliquely. In its course, different junctional specializations of the intercalated disc are evident. These include the macula adherens, fascia adherens and gap junction. It is principally the fascia adherens, and to some extent, the macula adherens which correspond to the intercalated disc of light microscopy.

The macula adherens in the upper left of the illustration has been enlarged in **inset 1**. It displays the typical features seen in macula adherentes in other tissues (referred to as desmosomes with the light microscope), namely, a thickening of the inner leaflet of the plasma membrane, a condensation of the adjacent cytoplasm and an intermediate dense line seen in the middle of the intercellular space. Typically, tonofilaments form loops in the adjacent cytoplasmic condensation and although the loops are not evident, the tonofilaments (**arrow**) can be seen in the macula adherens (**MA**) which has been sectioned obliquely on the right side of the illustration. The macula adherens is a plaque-like site of contact between cells. It is regarded to be a contact which provides for adhesion between the two cells.

The fascia adherens (**FA**) is more extensive than a macula, being disposed in a larger area of irregular outline. Thin sections showing the fascia adherens on edge (**inset 3**) reveals the plasma membrane of the neighboring cells to be separated by a space of 15 to 20 nm. In each cell, the fascia adherens is typified by a condensation of the subplasmalemma cytoplasm. The thin actin filaments of the myofibril are anchored in the cytoplasmic density of the fascia adherens. The fascia adherens of the intercalated disc corresponds to the zonula adherens of other tissues (see Plate 1-5).

The gap junctions (**GJ**) are seen in those

portions of the intercalated disc which are disposed longitudinally with respect to the direction of the myofilament. (This orientation may not be significant since gap junctions also appear cross-wise in some electron micrographs.) A gap junction consists of a thickening of the inner layer of the plasma membrane and a near fusion of the outer layer of the plasma membrane with that of the neighboring cell (see also Plate 5-3). Thus, in routinely prepared electron micrographs (**inset 2**) the gap junction appears as two dense lines, each representing a thickened inner layer of plasma membrane and a barely discernible intermediate line. The intermediate line represents the nearly fused outer layers of the plasma membranes of the two adjacent cells. Special stains are employed to reveal the gap between the nearly fused membranes. As noted earlier in reference to the nexus of smooth muscle, gap junctions are looked upon as sites where excitation spreads from one cell to another and where small molecules or ions pass readily from one cell to another.

Other features typical of striated muscle are also revealed in the illustration, namely mitochondria (**Mi**), sarcoplasmic reticulum (**SR**), and components of the sarcomere, namely Z lines (**Z**), M band (**M**), and myofilaments. This particular specimen is in a highly contracted state and consequently the I band is practically obscured.

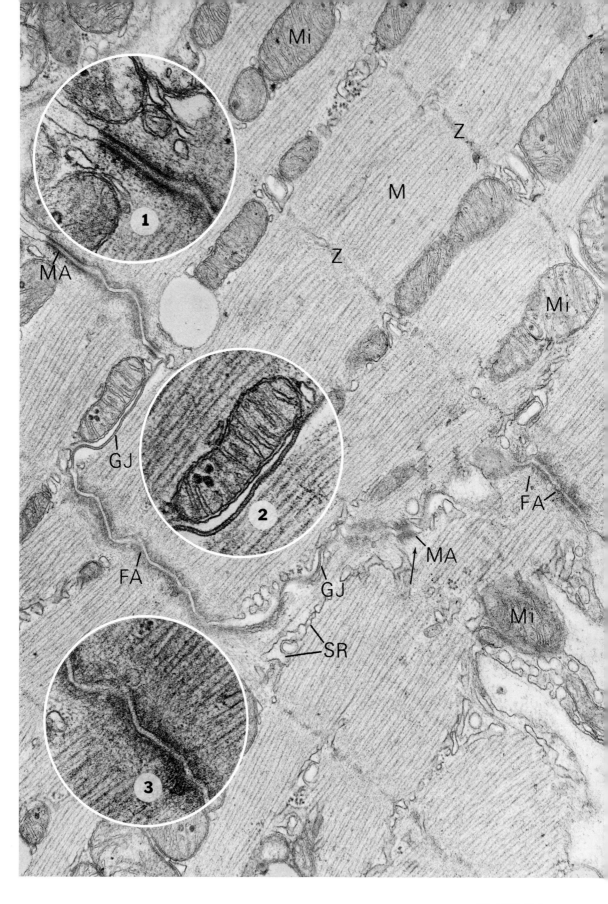

PLATE 5-8

Plate 5-9. CARDIAC MUSCLE, PURKINJE FIBERS

Some of the muscle cells within the heart are specialized to conduct impulses from the AV node through the ventricular septum and into the ventricles. These are the *Purkinje fibers*. Within the ventricular septum, they are grouped into a bundle, the AV bundle. This quickly branches into two main components, one going into each ventricle.

A cross section through cardiac muscle and Purkinje fibers is shown in Figure 1. This is a relatively low-power view and the cardiac muscle fibers (**CM**) appear small. They are at the periphery of the figure. The Purkinje fibers are in the center of the field. Connective tissue (**CT**) separates groups of Purkinje fibers from each other and from the cardiac muscle. Some small blood vessels (**BV**) are within the connective tissue.

The arrangement of Purkinje fibers is seen more advantageously at higher magnification (Fig. 2). They are arranged as groups of four or five fibers which are in intimate contact. These groups of Purkinje fibers are separated by connective tissue from other similar groups. The boundaries between the individual Purkinje fibers are not clear in most of the bundles that are shown in Figure 2; however, in some cases they are marked by small clefts (**arrows**). Because of their geometry, most cross sectioned Purkinje fibers do not show nuclei; only one nucleus (**N**) is evident in Figure 2. The cytoplasm of a Purkinje cell contains large amounts of glycogen. The glycogen-rich areas (**G**) appear homogeneous and frequently occupy the center portion of the fiber. The myofibrils (**M**) are located at the periphery of the cell and have a stippled appearance. Between the bundles of the Purkinje fibers is delicate connective tissue (**CT**).

A longitudinal section through Purkinje fibers is shown in Figure 3. The Purkinje fibers resemble swollen cardiac muscle cells and the myofibrils appear as the longitudinal subunits. The nuclei are in the homogeneous, glycogen-rich part of the cell.

KEY

BV, blood vessels
CM, cardiac muscle fibers
CT, connective tissue
G, glycogen-rich areas
M, myofibrils
N, nucleus of Purkinje cell
arrows, clefts between Purkinje cells

Fig. 1 (sheep), x 160; Fig. 2 (sheep), x 400; Fig. 3 (sheep), x 400.

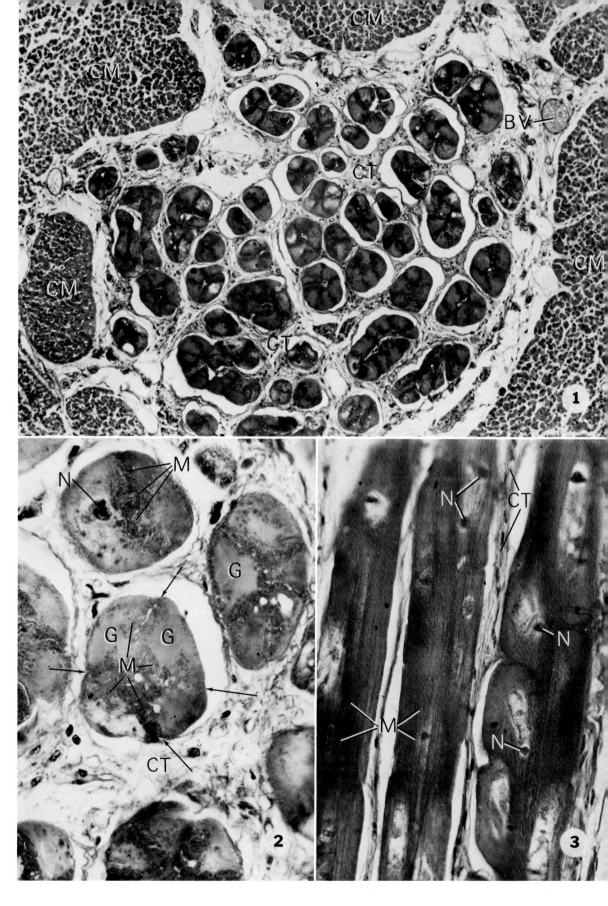

PLATE 5-9

6 NERVOUS SYSTEM

THE STRUCTURAL UNITS of the nervous system are the neurons or nerve cells. These cells are specialized to conduct impulses. Neurons vary greatly in shape in different parts of the nervous system. All of them, however, contain a cell body and cytoplasmic processes, called dendrites and axons. Neurons make contact with each other by means of specialized junctions referred to as synapses.

The cell body (*perikaryon*) is the part of the neuron which contains the nucleus. In many cases the cell body is extremely large. Typically, numerous dendrites extend from the cell body. These are relatively short and in a sense, they serve to increase the receptor surface of the neuron. In contrast, each nueron contains only one axon or axis cylinder. This is the conducting portion of the neuron, and in many neurons, the axon is extremely long allowing the neuron to conduct impulses from one part of the body to another.

The sensory neuron is the major exception to the typical organization of neurons wherein there are numerous dendrites and one axon. Instead of many processes, the sensory neuron has only one process joined to the cell body. This process is in fact a short stem which branches into a long peripheral process and a long central process. The peripheral process of the sensory neuron is a typical conducting axon and it is interposed between the peripheral dendritic arborization and the cell body. The peripheral process of the sensory neuron may also be called the dendritic branch (or process) because it conducts impulses toward the cell body.

The term nerve fiber is used extensively in neurohistology. In current usage, it refers to an axon and its enveloping cellular sheath (see below). The term fiber is also used to refer to the axon alone, without its sheath, and in the older literature, it may refer to dendrites especially if they are long.

Within the central nervous system, cell bodies are found in gray matter. The fibers are found both in the gray matter, and in the white matter. In many parts of the white matter the fibers are grouped and form discrete bundles whose origin and destination are known. In this case they are referred to as *tracts*. This is especially true in the spinal cord. The supporting cells, throughout the central nervous system, are called *neuroglia*. Three kinds of neuroglia are present: astrocytes, oligodendrocytes, and microglia. Microglial cells are capable of phagocytic activity. They develop from mesoderm. Astrocytes and oligodendrocytes are spoken of as supporting cells; however, they should not be thought of as providing only structural support, but rather as participating also in cooperative metabolic functions. The cells which line the cavity of the central nervous system are epithelial-like and are called *ependyma*. All of these cells, except the microglia, develop from the ectoderm.

Within the peripheral nervous system, cell bodies are located in *ganglia;* the nerve fibers constitute the conducting components of the nerves. The fibers are surrounded by a thin cellular tube called the *neurilemma* or *Schwann cell.* It is also called the *sheath of Schwann.* In most cases, the cell membrane of the Schwann cell is modified to form an additional cover of the nerve fiber called *myelin.* Nerve fibers which have such a cover are referred to as *myelinated;* fibers without a myelin cover are called *nonmyelinated* (fibers that go to the viscera are nonmyelinated). The myelin is an extension of the Schwann cell, it consists of layers of cell membrane wrapped around the fiber. The term "Schwann cell" or "sheath of Schwann" is meant to indicate the cytoplasmic part of the cell that is external to the myelin. In forming the cellular tube that surrounds the nerve fiber, each Schwann cell (and its myelin) covers a segment of the nerve fiber. The place where adjacent Schwann cells meet is called the *node of Ranvier.* Within the central nervous system, myelin is formed by oligodendrocytes.

Plate 6-1. SYMPATHETIC GANGLION

Sympathetic ganglia are peripheral motor ganglia which contain cell bodies of neurons (post-synaptic neurons) that conduct impulses to smooth muscle, cardiac muscle, and glands. Figure 1 is a low-magnification view of a sympathetic ganglion "stained" by a silver method. Numerous cell bodies (ganglion cells) (**CB**) and bundles of nerve fibers (**F**) are seen. In addition, some blood vessels (**BV**) and connective tissue (**CT**) are evident. The area enclosed within the **rectangle** includes a cell body which is shown at higher magnification in Figure 2.

The cell bodies in the ganglion appear as relatively large spherical structures. Because of the size of the cell body, the nucleus may not always be included in the section. The nucleus (**N**) shown in Figure 2 is typically large, spherical, and pale staining. The nucleolus appears as the smaller spherical body within the nucleus. The cytoplasm of this cell body contains a black deposit. This is due to a yellow pigment, *lipofuchsin* (**L**), which blackens in silver preparations. The lipofuchsin can also be seen in many of the cell bodies that are shown in Figure 1. Other components of the cytoplasm (Golgi, mitochondria, and Nissl bodies) are not evident in these preparations because each requires special methods for demonstration. The neuron in Figure 2 shows a number of *processes* (**P**) connected to the cell body. Because many processes join to the cell body, these neurons are designated as multipolar.

As noted above, numerous bundles of fibers are also demonstrated in the silver preparation (Fig. 1). They appear as the dark, threadlike structures (**F**). Although in this specimen it is not possible to distinguish the nerve fibers from the connective tissue fibers, most are actually nerve fibers. One can conclude with a reasonable degree of assurance that those fibers that are organized as discrete bundles are nerve fibers.

Figure 3 is an H & E preparation from the same block of tissue as seen in Figures 1 and 2, but several sections removed. The cell bodies (**CB**), some showing nuclei and nucleoli, are clearly seen. The dark structures which are in the immediate vicinity of the cell bodies (Fig. 3) are nuclei of supporting cells. These will be seen to greater advantage

KEY

BV, blood vessel
CB, cell body
CT, connective tissue
F, nerve fiber, longitudinal section
F¹, nerve fiber, cross section
L, lipofuchsin
N, nucleus
P, process

Fig. 1 (human), x 160; Fig. 2 (human), x 640; Fig. 3 (human), x 160.

in Plate 6-2. Supporting cells are also associated with the nerve fibers. The nuclei of these supporting cells stain with hematoxylin in an H & E preparation and give the bundles of nerve fibers a slightly different appearance from those of the silver preparation. When a bundle of fibers is cut longitudinally (**F**), and stained with H & E, the nuclei of the supporting cells appear elongated in the same direction as the fibers. When the nerve bundles are cut in cross section (**F**¹), the nuclei of supporting cells appear spherical. The nuclei of supporting cells are not evident in the silver preparation that is shown in Figure 1.

It should be noted that the multipolar nature of sympathetic ganglion cells is readily determined in the silver preparation, but not in the H & E preparation. One is hard pressed to find even a single process joined to the cell body of multipolar neurons in an H & E preparation.

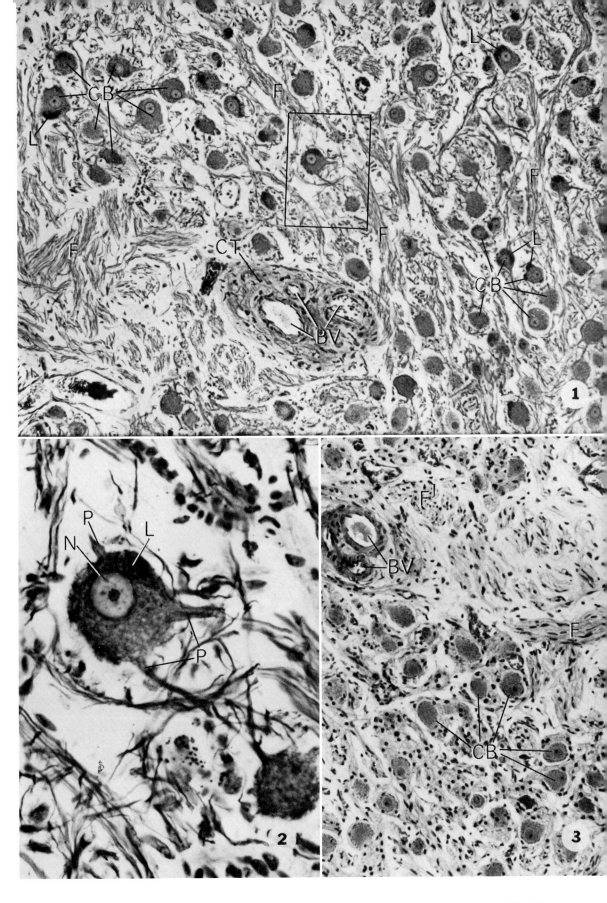

PLATE 6-1

Plate 6-2. SYMPATHETIC GANGLION I, ELECTRON MICROSCOPY

The specimen in the accompanying electron micrograph depicts a sympathetic ganglion similar to those seen in the light micrographs of the preceding plate. At the magnification utilized here the neuron cell bodies (**CB**) along with a myriad of nerve fibers (**NF**) can be readily identified. Two of the cell bodies were sectioned in a plane that includes the nucleus (**N**) and one also reveals the nucleolus (**Nu**). The neuron cell body and one of its processes (within the **rectangle**) is shown at higher magnification in Plate 6-3. Other cell elements present within the ganglion, but somewhat less easy to identify at this magnification, include fibroblasts (**F**), Schwann cells (**SCN**) and Satellite cells (**Sat N**). Surrounding the ganglion is a specialized connective tissue, the perineurium (**P**), part of which can be seen in the upper left corner of the micrograph. It is continuous with the connective tissue covering of the nerve bundles that enter the ganglion. Perineurium is considered in some detail with respect to nerve in Plate 6-5 and at the electron microscopic level in Plate 6-6. Also seen in the ganglion is a small blood vessel (**BV**). The intercellular matrix consists largely of collagen which together with the fibroblasts comprises the endoneurium of the ganglion.

A feature not appreciated with the light microscope, but evident in electron micrographs is the relationship of the satellite cells to the neuron cell bodies. Each cell body is surrounded by a thin sheath of satellite cell cytoplasm which covers not only the cell body, but may extend for a very short distance onto its processes. The attenuated satellite cell cytoplasm (**Sat**) is just barely recognizable at this low magnification. It can be seen best around the two cell bodies in the lower part of the micrograph. The cytoplasm of the satellite cell has slightly greater electron density than the neuron and thus gives the appearance of a thin rim around the neuron cell body. In the thin sections employed in electron microscopy the nuclear region of the satellite cell is infrequently included in the plane of section; in the preparation shown here only one satellite cell nucleus (**Sat N**), is present.

Typically, both myelinated and non-myelinated fibers are present in sympathetic

KEY

CB, neuron cell body
F, fibroblast (endoneurial cell)
My, myelin
N, nucleus
NF, nerve fibers
Nu, nucleolus
P, perineurium
Sat, satellite cell cytoplasm
Sat N, satellite cell nucleus
SCN, Schwann cell nucleus

Fig., x 4,200.

ganglia. However, only one of the many fibers included in the portion of the ganglion seen here is myelinated; it is just to the left of the blood vessel. The myelin sheath (**My**) surrounding the nerve fiber appears as the ovoid black ring. External to the myelin, one can identify the nucleus of the associated Schwann cell (**SCN**). In addition to a Schwann cell occurring in relation to the myelinated fiber, all of the non-myelinated nerve fibers are enclosed by Schwann cell cytoplasm. However, instead of a single axon being surrounded by Schwann cell cytoplasm as in the case of the myelinated fibers, the Schwann cells related to the unmyelinated nerve fibers will usually ensheath more than a single fiber — generally a number of sectioned fibers can be seen included within a Schwann cell. In effect the Schwann cell has the same relationship to the nerve fiber as the satellite cell has to the cell body. Both are disposed as an intimate cellular sheath around the neural element. Although Schwann and satellite cells are designated by different names, they probably have the same function and may differ only in terms of location. Both satellite cells and Schwann cells can be looked upon as peripheral neurologia.

As noted above, connective tissue occupies the interstices of the neural elements within the ganglion. In this illustration, several fibroblasts (**F**) are evident. Some fibroblasts are located in very close apposition to the neuron cell bodies and with the light microscope it would be most difficult, if not impossible, to distinguish such fibroblast nuclei from that of a satellite cell.

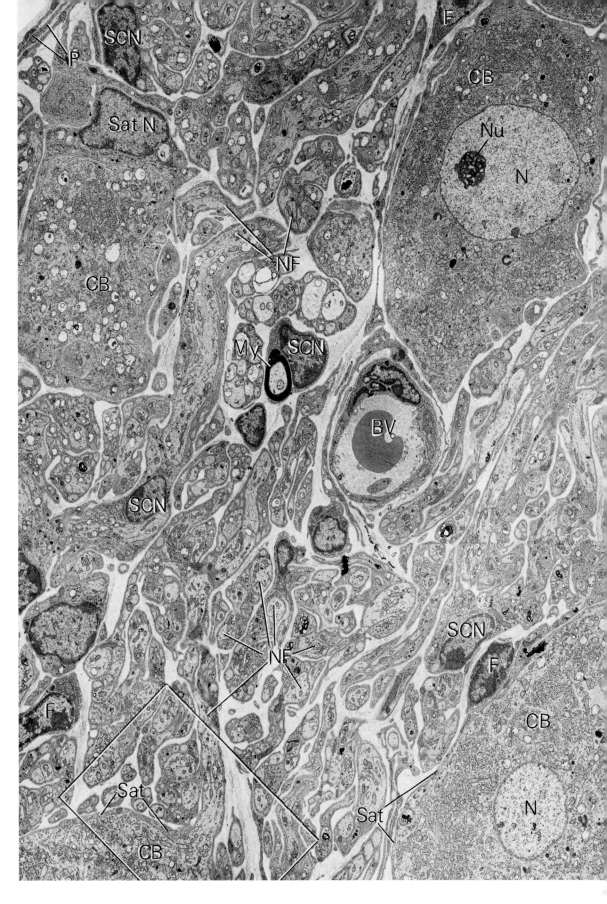

PLATE 6-2

Plate 6-3. Sympathetic Ganglion II, Electron Microscopy

The electron micrograph shown here reveals at higher magnification the rectangular area from the previous plate. The cytoplasm of the neuron cell body exhibits numerous mitochondria (**M**), clusters of free ribosome (polyribosomes) (**R**), and profiles of rough surfaced endoplasmic reticulum (**RER**). The ribosomes and elements of the endoplasmic reticulum tend to aggregate in recognizable masses. The limits of these ribosome-rich areas are not sharply defined. However, one such concentration is shown enscribed by the broken line. These localized regions of ribosome-rich cytoplasm may be visualized in the light microscope, after staining with a basic dye such as toluidine blue. The staining reaction results in the appearance of small colored bodies, referred to as Nissl bodies (see Fig. 3, Plate 6-9). Between the ribosome-rich areas, the microtubules, neurofilaments and mitochondria predominate, as they do throughout the cell process.

The satellite cell (**Sat**) can be distinguished from the neuron cell body simply by differences in cytoplasmic density; it appears conspicuously more electron dense than the neuron. As already noted, the satellite cell provides a complete covering sheath about the cell body. In some areas it may be extremely attenuated (**arrowheads**). Similarly, the nerve precess emanating from the cell body is ensheathed by cytoplasm, identical in appearance to that covering the cell body. The neuronal process is covered by cytoplasm of the Schwann cell (**SC**). (The site at which the Satellite cell terminates and the Schwann cell investment begins is not evident in the particular example shown here.)

The unmyelinated nerve fibers (**NF**) are sectioned in various planes. Each nerve fiber is surrounded by Schwann cell cytoplasm (**SC**) which displays the same electron opacity as the cytoplasm of the satellite cells. A few of these nerve fibers appear as singular profiles covered by Schwann cell cytoplasm (**asterisks**). Most of the nerve fibers however, are embedded in groups within the confines of the Schwann cell. Both the satellite cell and Schwann cell are surfaced by basement lamina (**BL**) (see **inset**). Thus, the neuron, by means of its associated cell cover, is isolated from the collagen matrix (**C**).

KEY

A, axon terminal
BL, basal lamina
C, collagen
D, dendrite
L, lysosome
M, mitochondria
NF, nerve fiber
R, ribosome clusters
RER, rough surfaced endoplasmic reticulum
Sat C, satellite cell
SC, Schwann cell
arrow, synaptic cleft
arrowheads, see text

Fig., x 22,000; inset, x 45,000.

With respect to the individual fibers, it is not always possible to distinguish an axon from a dendrite. However, a general rule is that if the fiber displays synaptic vesicles (**SV**) (the small round profiles) it is identified as an axon terminal (**A**); if it displays profiles of granular endoplasmic reticulum it is identified as a dendrite (**D**). Fibers which do not exhibit these specific characteristics are best referred to simply as nerve fibers. The axon (**A**) which has entered the satellite sheath of the neuron cell body contains numerous synaptic vesicles. Presumably it will make synaptic contact with the cell body in this vicinity (an axosomatic synapse).

The small circle encloses an axondendritic synapse which is shown at higher magnification in the inset. The axon (**A**) of this synapse reveals numerous synaptic vesicles most of which appear empty, but they contain the neurotransmitter acetylcholine. Vesicles with granules, several of which are seen in the inset, contain catecholamines. The space (**arrow**) between the axon (**A**) and dendrite (**D**) is called the synaptic cleft. It is across this space that the neurotransmitter substance passes to stimulate the membrane of the postsynaptic cell. The presence of ribosomes in the post-synaptic cytoplasm indicate a dendrite, thus the synapse is an axondendritic synapse.

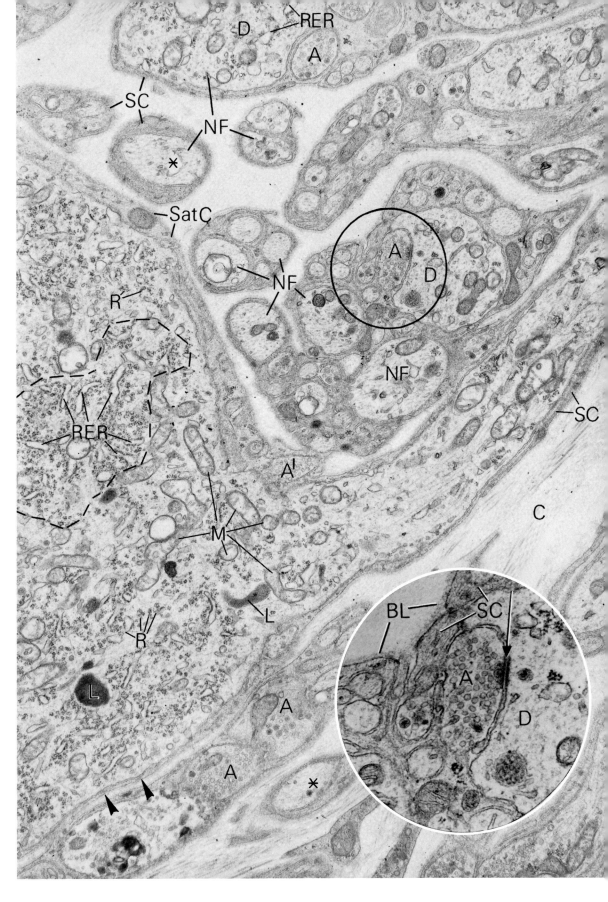

PLATE 6-3

Plate 6-4. Dorsal Root Ganglion

Dorsal root ganglia differ from autonomic ganglia in a number of ways. Whereas autonomic ganglia contain multipolar neurons and have motor synaptic connections, dorsal root ganglia contain unipolar neurons, are sensory, and have no synaptic connections.

Figure 1 shows a dorsal root ganglion and the nerve root (**NR**) at low power. Even at this magnification it is possible to identify the cell bodies (ganglion cells) (**CB**) which appear as the large spherical structures in the upper part of the figure. Surrounding the ganglion and nerve root are loose connective tissue (**CT**) and blood vessels (**BV**).

A higher magnification of the ganglion is shown in Figure 2. The cell bodies are generally spherical in shape. They also contain a large spherical nucleus. The nuclei are pale staining and usually show a densely staining round nucleolus. Many of the cell bodies are cut in such a plane that the nucleus and nucleolus are not included in the section. Again, the cytoplasmic organelles (Golgi, mitochondria, Nissl) are not revealed in routine H & E preparations. Frequently the ganglion cells are arranged so that rows of cell bodies are separated by bundles of fibers (**NF**). While this may not be a characteristic feature, when evident, it aids in distinguishing dorsal root ganglia from autonomic ganglia.

Figure 3 is an enlargement of the rectangle in Figure 2. A cell body is shown with a large spherical nucleus (**N**) and its darkly staining nucleolus (**Nl**). Surrounding the cell body are nuclei of supporting cells which are called *satellite cells* (**SC**). These nuclei are much smaller than the nuclei of nerve cells. The cytoplasm of satellite cells is usually not well delineated, so that the boundary between the satellite cell and the nerve cell cannot be identified. Other cells immediately beyond the satellite cells have elongated nuclei: these belong to fibroblasts (**F**).

In Figure 3, the large **arrowheads** show the centrally located axon, the small **arrows** show the neurilemma or where it should be. The clear region in between was occupied by myelin.

Dorsal root ganglion cells are designated unipolar neurons because only one process joins the cell body. It is however, extremely difficult to find the point where the cell body

and process join. A short distance from the cell body, the process divides into a long peripheral branch which is part of the peripheral nerve, and a long central branch which enters the spinal cord. Early in development, the two branches join the cell body separately as two processes. However, as development proceeds, these come closer together and ultimately they fuse into one. Because of this, the designation "pseudo-unipolar" is sometimes used for these neurons.

KEY

BV, blood vessels
CB, cell body
CT, connective tissue
F, fibroblasts
N, nucleus
Nl, nucleolus
NF, nerve fibers
NR, nerve root
SC, satellite cells
arrowheads, axon
arrows, neurilemma

Fig. 1 (cat), x 40; Fig. 2 (cat), x 160; Fig. 3 (cat), x 640.

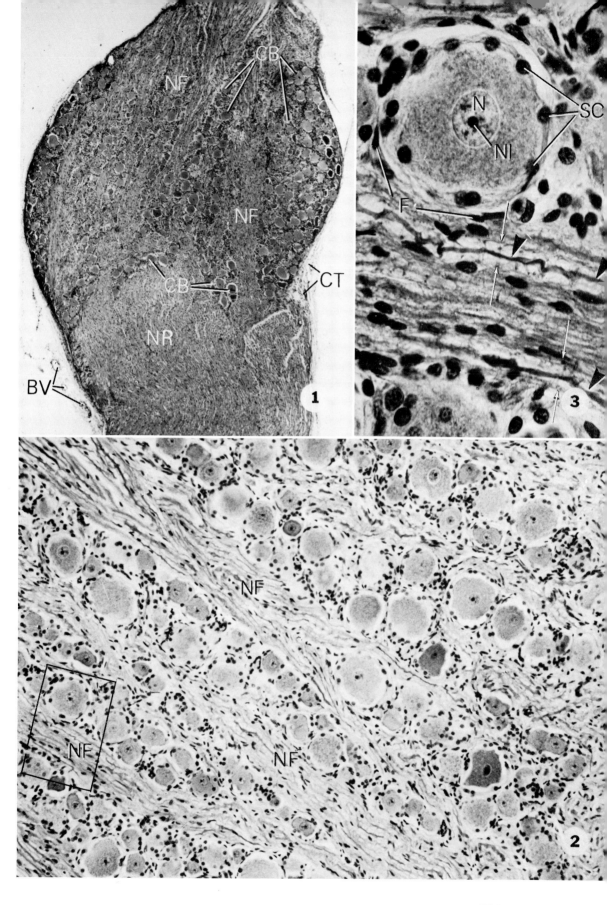

PLATE 6-4

Plate 6-5. PERIPHERAL NERVE

Nerves are comprised of bundles of nerve fibers held together by connective tissue. The nerve fibers consist of axons which are surrounded by a cellular investment called the *neurilemma,* or *sheath of Schwann.* In addition, the fibers may be myelinated or nonmyelinated. The myelin, if present, is immediately around the axon, and is in turn surrounded by the neurilemma.

The connective tissue that binds the nerve fibers together is designated as endoneurium, perineurium, and epineurium, according to its location. *Endoneurium* consists of the delicate connective tissue located between individual nerve fibers. The *perineurium* forms a sheath which surrounds a bundle of nerve fibers and its endoneurium. The *epineurium* separates and surrounds the perineurial bundles. Electron microscopic studies (see Plate 6-6) have shown that, unlike typical connective tissue, perineurial cells exhibit certain epithelial characteristics. In all but the smallest nerves, there are several layers of perineurial cells, each layer comprised of squamous cells in close apposition to their neighbors and separated from the extracellular connective tissue matrix by a distinct basement lamina. There is also some evidence that these cells have a contractile capability.

A cross section through a femoral nerve is shown in Figure 1. The nerve fibers are grouped in bundles (**NFB**) of different size and are separated from one another by epineurium (**Epn**). The latter contains some fat cells and blood vessels (**BV**), and is in turn surrounded by adipose tissue (**AT**) in which are larger blood vessels. The perineurium (**Pn**) is characteristically thin and may not be sharply delineated from the epineurium. The bundles of nerve fibers have separated somewhat from the perincurial sheath, causing a space to appear between the nerve fibers and its perineurium; this is a common occurrence in sections of nerves. The nerve fibers appear wavy, and in the section, some are cut in cross section, whereas others are cut longitudinally or obliquely.

The area that is marked by the rectangle in Figure 1 is examined at higher magnification in Figure 2. The axon (**A**) occupies a central position; it is surrounded by the myelin space (**M**). Most of the myelin is lost during the

preparation of the tissue and that which remains appears as radiations which extend from the axon to the neurilemma. The sheath of Schwann (**SS**) appears as the thin ring which surrounds the remains of the myelin. In some cases the nucleus of the Schwann cell is included in the section. These appear as the dark-staining objects (**arrows**) in the neurilemmal sheath. When the axon and its covers are sectioned longitudinally, the same relationship of axon (**A**), myelin (**M**), and neurilemma (**SS**) is to be seen, except that these appear as parallel tracts.

The endoneurium can be seen in some places. It appears as the delicate strands between the nerve fibers. The nuclei (**arrowheads**) of some endoneurial cells are also evident. Small blood vessels are frequently seen in the endoneurium.

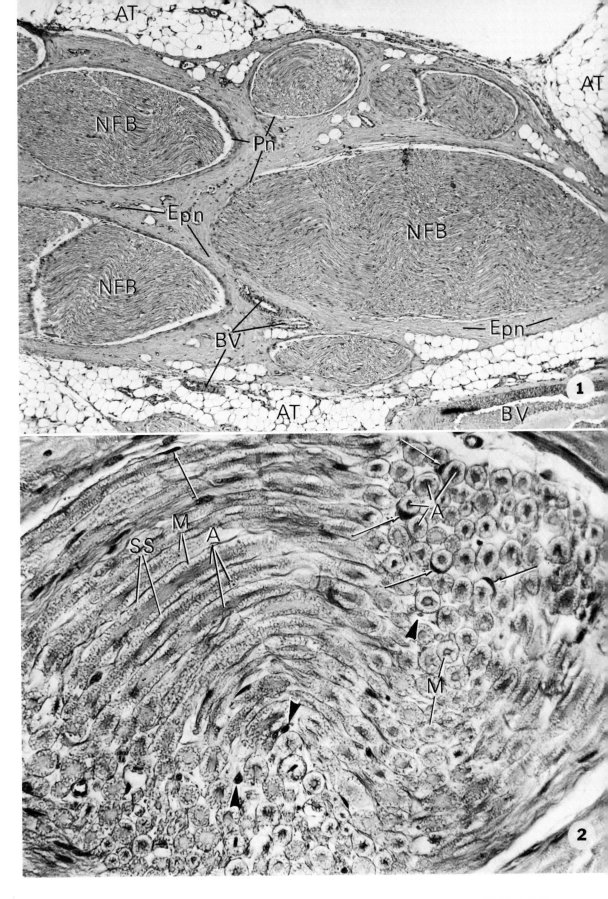

PLATE 6-5

Plate 6-6. PERINEURIUM, ELECTRON MICROSCOPY

As noted in the preceding plate perineurium has special characteristics which distinguish it from the connective tissue that comprises epineurium and endoneurium. Unlike the cells of the epineurium and those of the endoneurium, which are typical fibroblasts, perineurial cells exhibit epitheliod characteristics as well as myoid features.

The electron micrograph reveals the outer portion of a small nerve that has been longitudinally sectioned; an axon (**A**) that has been obliquely cut and its covering myelin sheath (**M**) is present in the upper right corner. The perineurium (**Per**) is to the left and appears as an orderly series of cellular layers. To the left of the perineurium is the epineurium which contains a moderate amount of collagen (**C**), fibroblast processes (**Epi F**), and elastic material (**E**). The epineurium, unlike the perineurium, is less well defined. It tends to blend with the connective tissue more removed from the nerve. Thus, there is no discrete boundary between the epineurium and the surrounding connective tissue.

In examining the perineurium at this low magnification the most notable feature is the relative uniformity of the individual cellular layers or lamellae. The cells that constitute each layer are in effect contiguous with one another. Typically the edge of one cell meets in apposition with its neighbors, thus forming a series of uninterrupted concentric sheathes, each of which completely surrounds the nerve bundle.

In contrast to the perineurial cells, a portion of another cell can be seen along the inner aspect of the perineurium. Though closely applied to the perineurium this cell exhibits characteristics of a typical fibroblast and as such represents an endoneurial fibroblast (**End F**). Note that it does not form a continuous sheath-like structure, but rather, exhibits a lateral margin (**arrowhead**) which does not meet on edge with another cell to provide continuity. This endoneurial cell is morphologically identical to the epineurial cell (**Epi F**); both are typical fibroblasts.

The cytological distinction between the fibroblasts of the epi- and endoneurium and the specialized perineurial cell can be better appreciated at higher magnification (**insets**). The upper inset reveals a small portion of the

KEY

A, axon
BL, basal lamina
C, collagen fibrils
CD, cytoplasmic density
E, elastic fibers
End F, endoneurial fibroblast
Epi F, epineurial fibroblast
M, myelin
Mi, mitochondrion
Per, perineurium
RER, rough endoplasmic reticulum
S, Schwann cell
arrowhead, margin of fibroblast

Fig., x 7,000; insets, x 26,000.

perineurial cell; the lower, an epineurial cell. The specific site from which each is taken is indicated by the small ovals. In comparing the two cells, note that the perineural cell exhibits basal lamina (**BL**) on both surfaces; the fibroblast typically lacks this covering material. Both cell types reveal pinocytotic vesicles as well as mitochondria (**Mi**). However, the remainder of the cytoplasm in these two micrographs shows an important difference. The perineural cell reveals numerous fine filaments, thought to represent myofilaments, and cytoplasmic densities (**CD**). Both are features characteristic of the smooth muscle cell. Again, the fibroblasts lack these elements. Although not evident here, the perineural cells also exhibit profiles of rough endoplasmic reticulum, but in lesser amount than that seen in the fibroblast (**RER**). The presence of rough endoplasmic reticulum in the perineurial cell suggests that it, like the fibroblast, produces collagen, and thus could account for the deposition of collagen (**C**) between the cellular laminae. The myoid nature of the perineurial cells, as evidenced by the microfilaments and cytoplasmic densities, explains the shortening of a nerve when accidentally or surgically cut. Finally, the epithelial-like arrangement of the perineurial cells is thought to serve as a selective permeability barrier.

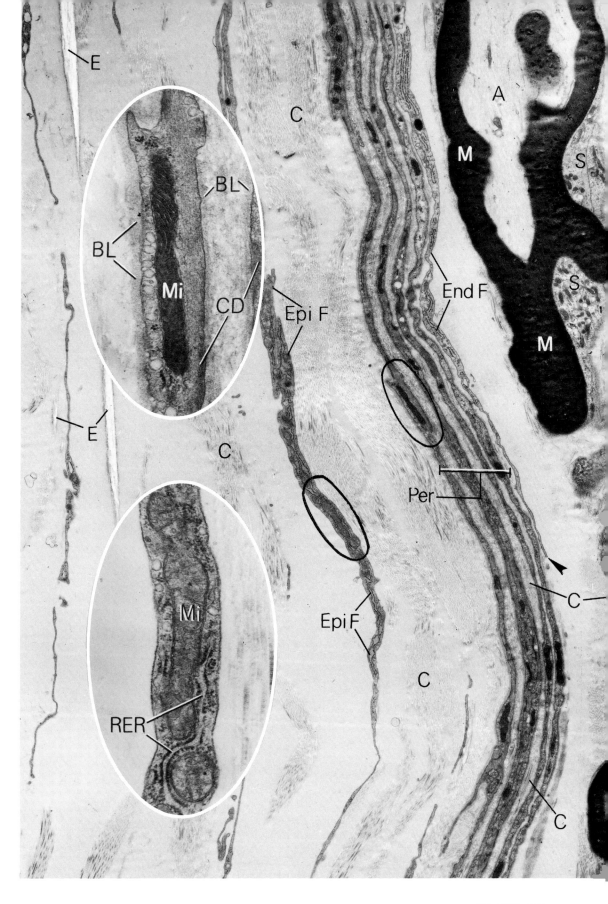

PLATE 6-6

Plate 6-7. CEREBRUM

The cerebral cortex is described as containing six distinguishable layers. No sharp boundaries separate these layers; rather, they are distinguished on the basis of predominance of cell type and fiber (axons and dendrites) arrangement. While the various layers can be recognized in H & E preparations, these preparations do not provide information regarding the fiber arrangement.

Figure 1 is a low-power view of the cerebral cortex and includes a small amount of white matter below the lowest broken line. At a glance, it is possible to recognize the two areas, inasmuch as the white matter contains many more nuclei than the cortex, and in addition, they are all of approximately the same size. These are nuclei of *neuroglial cells* (**NN**) and are shown at higher magnification in Figure 5. Figure 5 also shows that the cytoplasm of the neuroglial cells is not distinguishable and consequently the cells appear as naked nuclei in a "no man's land," referred to as the *neuropil* (**Np**). Small blood vessels (**BV**) are also evident in the white matter.

The six layers of the cortex are marked in Figure 1, and are best seen on the right side of the figure. None of these layers is sharply delineated; the horizontal lines represent only rough approximations. From the surface, the layers are: (**I**) The plexiform or molecular layer. This consists largely of fibers, most of which travel parallel to the surface, and relatively few cells. (**II**) The layer of small *pyramidal cells* (or outer granular layer). This consists mainly of small cells, many of which have a pyramidal shape. (**III**) The layer of medium pyramidal cells (or layer of outer pyramidal cells). This layer is not sharply marked from layer **II**. However, the cells are somewhat larger and possess a typical pyramidal shape. (**IV**) The granular layer (or inner granular layer). This is characterized by the presence of many small *stellate-shaped cells* (*granule cells*). (**V**) The layer of large pyramidal cells (or inner layer of pyramidal cells). This layer contains pyramidal cells which, in many parts of the cerebrum, are smaller than the pyramidal cells of layer **III**, but which, in the motor area, are extremely large and are called Betz cells. (**VI**) The layer of poly-

KEY

BV, blood vessel
Cap, capillary
NN, neuroglial cell nuclei
Np, neuropil
PC, pyramidal cell
Pol C, polymorphic cell body
arrow, cytoplasm of neuron

Fig. 1 (human), x 65; Figs. 2–5 (human), x 640.

morphic cells. This layer contains cells with diverse shapes, many of which have a spindle or fusiform shape. These cells are called *fusiform cells.*

Three cell types have been referred to above; pyramidal cells, stellate cells (or granule cells), and fusiform cells. Two other cell types are also present in the cerebral cortex, but are not illustrated. They are the horizontal *cells of Cajal*, which are present only in layer **I** and send their processes laterally, and *cells of Martinotti*, which send their axons toward the surface (opposite to that of pyramidal cells).

Layer **I** is illustrated at higher magnification in Figure 2 and reveals a blood capillary (**Cap**) and several nuclei. Most of these nuclei belong to neuroglial cells (**NN**). This conclusion is based on the fact that the cytoplasm belonging to these nuclei cannot be distinguished. One nucleus, however, is surrounded by cytoplasm (**arrow**) and is thus identified as part of a neuron cell body.

The **rectangle** in Figure 1 is examined at higher magnification in Figure 3. The pyramidal cells (**PC**) contain an oval nucleus in which is located a small intensely staining round nucleolus. The cytoplasmic limits of the cell body appear roughly triangular. The base of the cell faces the white matter and sends a single axon in that direction. This process, however, is not evident. The apex of each cell body shows a large dendritic process, the apical dendrite, that extends toward surface of the gray matter.

Figure 4 shows the small polymorphic cell bodies (**Pol C**) of layer **VI** and, again, neuroglial nuclei (**NN**).

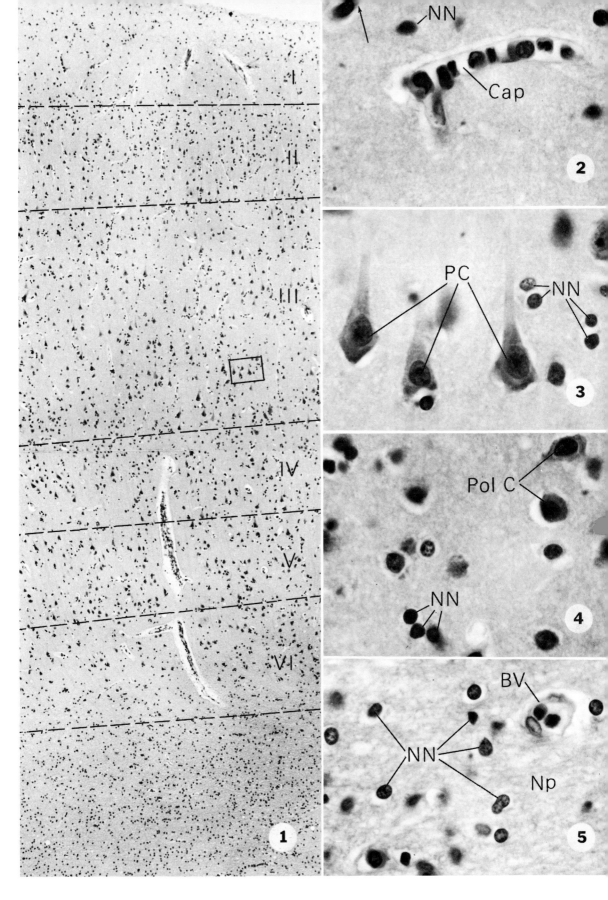

PLATE 6-7

Plate 6-8. Cerebellum

The cerebellar cortex is more or less the same in appearance, regardless of which region is examined. Figures 1 and 2 are low-power views of the cerebellum stained by H & E and toluidine blue, respectively. In both, the cortex can be seen to consist of an outer region, the *molecular layer* (**Mol**) (or plexiform layer), and an inner region, the *granular layer* (**Gr**). At the junction between the two are the large *Purkinje cells* (**Pkj**) which are characteristic of the cerebellum.

The **rectangle** in Figure 1 is examined at higher magnification in Figure 3. This shows the Purkinje cells between the molecular and granular layers. The cells of the molecular layer are widely spaced; in contrast, the cells of the granular layer are closely packed and result in the intensity of staining of this layer. The fibrous cover on the cerebellar surface is the pia mater (**Pia**). Some blood vessels (**BV**) can be seen in this layer. The white matter (**WM**), stains differently in the two preparations. Its fibrous nature can be recognized in Figure 1, owing to the light staining with eosin.

The Purkinje cells are large flask-shaped cells with extensively branched dendrites that extend into the molecular layer. A suggestion of the dendritic branching is obtained in the silver preparation (Fig. 5). A large nucleus with its nucleolus is evident in each cell body of the H & E preparation (Figs. 3 and 4). The Purkinje cell sends its axon through the granular layer into the white matter. The Purkinje cell axon represents the beginning of the outflow from the cerebellum. Most of the Purkinje cell axons will synapse in the intracerebellar nuclei and the outflow continues from these nuclei.

Several cell types are found in the molecular layer. Some of these are *basket cells* (**BC**). These characteristically show a small amount of cytoplasm around the nucleus. Basket cells have both axons and dendrites in the molecular layer. The axons travel parallel to the plane of the Purkinje layer and send basket-like nets around the cell bodies of a number of adjacent Purkinje cells. Some of these are probably among the fibers (**F**) that are shown in Figure 5. The molecular layer also contains *stellate cells* near the cerebellar surface, but they are not evident here. The processes

KEY

BC, basket cells
BV, blood vessel
F, fibers
G, Golgi II cell
Gr, granular layer
Mol, molecular layer
Pia, pia mater
Pkj, Purkinje cells
WM, white matter
arrows, glomeruli

Fig. 1 (human), x 40; Fig. 2 (human), x 40; Fig. 3 (human), x 160; Fig. 4 (human), x 400; Fig. 5 (cat), x 160.

of the stellate cells remain in the vicinity of the cell body. Some incoming (climbing) fibers synapse directly with dendrites of Purkinje cells within the molecular layer.

As noted previously, the granular layer contains numerous small cells called *granule cells.* They appear as the numerous small dark bodies. Granule cells receive incoming impulses from other parts of the central nervous system. They send axons into the molecular layer where they branch in the form of a T so that the axons contact the dendrites of several Purkinje cells and basket cells. The granular layer shows clear areas, called *glomeruli* (**arrows**), which are among the places where incoming (mossy) fibers contact granule cells. Only the glomeruli are evident; the details of fiber connection are not. The granular layer also contains another cell type, the *Golgi type II cell* (**G**). These are larger than the granule cells (Figs. 3 and 4). They have dendrites in the molecular layer and extensively branching axons in the granular layer. The cell bodies are usually near the Purkinje layer.

It should be emphasized that the details of fiber pathways and connections cannot be ascertained by examination of isolated unrelated sections. Only the location and some characteristics of the cell body can be learned from such sections. Fiber pathway and connection can only be established by a combination of experimental and special staining methods.

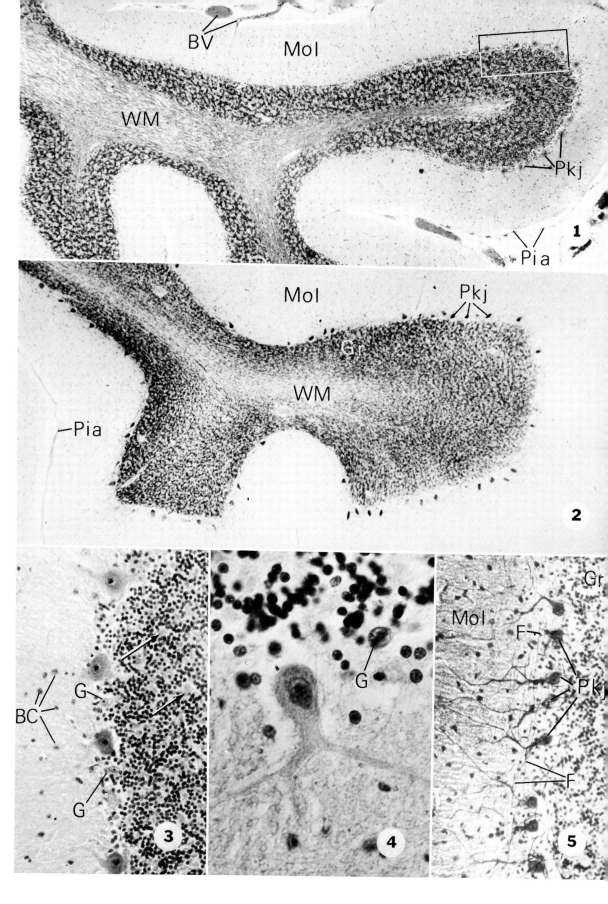

BV

Mol

WM

Pkj

Pia

1

Mol

Pkj

Gr

WM

Pia

2

BC

G

G

3

G

4

Gr

Mol

F

Pkj

F

5

PLATE 6-8

Plate 6-9. SPINAL CORD

The spinal cord is organized into two discrete parts. The outer part contains ascending and descending nerve fibers. This constitutes the white matter of the cord. The inner part contains cell bodies of neurons and nerve fibers. This is the gray matter of the spinal cord. Neuroglial cells are in both the white matter and the gray matter.

A cross section through the cervical region of the spinal cord (human) is shown in Figure 1. The preparation is designed to stain the myelin which surrounds the ascending and descending fibers. Although the fibers which have common origins and destinations in the physiological sense are arranged in tracts, these tracts cannot be distinguished unless they have been marked by special techniques such as causing injury to the cell bodies from which they arise.

The gray matter of the spinal cord appears roughly in the form of an H. The anterior and posterior prongs are referred to as anterior horns (**AH**) and posterior horns (**PH**), respectively. The connecting bar is called the gray commissure (**GC**). The neuron cell bodies that are within the anterior horns (anterior horn cells) are so large that they can be seen even at extremely low magnifications (**arrows**). The pale-staining fibrous material which surrounds the spinal cord is the pia mater (**Pia**). It follows the surface of the spinal cord intimately and dips into the large ventral fissure (**VF**) and into the shallower sulci. Blood vessels are present in the pia mater. Some ventral (**VR**) and dorsal (**DR**) roots of the spinal nerves are included in the section.

An H & E preparation showing a region of an anterior horn is illustrated in Figure 2. The nucleus (**N**) of the anterior horn cell appears as the large, spherical, pale-staining structure within the cell body. It contains a spherical, intensely staining nucleolus. The anterior horn cell contains many processes, two of which are seen in Figure 2. The illustration also shows a number of other nuclei (**NN**) which belong to neuroglial cells. The cytoplasm of these cells is not evident. The remainder of the field consists of nerve fibers and neuroglial cell cytoplasm whose organization is hard to interpret. This is called the neuropil (**Np**). A capillary crosses through the field below the cell body.

KEY

AH, anterior (ventral) horn
DR, dorsal roots
GC, gray commissure
N, nucleus of anterior horn cell
NB, Nissl bodies
NN, nuclei of neuroglial cells
Np, neuropil
PH, posterior (dorsal) horn
Pia, pia matter
VF, ventral fissure
VR, ventral roots
arrows, cell bodies of anterior (ventral) horn cells

Fig. 1 (human), x 16; Fig. 2 (human), x 640; Fig. 3 (human), x 640.

A toluidine blue preparation of the spinal cord (a comparable area to that of Fig. 2) is shown in Figure 3. This stains the Nissl bodies (**NB**) which appear as the large, dark-staining bodies in the cytoplasm. Nissl bodies do not extend into the axon hillock. (The axon leaves the cell body at the axon hillock.) The nuclei (**NN**) of neuroglial cells are evident; the cytoplasm is not. The neuropil stains very faintly.

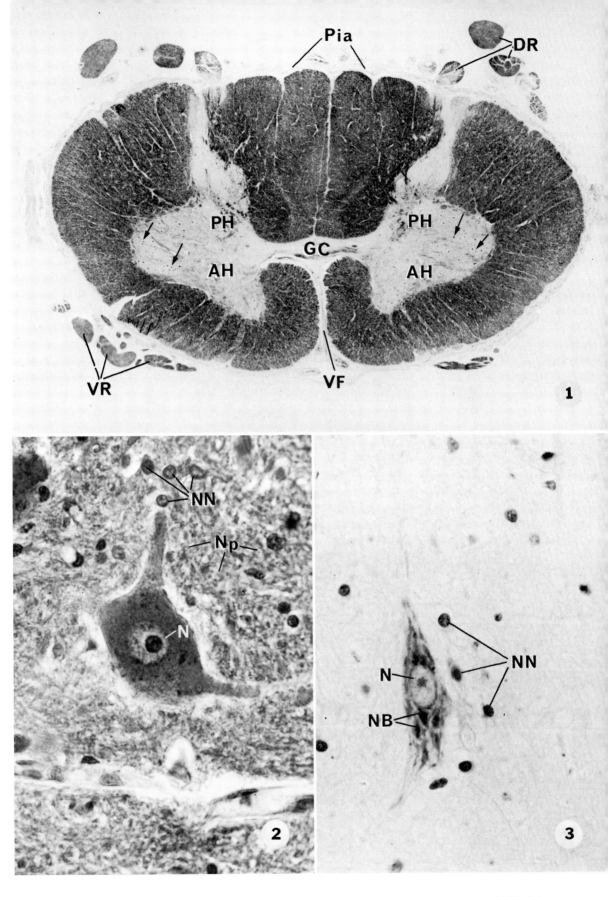

PLATE 6-9

7 CARDIOVASCULAR SYSTEM

THE CARDIOVASCULAR SYSTEM consists of the blood vessels, through which blood flows, and the heart, which pumps the blood. Arteries conduct blood away from the heart; veins return blood to the heart. Capillaries join the arterial system to the venous system; however, arteriovenous shunts which bypass capillaries also exist, and in some parts of the body the typical arrangement of artery → capillary → vein is modified so that a vein is interposed between two capillary networks. This arrangement occurs in the hepatic portal system and in the hypothalamic-hypophyseal portal system. In the kidneys there is an arterial portal system in that an efferent arteriole is interposed between the glomerular capillaries and the peritubular capillaries.

There are two circulations through which the heart pumps blood: the pulmonary circulation, to and from the lungs; and the systemic circulation, to and from all other tissues in the body.

The wall of the heart contains a large amount of muscle, the contraction of which forces blood into the arteries at high pressure. The pressure is dissipated as the blood flows through the vessels, so that in those vessels returning to the heart it is very low.

The arteries closest to the heart contain a large amount of elastic material and, because of this, they are called *elastic arteries*. The elastic material enables the vessel wall to be expanded by the blood which is ejected by the heart. The recoil of the expanded vessel during the time that the heart is relaxed contributes somewhat to the movement of blood. It also minimizes the extreme difference between systolic and diastolic pressure which would prevail if there were no elastic material within the arterial wall.

Further along the arterial tree, the elastic tissue is reduced and smooth muscle becomes more predominant. The arteries are then called *muscular arteries*. After their considerable branching and reduction in size, smooth muscle constitutes the bulk of the vascular wall and the vessels are called *arterioles*.

Arterioles are the major "stopcocks" which serve to shunt blood to one or other of the vascular territories of the body (skin, striated muscle, abdominal viscera, thoracic viscera, etc.). Moreover, arterioles constitute one of the major factors in the maintenance of blood pressure in that they are largely responsible for what is referred to as peripheral resistance.

Veins conduct blood under much lower pressure than is present in the arteries, and the walls of veins are significantly thinner than the walls of the arteries which they accompany. Small veins are called *venules*.

Capillaries are small tubular vessels whose wall consists of a single layer of squamous epithelium (endothelium) and a basement lamina. At isolated points along the length of some capillaries, the basement lamina splits to enclose perivascular cells called pericytes. The relationship of pericytes to the basement lamina requires the electron microscope for visualization. Other details of capillary structure are also revealed with the electron microscope and these are the basis for classifying capillaries as continuous or fenestrated. In certain locations (e.g., liver, spleen, red bone marrow, suprarenal glands) the smallest vessels are referred to as sinusoids. They are wider than capillaries and they have an irregular lumen and very thin walls. Among the lining endothelial cells of sinusoids in the liver there are phagocytic cells. The thinness of the capillary and sinusoidal wall lends itself to the passage of substances (gases, nutrients, cellular wastes etc.) through the wall.

The lymphatic vessels begin as *lymphatic capillaries* within connective-tissue spaces. These drain into larger lymphatic vessels, which ultimately open into the veins at the base of the neck. *Lymph nodes* are situated in the paths of the lymphatic vessels. The fluid within lymphatic vessels is called lymph.

Both veins and lymphatic vessels possess valves which serve to direct blood toward the heart (or lymph toward the large veins). Valves are especially important in the movement of fluid against gravity. It should be noted, however, that the veins of the portal system do not possess valves.

Plate 7-1. HEART

A section through the wall of the atrium is shown in Figure 1. The outermost part is the *epicardium* (**Epi**); the thick middle portion is the *myocardium* (**Myo**), and the inner part is called the *endocardium* (**Endo**). The myocardium is by far the thickest component. It consists of bundles of cardiac muscle. These do not all travel in the same direction; therefore, in most sections cardiac muscle fibers may be cut longitudinally, in cross section, or obliquely. Connective tissue (**CT**) separates the bundles of cardiac muscle. A large amount of connective tissue is in the vicinity of the blood vessel (**BV**) that is in the periphery of the myocardium. The myocardium is considered on pages 69 and 82.

The epicardium (**Epi**) is shown at higher magnification in Figure 2. It is surfaced by mesothelium. Under the mesothelium is the supporting connective tissue (**CT**), the fibrous elements of which are loosely arranged. Elastic fibers are present in the connective tissue; however, they are not evident in routine H & E preparations. A small nerve (**N**), which has probably just entered the myocardium, is present in the connective tissue between the muscle bundles. The nerve appears as a bundle of thin wavy fibers which are significantly thinner than the muscle fibers.

The endocardium (**Endo**) is shown at higher magnification in Figure 3. It can be divided into three layers: (**1**) an inner layer, which is comprised of endothelial cells that rest on a subendothelial layer of delicate collagenous fibers; (**2**) a middle layer, which is somewhat thicker and contains not only collagenous fibers, but also smooth muscle cells (**SM**) and elastic fibers (not evident); and (**3**) an outer layer, which consists of loose connective tissue and is called the subendocardial layer. The subendocardial layer is continuous with the connective tissue of the myocardium. The subendocardial layer contains blood vessels (**BV**), collagenous and elastic fibers, but no smooth muscle.

The ventricles have essentially the same structure as the atria except that the myocardium is much thicker. In addition, the subendocardial layer of the ventricles contains special muscle fibers which belong to the intrinsic conducting system of the heart (Purkinje fibers, see page 86).

KEY

BV, blood vessel
CT, connective tissue
Endo, endocardium
Epi, epicardium
Myo, myocardium
N, nerve
SM, smooth muscle
1, endothelium and subendothelial connective tissue
2, middle layer of endocardium
3, subendocardial layer

Fig. 1 (human), x 44; Figs. 2 and 3 (human), x 160.

The epicardium can be distinguished from endocardium in several ways. The larger blood vessels and nerves that supply the heart wall are in the epicardium; blood vessels in the endocardium are considerably smaller; the endocardium is layered and contains smooth muscle cells; the epicardium is not layered and contains large amounts of adipose tissue, particularly in the vicinity of the large vessels; and, finally, Purkinje fibers, when included in the section, are found in or near the subendocardial layer of the endocardium.

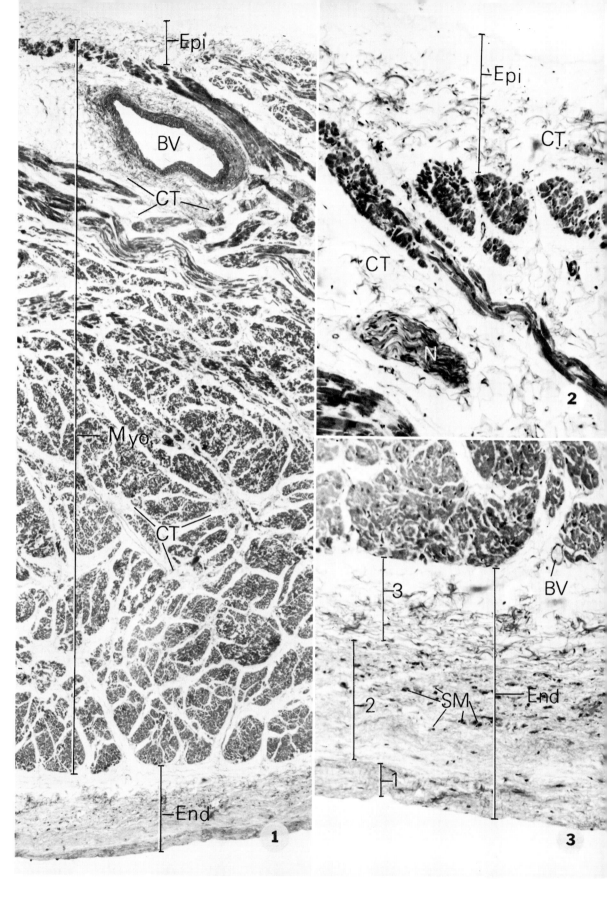

PLATE 7-1

Plate 7-2. THE AORTA

The aorta is the artery that carries blood away from the left ventricle. Because of the large amount of elastic tissue which it contains, it is referred to as an *elastic artery.* The elastic tissue, however, is not evident without special preparations (see page 30).

The layers which make up the wall of the aorta are shown in Figure 1. This is a longitudinal section through the entire thickness of the arterial wall near its origin. Three layers can be recognized. They are designated the *tunica intima* (**TI**), *tunica media* (**TM**), and *tunica adventitia* (**TA**). The adventitia is the outermost part. It consists mainly of connective tissue, and contains the blood vessels (**BV**) (vasa vasorum) and nerves (nervi vascularis) (**NV**) which supply the arterial wall.

The tunicae intima and media are shown at high magnification in Figure 2. The tunica intima consists of a lining of endothelial cells (**E**) which rest on a layer of connective tissue (**CT**). Both collagenous and elastic fibers are in the connective tissue. Some smooth muscle cells may also be in the intima of the aorta.

The tunica media contains an abundance of smooth muscle; however, the distinctive feature of the wall is the large amount of elastic material which is also present. The elastic material is present not in the form of fibers, but rather in the form of fenestrated "membranes." The smooth muscle cells are arranged in a closely wound spiral between the elastic membranes. In longitudinal sections through the wall of the aorta, the smooth muscle cells appear to be cut in cross section (**inset**). Therefore, the nucleus (**N**) is evident in some cells, whereas in others (**C**) it is not. This difference in appearance occurs because muscle cells are of considerable length, and when they are cross-sectioned, the nuclei are not included in every cell.

The smooth muscle cells of the tunica media are particularly evident when the aorta is cut longitudinally as it is in Figures 1 and 2. It should be noted that practically all of the smooth muscle in Figure 1 has been cut in cross section. This indicates that the smooth muscle cells are arranged in a circular fashion (actually a closely wound spiral).

In Figure 2 some of the smooth muscle cells have been cut longitudinally, indicating that they are not arranged in the spiral. This area

KEY

BV, blood vessels (vasa vasorum)
C, cytoplasm of smooth muscle cells
CT, connective tissue
E, endothelium
N, nuclei of smooth muscle cells
NV, nerves (nervi vascularis)
TA, tunica adventitia
TI, tunica intima
TM, tunica media
arrows, area showing longitudinally arranged smooth muscle

Fig. 1 (human), x 65; Fig. 2 (human), x 160; inset (human), x 640.

(**arrows**) is adjacent to the semilunar valve and is not typical of most of the aorta. It should be realized that in a cross section of the aorta, the smooth muscle cells are not as striking as in a longitudinal section, and indeed they may be difficult to distinguish from the connective tissue elements.

Other elastic arteries are the brachiocephalic, the subclavian, the beginning of the common carotid, and the pulmonary arteries. The elastic arteries are also called *conducting arteries.*

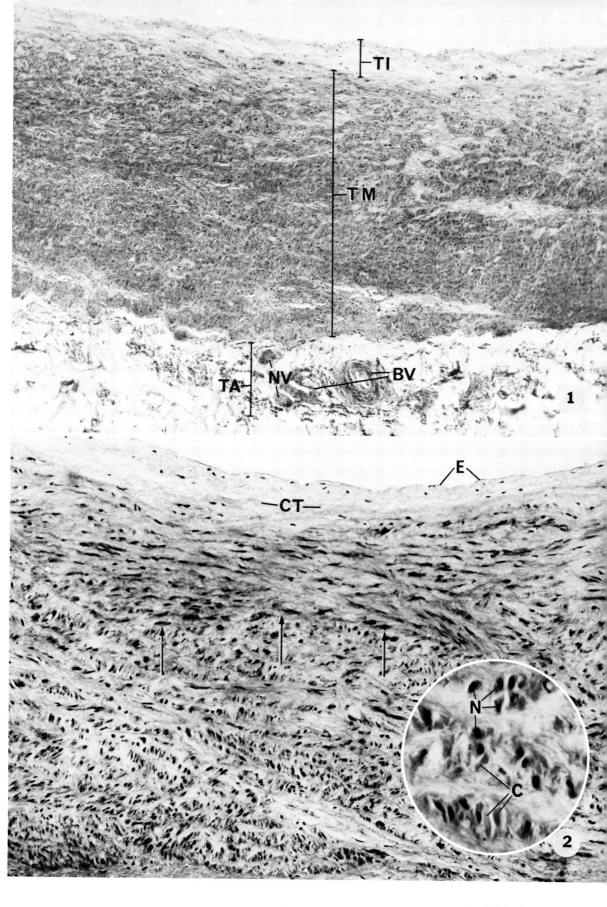

PLATE 7-2

Plate 7-3. MUSCULAR ARTERIES AND VEINS

As the arterial tree is traced further from the heart, the elastic tissue is considerably reduced in amount, and smooth muscle becomes the predominant component in the tunica media. The arteries are then called *muscular arteries* or arteries of medium caliber.

A cross section through a muscular artery is shown in Figure 1. Some blood cells are in the lumen. The wall of the artery is divided into three layers: tunica intima (**TI**), tunica media (**TM**), and tunica adventitia (**TA**).

Figure 2 is a higher magnification of the area included in the **rectangle** in Fig. 1. The tunica intima is comprised of an endothelial lining, its basal lamina (not evident), an extremely small amount of connective tissue, and the internal elastic membrane (**IEM**). The internal elastic membrane has a scalloped appearance and is highly refractile. The connective tissue is extremely scant and the endothelial cells appear to rest directly on the internal elastic membrane. The agonal contraction of the artery causes the internal elastic membrane to assume its scalloped formation and this contracts the endothelial cells so that the endothelial nuclei [**E(N)**] appear rounded and perched on the internal elastic membrane.

The tunica media consists mainly of circularly arranged smooth muscle cells. The nuclei of the smooth muscle cells [**SM(N)**] are elongated and oriented in the same direction. Their twisted appearance indicates that the smooth muscle cells are in a contracted state. The material between the nuclei is mainly cytoplasm of the muscle cells; however, the cytoplasmic boundaries are not evident. The refractile undulating material in the tunica media is elastic material (**EM**). Reticular fibers are also present, but they are not visualized in H & E preparations.

The tunica adventitia (**TA**) consists of connective tissue. The refractile scalloped sheet at the junction of the tunicae media and adventitia is the external elastic membrane (**EEM**). The nuclei [**F(N)**] of some fibroblasts can be seen; the cytoplasm of these cells cannot be distinguished from the extracellular material.

The walls of veins which accompany muscular arteries can be divided into tunica in-

KEY

AT, adipose tissue
BV, small blood vessels in surrounding connective tissue
E, endothelium
EEM, external elastic membrane
EM, elastic material
E(N), endothelial nuclei
F(N), fibroblast nuclei
IEM, internal elastic membrane
SM(N), smooth muscle nuclei
TA, tunica adventitia
TI, tunica intima
TM, tunica media

Fig. 1 (monkey), x 160; Fig. 2 (monkey), x 640; Fig. 3 (monkey), x 65; inset (monkey), x 640.

tima, tunica media, and tunica adventitia. Although there is elastic material in the wall, it is significantly less in amount than in the artery. Figure 3 enables one to compare a muscular artery with its accompanying vein. The lumen of the vein is larger than that of the artery, but the wall is thinner and the vessel frequently appears collapsed or flattened. The tunica intima (**TI**) is extremely thin (**inset**) and consists of a endothelial lining (**E**) that rests on a small amount of connective tissue. The tunica media (**TM**) is much thinner than that of the artery; the tunica adventitia (**TA**) is thicker. The tunica media consists largely of smooth muscle. The nuclei of the smooth muscle cells [**SM(N)**] are elongated and readily identified, but the cytoplasmic boundaries cannot be discerned.

The question of distinguishing between an artery and its accompanying vein or veins is simplified by their proximity, which enables one to compare histological features as in Figure 3.

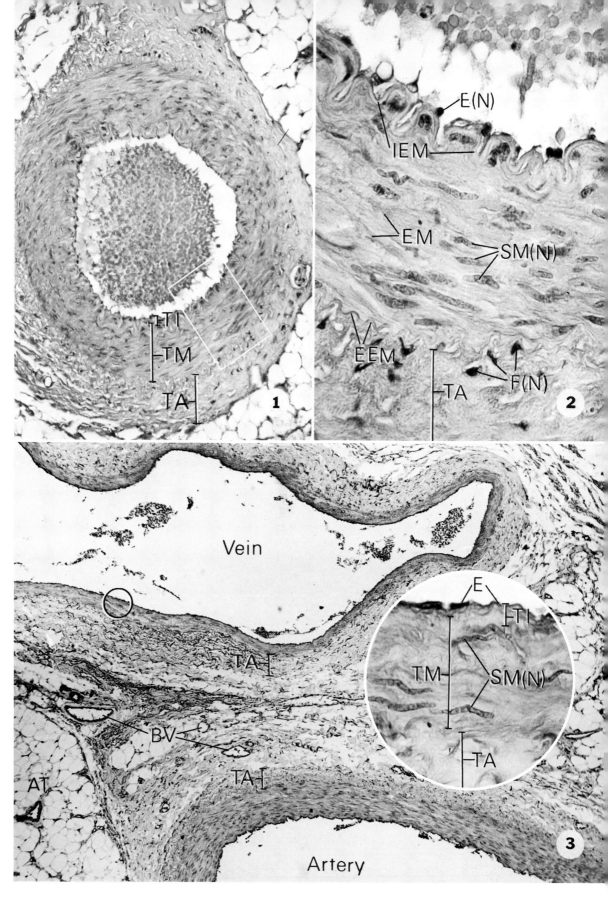

PLATE 7-3

Plate 7-4. ARTERIOLES AND LYMPHATIC VESSELS

Arterioles. The terminal components of the arterial tree, just before the capillary bed or the arteriovenous shunt, are the arterioles. Arterioles contain an endothelial lining and smooth muscle in the wall. The muscle component is limited in thickness to one or two cells. There may or may not be an internal elastic membrane, according to the size of the vessel.

A longitudinal section through an arteriole is shown in Figure 1. It branches on the right. The elongated nuclei which line the lumen belong to endothelial cells (**arrows**). An elastic membrane cannot be seen. The round nuclei located in the wall of this vessel belong to smooth muscle cells [**SM(N)**] which have been cut in cross section. They should not be confused with cuboidal cells. The **rectangle** in Figure 1 marks an area comparable to that seen in the electron micrograph in the following plate. Figures 2 and 3 show how, by changing the focus of the optical system, one can obtain information relevant to this point. In Figure 2 one sees the elongated nuclei of the endothelial cells (**arrows**) as in Figure 1. Round nuclei are aligned in rows in the wall of the vessel. Four nuclei (**A**) are indicated on the left and seven (**B**) on the right. Notice the "shadows" related to the four nuclei on the left. By changing the focus (Fig. 3) one comes to realize that the round-appearing nuclei are really elongated nuclei which are wrapped around the vessel wall in a circular fashion. Note how the length of the four nuclei in Figure 3 corresponds to the four nuclear "shadows" that are illustrated in Figure 2.

Lymphatic vessels have extremely thin walls. A lymphatic vessel from the mucosa of the pharynx is shown in Figure 4. It has been cut longitudinally and two valves (**V**) are included in the section. One of the valves is shown at high magnification in Figure 5. The wall of the lymphatic vessel consists of almost nothing but an endothelial lining. The nuclei (**arrows**) of the endothelial cells appear to be exposed to the lumen. This is because the cytoplasm is so attenuated. At the nuclear poles the cytoplasm continues as a thin thread. It is not possible to determine where one endothelial cell ends and the next begins. Connective tissue (**CT**) surrounds the lym-

KEY

A, smooth muscle cell nuclei at different focus levels in Figures 2 and 3
B, smooth muscle cell nuclei at different focus levels in Figures 2 and 3
CT, connective tissue
SM(C), smooth muscle cell cytoplasm
SM(N), smooth muscle cell nuclei
V, valves of lymphatic vessel
arrows, endothelial cell nuclei

Figs. 1–3 (monkey), x 640; Fig. 4 (human), x 160; Fig. 5 (human), x 640.

phatic vessel. Some lymphocytes and precipitated lymph are within the lumen of the vessel. As a general statement, lymphatic vessels possess lumens of very large caliber in comparison to the thickness of the wall (see also page 186, last paragraph).

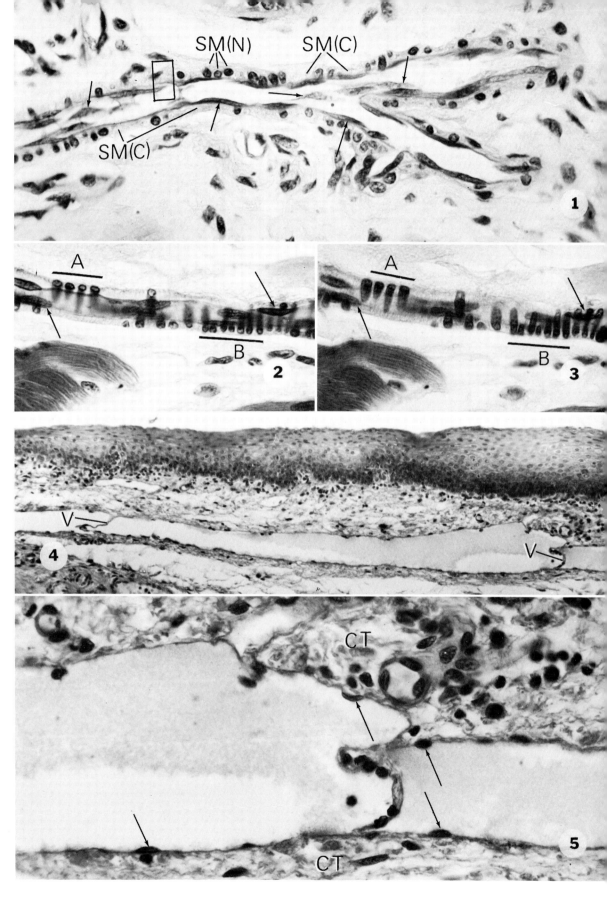

PLATE 7-4

Plate 7-5. ARTERIOLE, ELECTRON MICROSCOPY

The electron micrograph shown here reveals a portion of the wall of a longitudinally sectioned arteriole. The vessel is comparable in size and general structural organization to the arteriole shown in Figure 1 of the preceding plate. For purposes of orientation, the portion of the vessel wall seen in the electron micrograph would correspond to the area indicated by the small **rectangle** in Figure 1.

In comparing the light and electron micrographs note that with the light microscope, the endothelial boundaries are not delineated, only the nuclei are clearly evident. Also, the cytoplasm of the individual smooth muscle cells blend together, only their nuclei when present in the section are readily discernible. In contrast, the electron micrograph reveals the individual smooth muscle cells (**SM**) of the vessel wall; each cell is separated from its neighbor by a definable intercellular space. Evident in the micrograph are portions of two endothelial cells (**End**), one of which includes part of its nucleus. At the site of their apposition, the two endothelial cells are separated by a narrow (~ 20nm) intercellular space (**arrows**).

Between the endothelium and the smooth muscle cells is an internal elastic membrane (**IEM**). This is typically lacking in the smallest arterioles. The elastic membrane in this vessel is a continuous sheath which is permeated by irregularly shaped openings (**arrowheads**). Together with the endothelium it forms the tunica intima (**TI**). In sectioned material, the openings give the appearance of a discontinuous membrane, rather than a true sheath which simply contains fenestrations. The basal lamina (**BL**) of the endothelial and smooth muscle cells are closely applied to the elastic membrane; consequently, other than the elastic material, little extra-cellular matrix is present in the tunica intima of this vessel.

The tunica media is represented by the single layer of smooth muscle cells. The muscle cells are circumferentially disposed and appear here in cross section; none includes a nucleus. Each muscle cell is surrounded by basal lamina (**BL**). However, there may be focal sites where neighboring smooth muscle cells come into more intimate apposition to form a nexus or gap junction. At these sites of close membrane apposition the basal

KEY

BL, basal lamina
C, collagen fibrils
CD, cytoplasmic densities
E, elastic material
End, endothelial cell
F, fibroblast
IEM, internal elastic membrane
PV, pinocytotic vesicles
RBC, red blood cell
TA, tunica adventia
TI, tunica intima
arrows, endothelial cell intercellular space
arrowheads, openings in internal elastic membrane

Fig., x 12,000; inset, x 25,000.

lamina is absent. The cytoplasm of the muscle cell displays aggregates of mitochondria along with occasional profiles of rough endoplasmic reticulum. These organelles tend to be localized along the central axis of the cell at both ends of the nucleus. In addition, numerous cytoplasmic densities (**CD**) are present. They are adherent to the plasma membrane and extend into the interior of the cell to form a branching network. The cytoplasmic densities are regarded as attachment devices for the contractile filaments, analogous to the Z lines in striated muscle.

The tunica adventia (**TA**), is comprised of elastic material (**E**), numerous collagen fibrils (**C**), and fibroblasts (**F**). The elastic material is somewhat more abundant nearest the smooth muscle. If the vessel shown here could be traced back in the direction of the heart, the elastic material would quantitatively increase, ultimately forming a more continuous sheath-like structure, namely, an external elastic membrane. The bulk of the adventia consists of collagen fibrils, arranged in small bundles, separated by fibroblast processes.

The **inset** shows the area within the circle at higher magnification. It reveals with somewhat great clarity the cytoplasmic densities (**CD**) of the smooth muscle cells, the basal lamina (**BL**), and the collagen fibrils (**C**) and elastic material of the adventia. A series of pinocytotic vesicles (**PV**) along the plasma membrane are also evident.

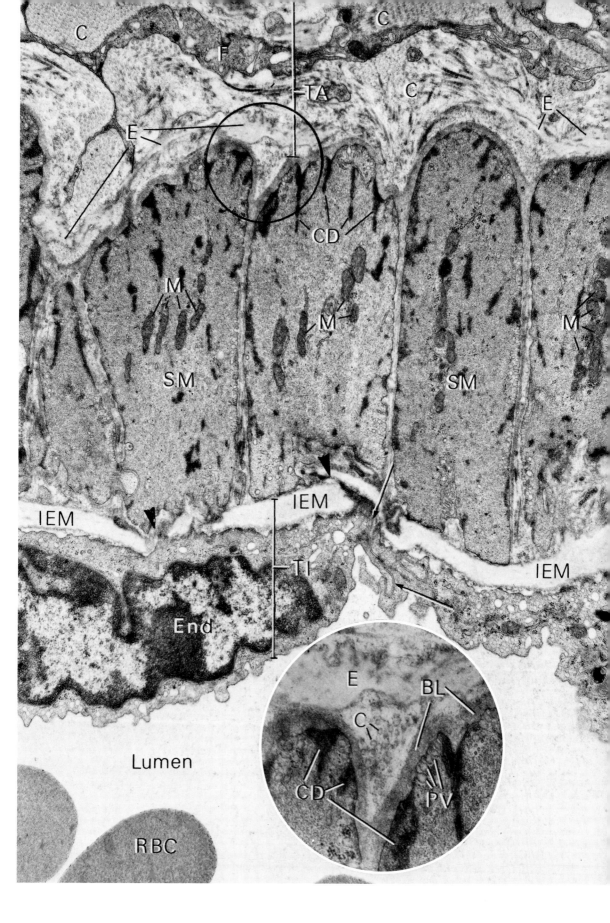

PLATE 7-5

8 LYMPHATIC TISSUE AND ORGANS

LYMPHATIC TISSUE, or lymphoid tissue, is a modified form of connective tissue characterized by the presence of large numbers of lymphocytes. In many locations, the lymphocytes are arranged as nodules. In histological sections, the nodules appear as circular or oval formations of closely packed cells, and frequently a lighter center is present. The lighter center is referred to as a germinal center.

Lymphatic tissue has traditionally been classified as dense and diffuse. Dense aggregations of lymphocytes (dense lymphoid tissue) occurs in the tonsils, nodules of the alimentary canal, lymph nodes, the spleen, bone marrow, and the thymus gland. Moreover, lymph nodules may be seen in the various loose connective tissues of the digestive and respiratory system. The mucosa of parts of the alimentary canal and respiratory tract contains a highly cellular lamina propria. Many of the cells within this lamina propria are lymphocytes. However, they are not organized in any characteristic pattern. This highly cellular lamina propria, containing large numbers of lymphocytes, is regarded by some as diffuse lymphoid tissue.

Whereas lymph nodules may be regarded as units of dense lymphoid tissue, the lymph nodes, spleen, and thymus should be regarded as lymphoid organs.

Except in the thymus gland, the stroma of lymphatic tissue consists of reticular fibers and closely associated reticular cells. Reticular cells are regarded to be concerned with the production of reticular fibers. In addition, some reticular cells have traditionally been described as being phagocytic. It is likely, however, that the phagocytic activity is due to macrophages which could not be distinguished from reticular cells with the light microscope. Moreover, it was formerly thought that reticular cells might give rise to lymphocytes, however, this view is no longer held. The "reticular cells" of the thymus gland differ from reticular cells in other lymphatic tissue. They develop from endoderm rather than mesenchyme, they are not closely associated with reticular fibers, they are not considered to be the source of reticular fibers, and they retain an epitheloid character by forming a cytoreticulum within the thymus gland. They are also called epithelio-reticular cells.

Lymphocytes circulate between the various lymphatic tissues and organs, using the blood vessels and lymphatic vessels as major channels for their transport. Although morphologically similar when viewed with the light microscope, lymphocytes are nevertheless a functionally heterogeneous group of cells. Functionally competent lymphocytes are designated as T-lymphocytes (thymus dependent) and B-lymphocytes (bursa or bone marrow dependent; thymus independent). T-lymphocytes from the thymus and B-lymphocytes (from the bone marrow) colonize the various lymphatic tissues of the body and under the proper stimulus they proliferate and participate in immunologic reactions. B-lymphocytes are functional in humoral immunity which involves the production of antibodies. T-lymphocytes are functional in cellular immunity, in which microbes and cells recognized as "nonself" are destroyed.

T- and B-lymphocytes work in cooperation with each other; they also work with plasma cells (transformed B-lymphocytes which specialize in antibody formation) and with macrophages. The macrophages derive from mono-cytes. In addition to their role as phagocytes, macrophages facilitate the initial stimulation of lymphocytes by antigen.

Plate 8-1. Tonsil and Lymph Node I

Tonsil. The palatine tonsils (fauceal tonsils) (Fig. 1) consist of dense accumulations of lymphocytes in the mucous membrane of the fauces (the junction of oral cavity and oropharanx). The epithelium (**Ep**) that forms the surface of the tonsil dips into the underlying connective tissue (**CT**) in numerous places, forming crypts, the *tonsillar crypts.*

A number of lymph nodules (**LN**) are shown in Figure 1. Each has a *germinal center* (**GC**). Between the nodules are territories which are more or less densely packed with lymphocytes. An epithelial crypt (**arrow**) appears in the center of the illustration. This retains a surface of stratified squamous epithelium. However, in this specimen, and as is often the case, the epithelium is heavily infiltrated with lymphocytes and is difficult to identify. This process of lymphatic invasion of the epithelial surface is illustrated more effectively in Figure 2.

The epithelial surface (**Ep**) is clearly evident on the right side of Figure 2 and is easy to distinguish from the underlying connective tissue (**CT**). On the left, however, lymphocytes have invaded the epithelial surface and have obscured the epithelial-connective tissue boundary. The **arrowheads** indicate areas where the base of the epithelium can still be recognized.

In addition to the palatine tonsils, similar aggregations of lymphatic tissue are present beneath the epithelium of the tongue (called *lingual tonsils;* see Plate 11-2), under the epithelium of the roof of the nasopharanx (called *pharyngeal tonsils*), and in smaller accumulations around the openings of the Eustachian tubes.

Lymph node I. Lymph nodes are small lymphatic organs that are located in the path of lymph vessels; they are exposed to the lymph as it passes through. A section through a lymph node (Fig. 3) illustrates the following characteristic features. A connective tissue capsule (**Cap**) surrounds the entire mass of lymphoid tissue. Trabeculae extend from the capsule into the substance of the lymph node to form part of the supporting stroma. Part of the surface of the lymph node is slightly concave and contains a hilus (**arrowhead**). At this point, blood vessels (**BV**) enter and leave, and efferent lymphatics leave the lymph node.

KEY

BV, blood vessels
Cap, connective tissue capsule
CS, cortical sinus
CT, connective tissue
Ep, epithelium
GC, germinal center
LN, lymph nodule
arrow, tonsillar crypt
arrowhead (Fig. 2), epithelial-connective tissue junction
arrowhead (Fig. 3), hilus of lymph node
asterisk, deep cortex

Fig. 1 (human), x 40; Fig. 2 (human), x 65; Fig. 3 (monkey), x 40.

The outer part of the lymph node, the *cortex* (Fig. 3), has a greater concentration of cells than the inner part, the *medulla*. Some lymph nodules with germinal centers can be recognized in the cortex (**rectangle**). This area will be examined at higher magnification in Plate 8-2. In some regions the cortex extends more deeply into the center of the node (**asterisk**), deeper than the territory of the cortical nodules. This deeper portion of the cortex (usually nodule free) is referred to as the deep cortex. It is of significance because this is the region which contains postcapillary venules through which lymphocytes enter the lymph node from the blood stream. T-lymphocytes, labeled with radioactive isotopes for identification, are found to preferentially locate in the deep cortex.

Immediately under the capsule (**Cap**) is an area where there are fewer cells than in the densely packed region of the cortex. This is a lymph sinus which, because of its location, is designated as the *cortical sinus* (**CS**) (or subcapsular sinus). Lymph enters the cortical sinus via afferent vessels, it passes through the node, and leaves via efferent vessels near or at the hilus.

The medulla contains both cords of lymphocytes and channels of lymph sinuses. The lymph sinuses (also called *medullary sinuses*) appear lighter than the cords of tissue (medullary cords), and communicate with the cortical sinus.

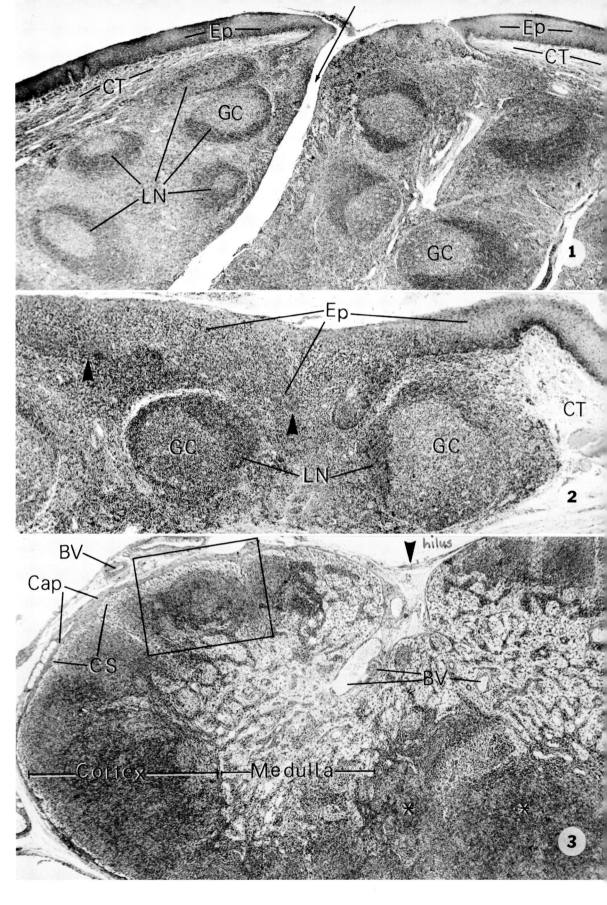

PLATE 8-1

Plate 8-2. Lymph Node II

The cortical region of the lymph node (from **rectangle** on Plate 8-1) is examined at higher magnification in Figure 1. A lymph nodule (**LN**) with a germinal center (**GC**) occupies the center of the field. Above this is the cortical sinus (**CS**), and the capsule (**Cap**). A trabecula (**T**) is shown extending from the capsule to form part of the supporting stroma of the lymph node. The cortical sinus follows the trabecula into the substance of the lymph node; thus the trabecula will be separated from the dense aggregation of lymphocytes in the cortex and medulla by a lymph sinus on all sides. **Arrowheads** indicate the sinus on each side of the trabecula.

The area within the **rectangle** in Figure 1 is examined at higher magnification in Figure 2. It shows the cortical sinus (**CS**), the outer part of the cortex and the capsule (**Cap**). The stroma of the lymph node consists of reticular fibers and their associated reticular cells, and trabeculae. Reticular cells, though present throughout the node, are readily identified in the cortical sinus since, here, they are not obscured by large numbers of lymphocytes. The nuclei of reticular cells (**RC**) are usually elongated and pale staining. A small amount of cytoplasm can be seen immediately surrounding the nucleus, and this sends out cytoplasmic processes which extend beyond the vicinity of the nucleus. Actually the cytoplasmic extensions of reticular cells are closely associated with the delicate reticular fibers and it is not possible in H & E preparations to determine where the reticular cell cytoplasm ends and the fiber begins. Reticular cells are fixed cells. The lymphocytes appear as the free, unattached cells with densely staining nuclei and a thin but evident ring of surrounding cytoplasm. Recent findings indicate that the lymph sinus has two kinds of lining cells: endothelial cells and macrophages. These cells are evidently distinct from the reticular cells in that there is no convincing evidence that either one plays a role in the production of reticular fibers. Formerly it was thought that these three cells represented different functional forms of one cell type, namely, the reticular cell. However, the tendency now is to use the term "reticular cell" for the cell which is associated with reticular fibers.

KEY

Cap, capsule
CS, cortical sinus
GC, germinal center
LN, lymph nodule
RC, reticular cells
T, trabecula
arrowheads (Fig. 1), lymph sinus
arrowheads (Fig. 3), large lymphocytes
black circle, medium-sized lymphocytes
white circle, small lymphocytes

Fig. 1 (monkey), x 170; Figs. 2 and 3 (monkey), x 640.

Part of the lymph nodule and its germinal center are examined at higher magnification in Figure 3. The outer part of the nodule is shown at the top of the figure; the germinal center is at the lower half. At least three types of lymphocytes can be distinguished: (1) Small lymphocytes (**white circle**). These are closely packed at the outer part of the nodule, but are also found throughout the node. They have small nuclei which stain intensely with hematoxylin. (2) Medium-sized lymphocytes (**black circle**). These are the most numerous cell type in the germinal center; they have pale-staining nuclei somewhat larger than those of the small lymphocytes and often show distinct nucleoli. (3) Large lymphocytes (**arrowheads**). These are not as numerous as the medium-sized cells and have nuclei that may be twice as large as those of the medium lymphocytes. Intermediate cell types are also present but are difficult to classify.

Germinal centers are a site where lymphocytes are being produced. A portion of the newly formed lymphocytes also die locally. These dying lymphocytes are disposed of by macrophages and in large germinal centers it is easy to find macrophages with cellular debris. Plasma cells are also produced in germinal centers.

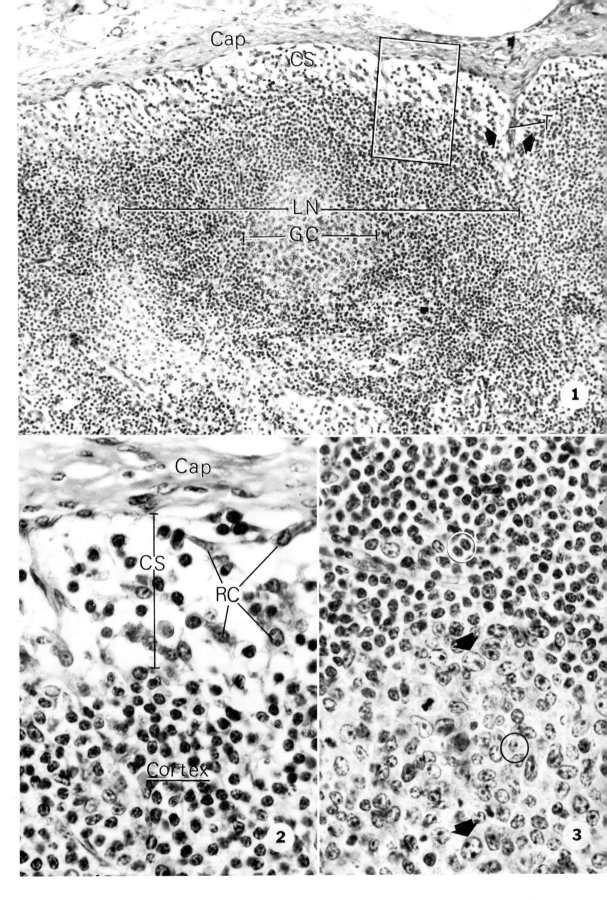

PLATE 8-2

Plate 8-3. Lymph Node III, Electron Microscopy

Some of the more significant aspects relating to the structural organization of the lymph node and its cells are evident in the accompanying electron micrograph. The region of the node shown here corresponds to the light microscopic picture in Plate 8-2, Figure 2.

The capsule of the lymph node is on the left side of the micrograph. It consists largely of collagen bundles (**C**), and some fibroblasts. The cortical sinus (**CS**), which lies just below the capsule, can be recognized at the electron microscopic level as a lymphatic channel. It is lined by endothelial cells (**En**) which, in effect, represent a continuation of the lining of the afferent lymphatic vessels that enter the node. The **inset** shows at higher magnification the area within the oval in the upper left of the micrograph. Evident within the inset are portions of two continguous endothelial cells (**En**) separated by a narrow intercellular space (**arrow**). The connective tissue of the capsule (**Cap**) is to the left of the endothelium and a portion of a lympocyte (**L**) within the sinus is seen on the right. In contrast to the continuous nature of the endothelium which faces the capsule, the portion of the endothelium facing the deep surface of the sinus frequently shows discontinuities. Macrophages located within the parenchyma of the node may abut on the sinus wall, or actually project into the sinus through these discontinuities. When interposed in this way, the macrophages can be regarded as a component of the sinus wall. However, it is not clear if these macrophages are actually fixed components of the wall, or if they are more transient elements. An example of a macrophage (**M**) situated at the interface of the sinus and parenchyma is seen at the site of the curved arrow. Here the endothelium (**En**) shows a gap, and an extension of the macrophage reaches the sinus in the vicinity of the gap. Conceivably this macrophage is in a position to monitor and phagocytize substances within the sinus.

A second type of endothelial discontinuity is seen in the lower right of the micrograph (**arrowheads**). Here a lymphocyte is in the process of leaving the sinus and entering the parenchyma of the lymph node. The lack of contiguity of the endothelium in this instance

is clearly transitory, since the endothelium is parted only during the interval that the lymphocyte is moving across the sinus wall.

In addition to the macrophages, and the lymphocytes which constitute the bulk of the parenchyma of the node, reticular cells are also a conspicuous cell component when viewed at the electron microscopic level. In identifying these various cell types, the lymphocyte (**L**) is readily recognized by virtue of the dense chromatin (heterochromatin) pattern of its nucleus and relative paucity of cytoplasm. On the other hand, the nuclei of both the macrophage and reticular cell display mostly diffuse chromatin and only a small amount of chromatin is in the condensed form. It is this feature which accounts for the relatively pale staining of reticular cells and macrophage nuclei as seen in the light microscope. In the electron micrograph the reticular cell is distinguished from the macrophage by its relative lack of lysosomal granules. With the light microscope it is difficult to distinguish macrophages from reticular cells of the parenchyma. However, the macrophages can be identified if their cytoplasm contains recognizable phagocytosed substances. An additional feature serves to aid in the identification of these cells in the light microscope, namely, macrophages are rarely seen in the cortical sinus. Thus those cells in the sinuses which exhibit lightly stained nuclei can be regarded as reticular cells, particularly if they also exhibit recognizable cytoplasmic processes.

The area within the rectangle in the upper right of the macrograph is shown in the next plate at higher magnification.

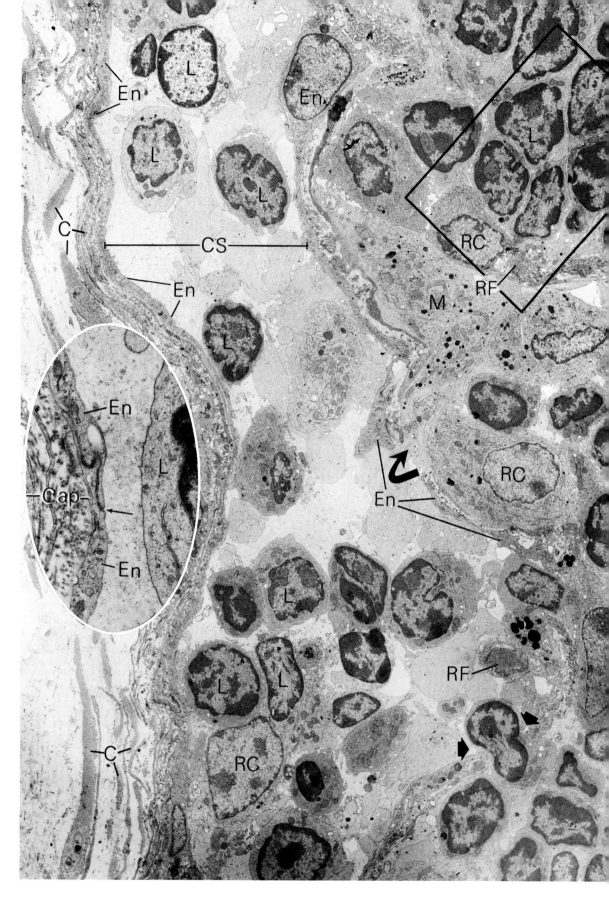

PLATE 8-3

Plate 8-4. LYMPH NODE IV, ELECTRON MICROSCOPY

The electron micrograph shown here illustrates the character of lymphocytes and reticular cells, and their relationship to the reticular fibers.

Lymphocytes (**L**) possess large numbers of ribosomes distributed throughout the cytoplasmic matrix which give the cytoplasm a stippled appearance. The Golgi area (**GA**) is relatively small and consequently inconspicuous. Mitochondria (**M**), though not numerous in terms of absolute numbers, occupy a relatively substantial portion of the available cytoplasmic volume. Profiles of rough surfaced endoplasmic reticulum are rare; also, occasional granules are present. In paraffin sections prepared for the light microscope, the cytoplasm of the lymphocyte is inconspicuous, often appearing as nothing more than a light halo around a dense nucleus. However, in blood smears where the cell is flattened, the cytoplasm is more evident. In such preparations the cytoplasm is stained pale blue due to the ribosomes.

As already mentioned, the reticular cell can be distinguished from the lymphocyte by the relatively small amount of condensed chromatin in the nucleus. The cytoplasm of the reticular cell (**RC**) resembles that of the fibroblast in that it contains moderate numbers of mitochondria (**M**), a relatively extensive Golgi apparatus (**GA**) and profiles of rough surface endoplasmic reticulum. The most distinctive and unique feature of the reticular cell is its relationship to the reticular fibers. Unlike the fibroblast the reticular cell virtually ensheaths the fiber. Cross sections of the reticular fibers (**RF**) show that it is surrounded by cytoplasmic extensions (**arrows**) of the reticular cell. By virtue of this ensheathing, the reticular cell cytoplasm is interposed between the reticular fiber and the lymphocytes. It should be noted that the lymphocytes are tightly packed with little intercellular space separating the cells. As seen in the illustration, collagen fibrils are conspicuously absent from the space between the lymphocytes.

The reticular fiber of the lymph node consists of a bundle of collagen fibrils imbedded in and surrounded by a variable amount of matrix. The matrix contains specific polysaccharides which accounts for the special

KEY

GA, Golgi area
L, lymphocytes
M, mitochondria
RC, reticular cell
RF, reticular fiber
arrows, reticular cell process

Fig., x 18,500.

silver staining reactions that distinguishes reticular fibers from collagen fibers.

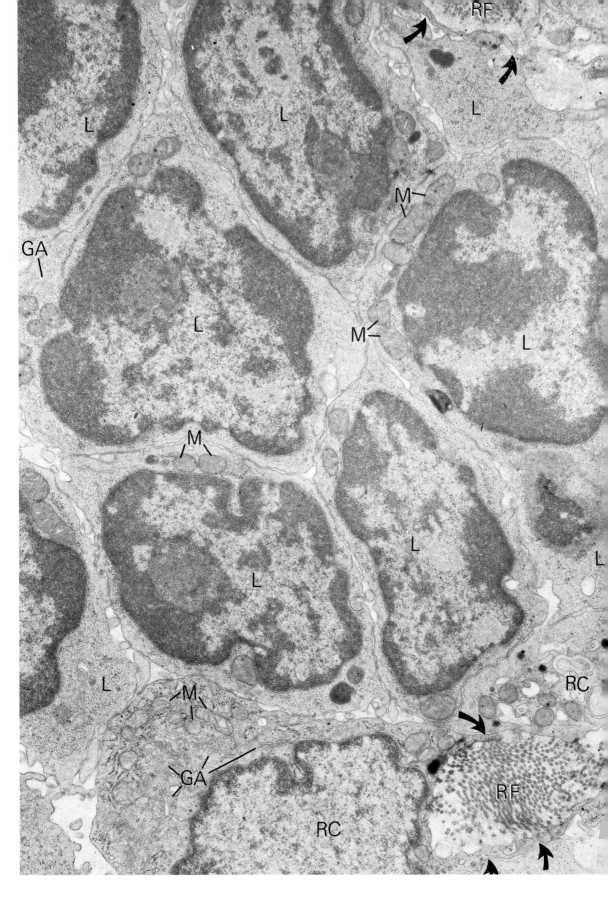

PLATE 8-4

Plate 8-5. SPLEEN I

The spleen is a lymphoid organ surrounded by a capsule and placed in the path of the blood stream (splenic artery and vein). Two major territories are evident in a low-magnification view of a spleen section, *red pulp* and *white pulp* (Fig. 1). The *red pulp* (**RP**) presents an overall red-staining response because of the large numbers of red cells that are present. The white pulp (**WP**), on the other hand, consists of many closely packed lymphocytes. The predominant components of the red pulp are the *venous sinuses*, and "cords" of splenic tissue, called *Billroth's cords*. It is not always easy to distinguish the venous sinuses from the Billroth's cords at low magnification. For example, in those parts of the specimen indicated by the **question marks** (Fig. 1) this cannot be done with assurance. In the lower left, however, the sinuses (**VS**) are dilated and the contents are somewhat separated from the walls, thereby highlighting the profiles of some sinuses. When the venous sinuses are delineated as they are in the lower left, the Billroth's cords can be identified as the tissue between the sinuses. Red blood cells are typically present in both the venous sinuses and the Billroth's cords.

The red pulp is viewed at higher magnification in Figure 2. Some sinuses (**VS**) are evident because the luminal contents appear to be separated from the vessel wall. Billroth's cords (**BC**) are between the venous sinuses. In some preparations, the venous sinuses may be packed with red cells, and in these cases the islands of predominantly red cells direct attention to the location of the sinuses.

The large number of cells in the *white pulp* (Fig. 3), and the intense nuclear staining makes the white pulp appear as islands of spotted blue in H & E preparations. The cells of the white pulp are actually grouped around an artery, and this formation of lymphocytes is referred to as the periarterial lymphatic sheath. The cells surround the artery along its length after the artery has left the trabecula. Therefore, in each island, or cylinder, of white pulp an artery, called the *central artery* (**CA**) may be seen. This is usually eccentrically located. The cluster of lymphocytes surrounding the arteries expands at intervals and the expansions are referred to as *splenic*

KEY

BC, Billroth's cords
CA, central artery
Cap, capsule
RP, red pulp
T, trabeculae
VS, venous sinuses
WP, white pulp
?, areas of red pulp where venous sinuses and Billroth's cords are difficult to distinguish

Fig. 1 (monkey), x 65; Fig. 2 (monkey), x 160; (inset), x 640; Fig. 3 (monkey), x 640.

nodules, or *Malpighian corpuscles*. The splenic nodules may contain germinal centers.

The capsule (**Cap**) of the spleen consists of fibroelastic tissue and scattered smooth muscle cells. On its surface is a layer of mesothelial cells (**circular inset**). Trabeculae (**T**) extend from the capsule into the substance of the spleen. These also contain fibroelastic tissue and smooth muscle. The capsule and trabeculae bring about changes in the size and volume of the spleen due to the contraction of the muscle.

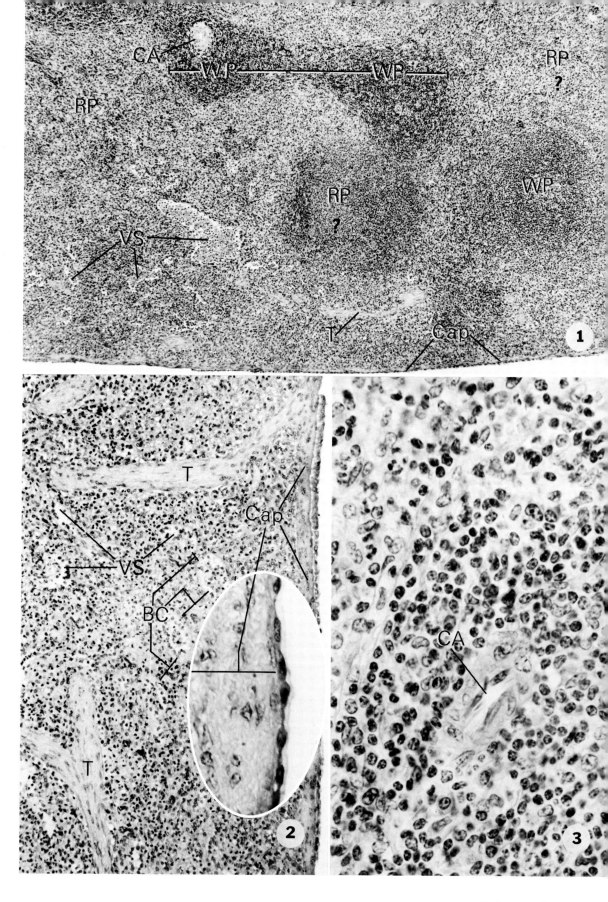

PLATE 8-5

Plate 8-6. SPLEEN II

The red pulp of the spleen is shown in greater detail in Figure 1. Venous sinuses (**VS**) and Billroth's cords (**BC**) fill the field. The venous sinuses can be recognized by their outline. They are unique vascular channels that are shaped like a sausage or elongated balloon and present circular profiles when cross sectioned. Their walls consist of elongated rod-like cells which are oriented parallel to each other in the long axis of the sinus. Therefore, when the venous sinus is cut in cross section, as a number of them are in Figure 1, the rod-shaped lining cells are also cut in cross section, and the cut edges form a ring that constitutes the profile of the sinus (**arrows**). Occasionally a nucleus is included in the cross section through a lining cell. The nucleus protrudes into the lumen and it is sometimes difficult to distinguish the nucleus of a lining cell from the contents of the sinus. Billroth's cords can be identified as the territories between the venous sinuses. The cords can be delineated best by locating the boundary of neighboring sinuses. The cords are filled with a variety of cell types, among which are numerous red blood cells. These red cells have obviously left the vascular channels, i.e., they are extravascular.

The framework of the spleen consists of a capsule, trabeculae, and a reticular stroma. The reticular stroma is illustrated in Figures 2 and 3 (silver preparations). In the red pulp (**RP**), the reticular fibers are arranged in ring-like formations around the venous sinuses. These fibers appear as irregular but characteristic ladders when cut longitudinally. (Although these ringlike structures surrounding the venous sinuses are referred to as reticular fibers, the electron microscope reveals that they consist mostly of basement membrane-like material in which there are relatively few collagen fibrils). This ringlike arrangement is not present in the white pulp (**WP**) where there are no venous sinuses. In the white pulp, the reticular stroma consists of a delicate irregular network of typical reticular fibers.

It is still not known whether an open or closed circulation prevails in the spleen. A brief outline of the splenic circulation will pinpoint this problem and be of help in understanding splenic structure. The splenic

KEY

BC, Billroth's cords (pulp cords)
RP, red pulp
VS, venous sinus
WP, white pulp
arrows, cross sections of venous lining cells

Fig. 1 (monkey), x 640; Fig. 2 (human), x 160; Fig. 3 (human), x 640.

artery enters the spleen at the hilus. Branches travel via trabeculae until as a consequence of branching, the arteries are reduced in diameter. They leave the trabeculae to be surrounded by lymphocytes. The accumulations of lymphocytes around these arteries constitute the white pulp, and the artery is called the central artery. Upon further reduction in size the arteries become arterioles. These then enter the red pulp and form a cluster of branches, which is called a penicillus. While in the red pulp, three successive segments of each branch are described: (1) arteries of the pulp, (2) sheathed arteries (they are only slightly developed in man, but are conspicuous in the dog and certain other vertebrates), and (3) terminal capillaries (also called arterial capillaries). At this point there is still uncertainty as to whether the arterial capillaries continue directly into the venous sinuses (closed circulation) or open into splenic cords (open circulation), or whether both situations prevail. The venous sinuses are large channels which flow into veins that ultimately enter the trabeculae and leave the spleen as the splenic vein. It should be noted that the venous sinuses are extremely numerous, whereas arterioles of the red pulp are fewer in number and more difficult to find.

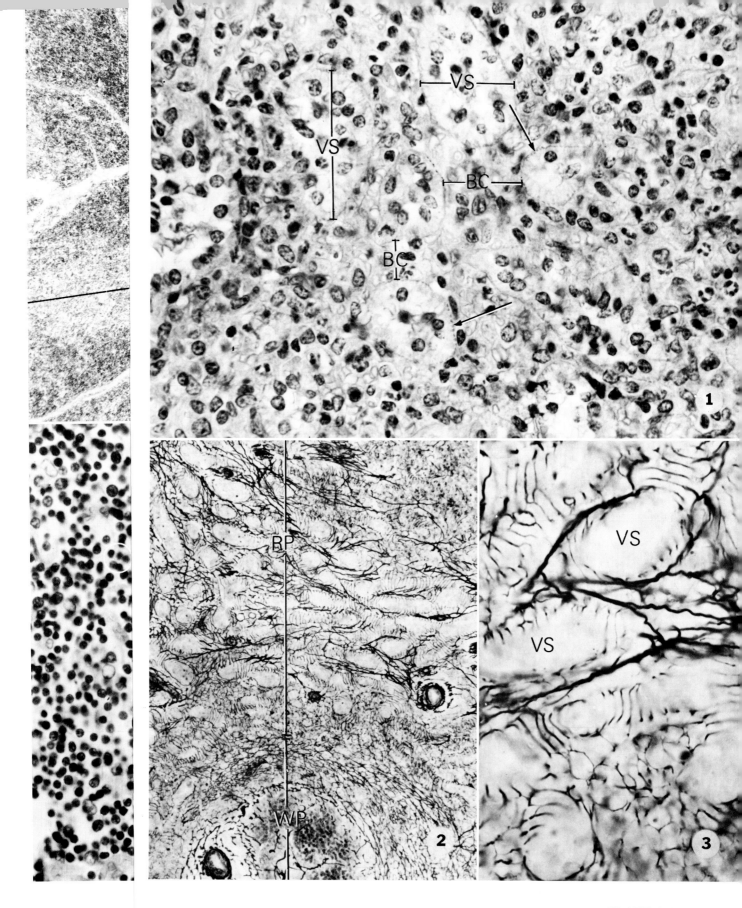

PLATE 8-6

9 INTEGUMENT

The thyr
with specia
supporting (
ing elemen
consists of
reticular ce
within the t
from entode
not phagocy
not associat
cytes migra
during em
yolk sac an
Upon enter
proliferate.
migrate to
them also d
    The thyr
tains dens
medulla in
packed. As
darker in
(**Cap**) surr
lobes) of th
the substa
The lobul
inasmuch
tinuous inn
into the cc
and capsu
possesses
thymic or
are large
epithelio-r
with eosi
guished w:
    The ma
mus are (
characteris
nuclei (**wh**
supporting
dented, p
Both of th
is a high-p
cortex an
tains mac
tinguish
A few plas
periphery
voluting th
    The thy
ture until

THE INTEGUMENT, OR SKIN, consists of two major layers, the *epidermis* and the *dermis*. Under the dermis is a layer which contains large amounts of adipose tissue, the *hypodermis* (also called the tela subcutanea or superficial fascia). The skin serves a variety of functions, and variations in the character of the dermis and epidermis occur according to functional demands.

The epidermis consists of stratified squamous epithelium. The deepest layer of cells in the epidermis is called the stratum germinativum. Cells from this layer migrate to the surface to replace those which are constantly being lost. As the cells move toward the surface they engage in the synthesis of an intracellular protein, called *keratin.* The cells ultimately become a keratinized mass. Collectively the keratinized cells constitute the *stratum corneum.* This serves as a thin but tough protective coat on the outer surface of the skin. Certain epidermal cells, called melanocytes, produce melanin. This is a pigment that protects against ultraviolet irradiation. Melanocytes are difficult to identify in H & E preparations; they do not undergo keratinization. They can however be visualized by specialized techniques. The epidermis also contains two other cell types which require special procedures for their demonstration: Langerhans cells and Merkel cells. Merkel cells are thought to have a sensory function; the function of Langerhans cells is not known.

The epidermis gives rise to nails, hairs, sebaceous glands, sweat glands, and the parenchyma of mammary glands. Sweat glands and hairs develop from the epidermal surface and grow into the underlying dermis. Very frequently they extend as far as the dermo-hypodermal junction or into the hypodermis itself. Sebaceous glands arise from developing hair follicles (a hair follicle is the epithelial sheath that surrounds the hair shaft) and remain associated with them. In a few places sebaceous glands exist without hair follicles, for example, at epidermomucosal junctions. However, in these cases the development of the sebaceous glands probably occurs in association with a hair follicle which subsequently disappears. Each hair follicle is also associated with a bundle of smooth muscle cells, the *arrector pili.* Hairs are not found on the palms of the hands and the soles of the feet, and these areas have no sebaceous glands. Sweat glands are, however, found in these two regions.

INTEGUMENT

The dermis consists largely of dense irregular connective tissue. It contains nerve endings, blood vessels, and lymphatic vessels. Two kinds of nerve endings can be seen in routine H & E preparations: *Meissner's corpuscles* and *Pacinian* or *lamellated corpuscles*. Meissner's corpuscles are for tactile discrimination; they are immediately under the epidermis. Pacinian corpuscles are for deep pressure: they are deeply situated in the dermis and may also be in the hypodermis. Whereas Meissner's corpuscles are confined to the skin, Pacinian corpuscles are distributed more widely throughout the body.

Plate 9-1. SKIN I

A section from the skin of the face is shown in Figure 1. The epidermis (**Epi**) is the surface layer; the dermis (**Derm**) is the underlying connective tissue. Figure 1 provides general orientation regarding the location of sweat glands (**Sw**) and their ducts, (**D**), hair follicles (**HF**), sebaceous glands (**Seb**), and the arrector pili muscle (**AP**).

The epidermis (**Epi**) and dermis (**Derm**) from the anterior abdominal wall are shown at higher magnification in Figure 2. The epidermis is relatively thin. The deep part is called the Malpighian layer. It consists of a *stratum germinativum* (**SG**), and a *stratum spinosum* (**SS**). As the cells from the stratum germinativum move toward the surface, they synthesize the intracellular protein, keratin. Just before the cells became keratinized, granules (keratohyaline granules) appear in the cytoplasm of the cells. These granules stain with hematoxylin, giving the cells a dark appearance. The layer of cells which contains the keratohyaline granules is referred to as the *stratum granulosum* (**SGr**). In places where the skin is not particularly thick, as in the anterior abdominal wall, this layer is not very striking. On the surface, the epidermis consists of a layer of keratinized cells, called the *stratum corneum* (**SC**). This layer looks more fibrous than cellular. The nuclei of the cells have been disrupted and they can no longer be seen.

In contrast to the epidermal cells which are closely applied, the cells of the dermis are widely separated. Like fibroblasts in other sites, the cytoplasm of these cells cannot be distinguished from the intercellular fibrous material, so that the dermis appears to consist of nuclei that are separated by fibers. Most of these fibers are collagenous, but elastic fibers are also present. Immediately under the epithelium, the dermis is less dense. This part of the dermis is called the *papillary layer* (**PL**). The deeper part of the dermis is less cellular, and contains more numerous and thicker bundles of collagenous fibers. This part of the dermis is called the *reticular layer* (**RL**). The elastic fibers are more coarse in the reticular layer than in the papillary layer (see Fig. 1, Plate 2-6).

A section through the skin of the palmar surface of the hand is shown in Figure 3. The

KEY

AP, arrector pili muscle
D, ducts
Derm, dermis
DP, dermal papillae
Epi, epidermis
HF, hair follicle
PL, papillary layer
RL, reticular layer
SC, stratum corneum
Seb, sebaceous gland
SG, stratum germinativum
SGr, stratum granulosum
SL, stratum lucidum
SS, stratum spinosum
Sw, sweat gland
arrowheads, spiral portion of sweat ducts
arrows, Meissner's corpuscles

Fig. 1 (human), x 65; Fig. 2 (human), x 120; Fig. 3 (human), x 65.

epidermis (**Epi**) is especially thick and five layers can be recognized: the stratum germinativum (**SG**), the stratum spinosum (**SS**), the stratum granulosum (**SGr**), the stratum lucidum (**SL**), and the stratum corneum (**SC**). The stratum lucidum is present in epidermis only if the stratum corneum is exceptionally thick, as it is in the palms and soles. The epidermal—dermal junction is irregular, owing to the presence of numerous connective tissue papillae (dermal papillae) (**DP**) which project into the undersurface of the epidermis. The **arrows** indicate structures just under the epidermis which are likely to be Meissner's corpuscles. Although their identification is not clear at this magnification, the horizontal disposition of nuclei in these areas suggests that they are. Note that the papillary layer (**PL**) of the dermis is more cellular than the reticular layer (**RL**). Two ducts (**D**) from sweat glands are shown as they enter the undersurface of the epidermis. The ducts are slightly curved (**D**, Fig. 1) as they travel through the dermis; they take a spiral course (**arrowheads**, Fig. 3) as they penetrate the epidermis.

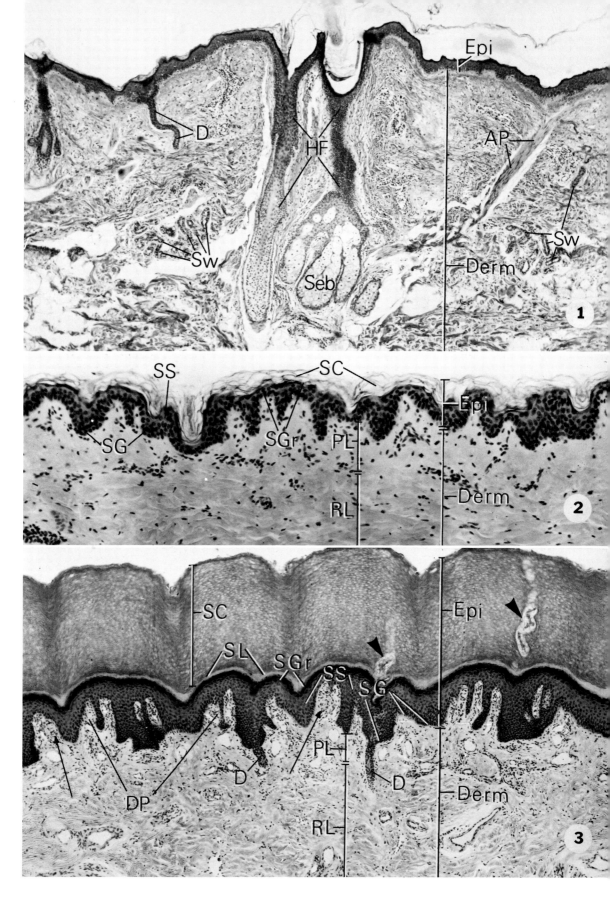

PLATE 9-1

Plate 9-2. SKIN II

Two sebaceous glands opening into a hair follicle are shown in Figure 1. The sebaceous glands (**Seb**) appear as a thick cluster of cells that are closely applied to each other. The cytoplasm appears empty because it contains much lipid material which is lost during the preparation of the tissue. The cells at the periphery of the sebaceous gland are small and flat. They contain only a small amount of cytoplasm, and are capable of dividing. As the cells move away from the peripheral location, they begin to elaborate their product and the cytoplasm becomes filled with lipid. The synthetic activity continues until the cell is filled with the lipid product. At this point the nucleus becomes pyknotic (**arrows**), the cell is disrupted, and the oily product is discharged into the hair follicle (**HF**) and ultimately onto the skin surface. Because the cell is sacrificed during the secretion, sebaceous glands are classified as *holocrine glands*.

The hair follicle is in a resting stage and does not show the various layers that are evident in an active follicle. The hair shaft (**HS**) is in the center of the follicular tube. It stains very lightly.

Sweat glands develop from the epidermis. They are simple, coiled tubular glands. The secretory portion of the gland is a coiled tube deep in the dermis or in the upper part of the hypodermis. The duct portion travels through the dermis as a slightly curving tube, and as it penetrates the epidermis it spirals. A section through the terminal portion of a sweat gland (**Sw**) is shown in Figure 2. This is only one tube, but because it is coiled, it is cut in a number of places. The secretory portion of the gland consists of columnar cells (**lower inset**). The round nuclei at the basal part of the glandular epithelium belong to myoepithelial cells. The duct (**D**) portion of the gland is narrower; it consists of two layers of cuboidal cells, but no myoepithelial cells. The duct cells stain more intensely than the cells of the secretory part of the gland. The lumen of the duct portion is evident in the **upper inset**. The field (Fig. 2) also includes some adipose tissue (**AT**).

Pacinian corpuscles (**PC**) are located deep in the dermis or in the outer portion of the hypodermis. They are pressor receptors. In histological sections (Fig. 3), they resemble

KEY

AT, adipose tissue
D, duct
HF, hair follicle
HS, hair shaft
MC, Meissner's corpuscle
PC, Pacinian corpuscle
Seb, sebaceous gland
Sw, sweat gland
arrows, pyknotic nuclei

Fig. 1 (monkey), x 160; Fig. 2 (human), x 160; (insets), x 400; Fig. 3 (human), x 160; Fig. 4 (human), x 640.

the cut face of an onion. Successive concentric layers of cells and delicate collagenous fibers account for this appearance. The nuclei of some of the extremely flat cells can be seen. The nerve component is located in the center.

Meissner's corpuscles (**MC**) are located immediately under the epidermis. They are tactile receptors. In histological section (Fig. 4), they have an elongated shape. The internal structure consists of cells and supporting elements that are oriented at right angles to the long axis of the corpuscle. The corpuscle is separated from the epidermal cells by a small amount of connective tissue.

"Intercellular bridges" appear as the faint ladderlike striations seen between the epidermal cells in Figure 4. These "bridges" are not cytoplasmic continuities between neighboring cells but rather places where short spinous projections of one cell meet and contact similar projections from the adjacent cell.

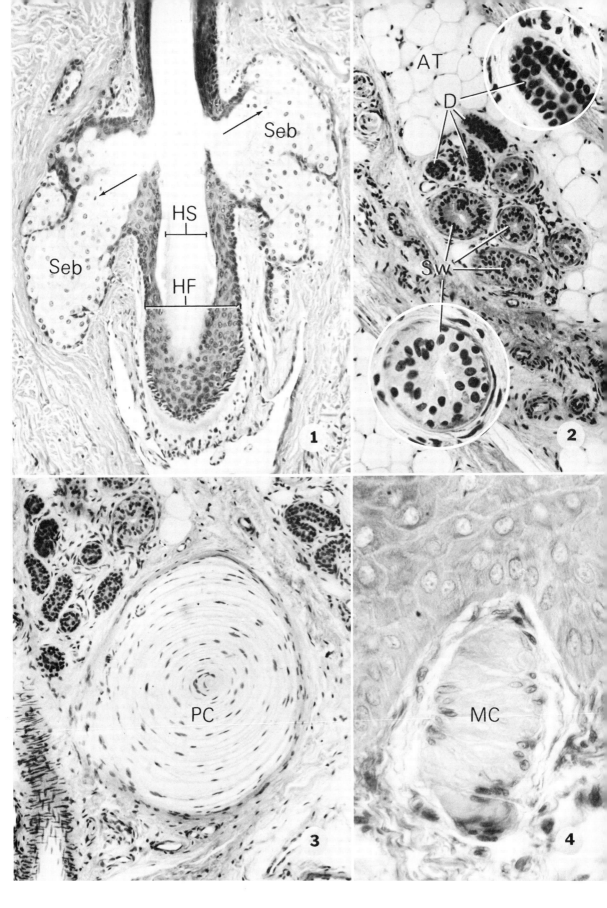

PLATE 9-2

10 DIGESTIVE SYSTEM

THE DIGESTIVE SYSTEM consists of the alimentary canal and a number of glands associated with the canal. From the esophagus to the anus, the alimentary canal is a tube whose wall can be recognized as comprising four layers designated the mucosa, submucosa, muscularis externa, and serosa (or adventitia). The oral cavity and pharynx are not only engaged in the early aspects of alimentation, but also serve the respiratory system and consequently have special structural features which reflect these overlapping functions.

The *mucosa* is the inner lining of the four layers of the alimentary canal. It consists of an epithelial surface, a cellular connective tissue called the *lamina propria,* and a thin layer of smooth muscle, called the *muscularis mucosae.* From the stomach to the anal canal, the mucosa contains glands. The esophagus also has mucosal glands, but only at its upper and lower ends, not in the intermediate portion. Moreover, from the stomach to the anal canal, the lamina propria contains large numbers of lymphocytes and other cell types characteristic of lymphoid tissue. The lymphocyte rich lamina propria is sometimes referred to as diffuse lymphoid tissue. In addition, lymphatic nodules are present in the mucosa of the alimentary canal. Progressing down the small intestine, the nodules are present in increasingly larger aggregations. These aggregations of lymphatic nodules are called Peyers patches.

The *submucosa* is made up of irregular connective tissue. It serves as the major route for the larger blood vessels that are within the wall of the alimentary canal. In the esophagus and upper part of the duodenum, the submucosa contains glands. Autonomic ganglion cells are also present in the submucosa (*Meissner's plexus*).

The *muscularis externa* consists of smooth muscle, except in the upper part of the esophagus. The smooth muscle is arranged in layers. Between the layers of smooth muscle, especially in the intestine, the muscularis externa contains autonomic ganglion cells which are part of *Auerbach's plexus.* The upper part of the esophagus contains striated muscle; the middle region contains both smooth muscle and striated muscle; and the lower part contains smooth muscle.

The *serosa* (visceral peritoneum) consists of a layer of simple squamous epithelium (mesothelium) and a small amount of supporting connective tissue. The esophagus and bare areas of the alimentary tube do not possess a serosa. In these places, the outer layer consists of connective tissue and is called the *adventitia*.

A large number of glands are associated with the alimentary canal. They develop from the epithelial lining of the canal. Some of these (the gastric glands and intestinal glands) are confined to the mucosa; some extend into the submucosa (esophageal and duodenal glands); and some extend beyond the wall of the tube (the salivary glands and pancreas).

The mucosal glands are simply tubular invaginations from the surface epithelium into the underlying connective tissue. The submucosal and extramural glands develop into a branching system of ducts which have a ball-like arrangement of cells (the *acini* or *alveoli*) at their terminals. The duct system allows the secretions to reach the lumen of the alimentary canal. In addition to its acinar components the pancreas contains the *islets of Langerhans*, which are endocrine components.

The liver is also a gland that is related to the alimentary canal. It develops from the epithelial lining of the alimentary canal and retains a connection with the lumen via the hepatic duct and common bile duct. However, the liver is significantly different from the other glands in structural organization and function and will be dealt with specially. The gall bladder is a sac-like structure which stores and concentrates the bile (a liver product) until it is needed.

Plate 10-1. TONGUE I

The tongue is a muscular organ covered by mucous membrane. The mucous membrane consists of stratified squamous epithelium (**EP**) resting on a loose connective tissue (**CT**). The undersurface of the tongue is relatively uncomplicated (Fig. 4); however, the dorsal surface is modified to form three types of papilla (Figs. 1-3): *filiform, fungiform,* and *circumvallate.* These are organized as follows: the circumvallate papillae form a V-shaped row which divides the tongue into a body and a root. The dorsal surface of the body, i.e., anterior to the circumvallate papillae, contains filiform and fungiform papillae. The filiform papillae (**Fil P**) are more numerous. These are bent conical elevations of the epithelium, with the point of the elevation directed posteriorly (Fig. 1). These papillae do not possess taste buds.

Fungiform papillae (**Fun P**) are scattered about as isolated, slightly rounded, and elevated structures situated between the filiform papillae. A large connective tissue core (primary connective tissue papilla) forms the center of the fungiform papilla, and smaller connective tissue papillae (secondary connective tissue papillae) project into the base of the surface epithelium (**arrowhead**, Fig. 2). Fungiform papillae contain one or more taste buds (**TB**) on their free surface. None is included in Figure 2, but at least five are shown in Figure 3. Taste buds extend throughout the whole thickness of the epithelium. This is not evident when the taste bud is cut obliquely, in which case the taste bud may appear as an oval or circular structure. The filiform papillae in Figure 2 have an appearance different from those in Figure 1 because they are cut in a different plane and the bent conical nature of the papilla is not evident. The epithelium on the dorsal surface of the tongue is keratinized. The keratinized layer is usually thin.

The undersurface of the tongue is shown in Figure 4. The smooth surface of the stratified squamous epithelium (**Ep**) contrasts with the irregular surface of the dorsum of the tongue. Connective tissue (**CT**) is immediately deep to the epithelium, and deeper still is the striated muscle (**M**). The epithelial surface on the underside of the tongue is not usually keratinized.

KEY

BV, blood vessel
CT, connective tissue
Ep, epithelium
Fil P, filiform papillae
Fun P, fungiform papillae
M, muscle
TB, taste buds
arrowhead (Fig. 2), secondary connective tissue papilla
arrows, connective tissue, papillae

Figs. 1–4 (monkey), x 65.

The numerous connective tissue papillae that project into the base of the epithelium of the entire tongue give the epithelial-connective tissue junction an irregular profile. Often connective tissue papillae are cut obliquely and then appear as islands of connective tissue within the epithelial layer (**arrows**, Figs. 1-3). These should not be confused with taste buds which may also appear as light areas within the epithelium. The epithelium that immediately surrounds the connective tissue "island" consists of basal cells. They stain differently from the cells which surround the taste bud.

The connective tissue extends as far as the muscle without change in character, and no submucosa is recognized. The muscle of the tongue is striated, and is unique in its organization in that the fibers travel in three planes. Therefore, most sections will show muscle fibers cut longitudinally, at right angles to each other, and in cross section. In Figure 4, fibers that are cut longitudinally and in cross section are shown.

The surface of the tongue behind the vallate papillae (namely, the root of the tongue) contains lingual tonsils (see page 188).

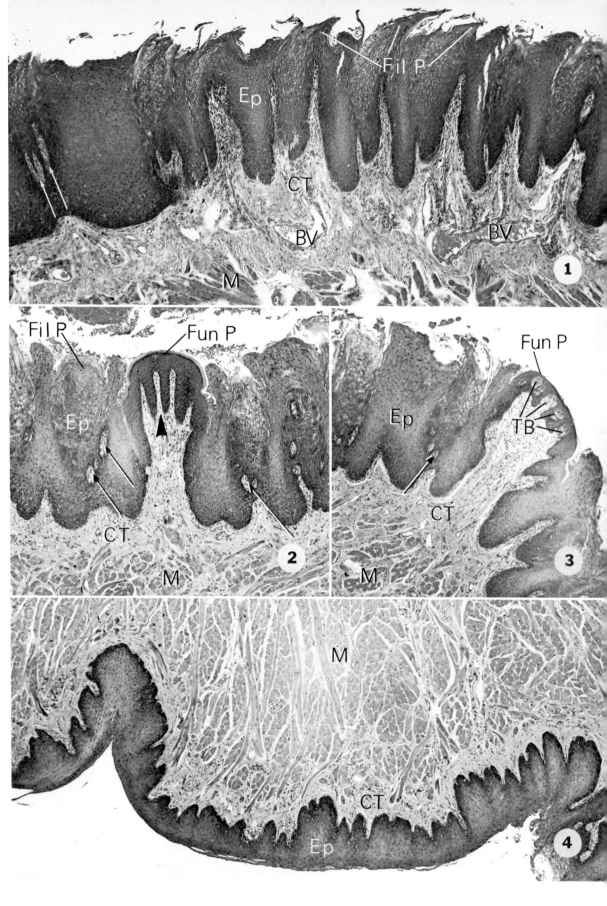

PLATE 10-1

Plate 10-2. Tongue II

The sides of the tongue contain a series of ridges that bear taste buds. When these ridges are cut at right angles to their long axis, they appear as a row of papillae (Fig. 1). These ridges, called *foliate papillae,* can immediately be distinguished from fungiform papillae because they appear in rows, whereas fungiform papillae appear alone. Moreover, numerous taste buds (**TB**) are present on adjacent walls of neighboring foliate papillae. In contrast, fungiform papillae have taste buds on the dorsal surface. The foliate papillae are covered by stratified squamous epithelium that is usually not, or is only slightly, keratinized. The part of the epithelium (**Ep**) that is on the free surface of the foliate papillae is thick and has a number of secondary connective tissue papillae (**arrowheads**) projecting into its undersurface.

The connective tissue within and under the foliate papillae contains serous type glands (**GI**), called *von Ebner's glands,* which open via ducts (**D**) into the cleft between neighboring papillae. Occasionally, the ducts are dilated (**D′**). The darker patches (**arrows**) within the connective tissue represent accumulations of round cells, which are probably lymphocytes. Foliate papillae are not conspicuous in the adult human tongue, but are more evident in the infant tongue.

Of the true papillae found on the dorsal surface of the tongue—filiform, fungiform, and circumvallate (vallate)—the circumvallate are the largest. About seven to eleven of these form a "V" between the body and root of the tongue. *Circumvallate papillae* are covered by stratified squamous epithelium which may be slightly keratinized. Each circumvallate papilla (Fig. 2) is surrounded by a trench or cleft. Numerous taste buds (**TB**) are on the lateral walls of the papillae; moreover, the tongue epithelium facing the papilla within the cleft may contain some taste buds. The dorsal surface of the papilla is rather smooth; however, numerous secondary connective tissue papillae (**arrowheads**) project into the underside of the epithelium. The deep trench surrounding the circumvallate papillae and the presence of taste buds on the sides rather than on the surface are features which distinguish circumvallate from fungiform papillae.

The connective tissue near the circumvallate papillae contains many serous type glands (**Gl**), von Ebner's glands, which open via ducts (**D**) into the bottom of the trench.

The taste buds extend through the full thickness of the stratified squamous epithelium (Fig. 3) and open at the surface at a small pore (**arrowheads**). The cells of the taste bud are chiefly spindle shaped and oriented at a right angle to the surface. The nuclei of the cells are elongated and mainly in the basal two-thirds of the bud. Nerve fibers enter the epithelium and end in close contact with the cells of the taste bud, but they cannot be identified in routine H & E preparations. Several cell types are present in the taste bud; some are special receptor cells. Note the intercellular "bridges" between the cells in the stratified squamous epithelium (**arrow**).

In addition to von Ebner's glands, which are entirely of the serous type, the tongue contains mixed (serous and mucous) glands near the apex and mucous glands in the root (not illustrated).

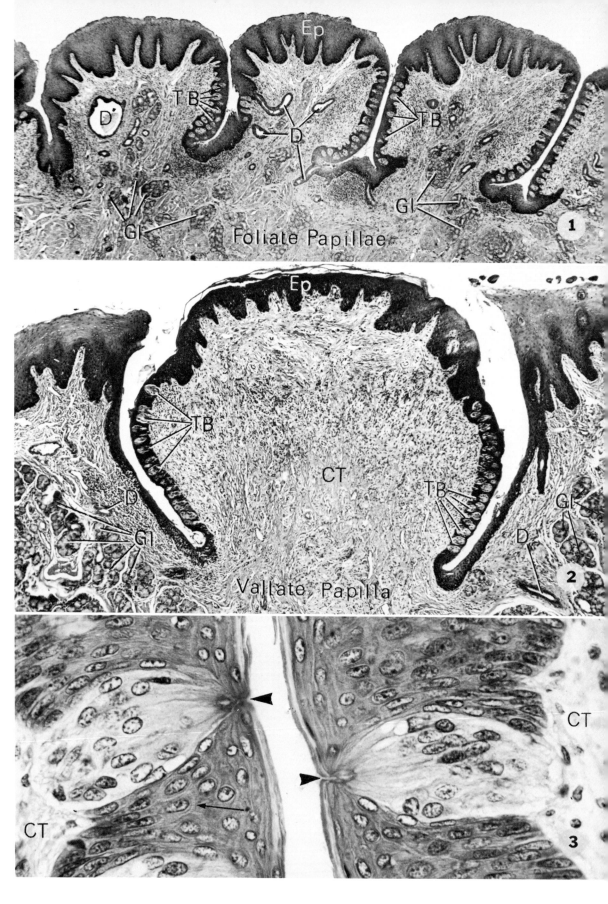

1 Ep

TB

D

Gl

Foliate Papillae

2 Ep

TB

CT

TB

D

Gl

Gl

D

Vallate Papilla

3 CT

CT

PLATE 10-2

Plate 10-3. SOFT PALATE

The *soft palate* is the posterior part of the roof of the mouth. Instead of bone, as in the *hard palate*, it contains striated muscle between the nasal and oral surfaces. During swallowing, the soft palate separates the nasopharynx from the oropharynx.

A section through the entire thickness of the soft palate is shown in Figure 1. From top to bottom, the following components can be recognized: (1) the epithelial (**Ep**) lining of the nasal surface (a small polyp (**P**) is connected by a stalk to the surface); (2) the lamina propria (**LP**) of nasal mucosa; (3) glands (**Gl**); (4) striated muscle (**StM**); (5) mucous glands (**MGl**); (6) lamina propria (**LP**) of oral mucosa; and (7) epithelial (**Ep**) lining of the oral surface.

The epithelium (**Ep**) lining the nasal surface consists of ciliated pseudostratified columnar cells (Fig. 2). Goblet cells (**GC**) are also present in this layer. The epithelium rests on a thick basement membrane (**BM**). The lamina propria (**LP**) is loose and cellular. It contains an aggregation of lymphocytes (**Lym**) and mixed sero-mucous glands. Some of the nuclei of the cells which make up these glands are oval in appearance (**arrows**), whereas others are flattened against the basal part of the cell. The glands may also invade the muscular layer (see Fig. 1).

The muscle of the soft palate is striated. Although striations are not evident at the magnification in Figure 1, it is possible on the basis of other characteristics (see page 156) to conclude that it is striated and not smooth. Connective tissue is between the muscle bundles.

The oral side of the soft palate contains numerous mucous glands. The nuclei of the mucous cells are pressed against the basal part of the cell (**arrowheads,** Fig. 3) thereby outlining the mucous alveoli. A duct (**D**) through which these glands empty their secretions onto the surface is seen in Figure 3.

The epithelium on the oral surface is stratified squamous. Numerous connective tissue papillae (**asterisks**) project into the undersurface of the epithelium. The dark staining of the deepest part of the epithelium is due in part to the cytoplasmic staining of the basal cells. New cells which will migrate to the surface are produced in this layer. As the cells

KEY

BM, basement membrane
D, duct
Ep, epithelium
GC, goblet cells
Gl, glands
LP, lamina propria
Lym, lymphocytes
MGl, mucous glands
P, polyp
StM, striated muscle
arrowheads, flat nuclei of mucous cells
arrows (Fig. 2), oval nuclei of serous cells
arrows (Fig. 3), lymphocytes in epithelial layer
asterisks, connective tissue papillae

Fig. 1 (monkey), x 40; Figs. 2 and 3 (monkey), x 160.

approach the surface, the nuclei become flattened and oriented in a plane parallel to the surface. In this specimen, the presence of nuclei in the surface cells indicates that the epithelium is not keratinized.

Stratified squamous epithelium is also present on the posterior edge and on part of the adjacent "nasal" surface of the soft palate. At some distance from the posterior edge, the stratified squamous epithelium is replaced by pseudostratified ciliated columnar epithelium. However, at the junction between the two, there is a narrow band of stratified columnar epithelium.

Stratified columnar epithelium does not have a wide distribution. It is present where stratified squamous epithelium meets columnar or pseudostratified columnar epithelium as, for example, in large ducts, in the larynx, at the junction of the naso- and oropharynx, and on the upper surface of the soft palate.

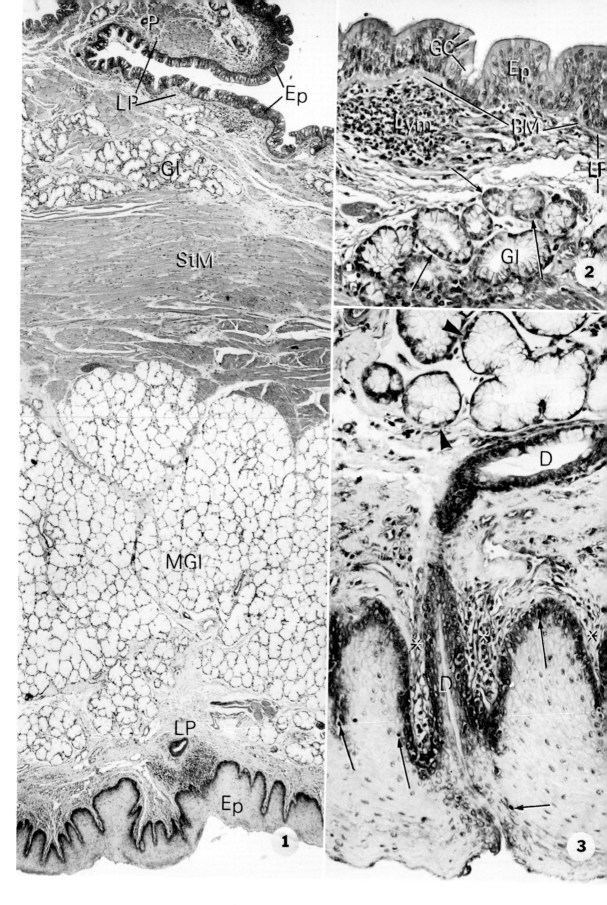

PLATE 10-3

Plate 10-4. SALIVARY GLANDS I

The salivary glands are compound (branched) tubulo-alveolar glands. Acini of salivary glands are made up of either serous cells (*serous acini*) or mucous cells (*mucous acini*). When they have just discharged their products, it is sometimes difficult to distinguish between mucous and serous cells. However, the nondepleted cells are relatively easy to distinguish. For example, the cytoplasm of serous cells is typically evident whereas the cytoplasmic part of the mucous cell regularly appears empty. This is because the mucus is usually lost during the preparation of routine H & E sections. In addition to cytoplasmic appearance, consideration of the shape and location of the nucleus may be of assistance in distinguishing between mucous and serous cells. The nuclei of mucous cells usually appear flattened and pressed against the base of the cell; the nuclei of serous cells, on the other hand, are more often oval or spherical and not pressed against the base of the cell. The most definitive way to distinguish between mucous and serous cells is to stain the mucus. This requires special methods.

The ducts of salivary glands are designated as *intercalary*, *secretory*, and *excretory*. The smallest ducts are the intercalary ducts. These are comprised of low cuboidal or flattened cells. They empty into larger ducts called secretory or striated ducts. The latter are lined by columnar cells whose cytoplasm stains with eosin and contains basal striations. (The electron microscope shows that the basal striations are due to mitochondria oriented parallel to basal infoldings of the plasma membrane.) The largest ducts are the excretory ducts. They are usually surrounded by a large amount of connective tissue.

The *submandibular glands* contain both serous and mucous acini (Fig. 1). In man the serous components predominate. The mucous acini (**MA**) appear as the light areas; the serous acini appear as the darker areas. The nuclei of the cells that constitute the serous acini occupy a peripheral location and suggest the extent of the acini. The duct (**ED**) that is surrounded by a large amount of connective tissue (**CT**) is an excretory duct. A large number of striated ducts (**SD**) are within the substance of the gland. These are smaller than the excretory duct but they also have a rela-

KEY

CT, connective tissue
ED, excretory duct
ID, intercalary duct
L, lumen
MA, mucous acinus
S, septa
SA, serous acinus
SD, striated duct
arrows, serous demilunes

Fig. 1 (human submandibular gland), x 65; Fig. 2 (human submandibular gland), x 160; (inset), x 400.

tively large patent lumen and thus they can be readily distinguished from the surrounding acini. The nuclei of the duct cells appear as a ring around the lumen. Connective tissue septa (**S**) are seen throughout the field.

Figure 2 shows the submandibular gland at higher magnification. A large striated duct (**SD**) occupies the center of the field. An intercalary duct (**ID**) is seen where it joins the striated duct. Serous acini (**SA**) and mucous acini are present throughout the field. Not all of the serous cells are organized as acini. Many of them form a cap on the mucous acini (**arrows**). These caps of serous cells are called demilunes. A demilune capping a mucous acinus is shown in the **inset**. Note how the nuclei of the mucous cells are flattened and are at the basal end of the cell; the nuclei of the serous cells are spherical. The lumen (**L**) of the mucous acinus is clearly evident.

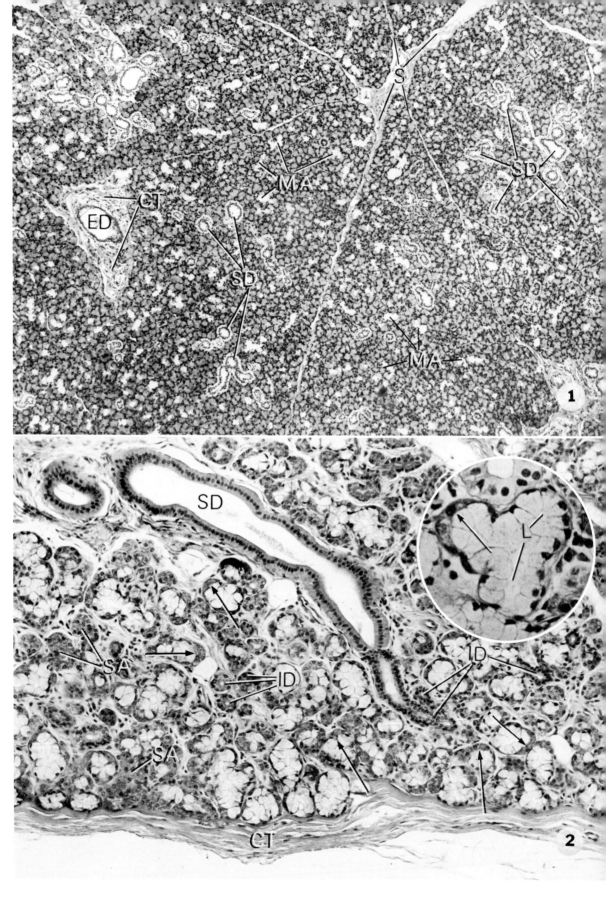

PLATE 10-4

Plate 10-5. SALIVARY GLANDS II

The *sublingual glands* resemble the submandibular glands in that they contain both serous and mucous elements. However, in man, the *mucous acini* predominate. *Intercalary ducts* are not usually present, or if they are, they are extremely short and thus difficult to find. The sublingual gland is shown in Figure 1. The mucous acini are the most conspicuous components. They are the light groups of cells; the darker groups are *serous acini* (**SA**) or *demilunes* (**arrows**). Many of the mucous acini are not really a spherical arrangement of cells, but rather tubular channels of mucous cells. In this respect they differ from serous acini. A large excretory duct (**ED**) is located in the center of the field, surrounded by connective tissue. The lining of the duct consists of low columnar epithelium.

The *parotid gland* in the human consists of *serous acini* (Fig. 2). Intercalary (**ID**), *striated* (**SD**), and *excretory ducts* are typically evident. The section was stained to reveal the granules that are present in serous cells. The septa (**S**) and stroma are also highlighted in this preparation by special stains. The striated ducts can be readily identified because they possess clearly evident, patent, lumens and a lining of columnar cells. The lumens of the acini are not conspicuous and the organization of the acini may not always be clear. However, in many cases the nuclei of the acinar cells appear to be disposed in a circular pattern, thereby suggesting the extent of the acinus.

A higher magnification of the stromal connective tissue that borders several acini is shown in the **inset.** The nuclei are in the basal part of the cell; the lumens (**arrows**) are beyond the apex. Many of the cells contain secretory granules (the secretory granules of gland cells which produce digestive enzymes are called *zymogen granules*). Some of the flattened nuclei that appear to be at the junction of the connective tissue and the base of the serous cells are nuclei of myoepithelial cells. These cells are also present in the other salivary glands and in the ducts of salivary glands.

Fat cells are usually present in the connective tissue of the larger septa within the salivary glands. These appear empty in H & E sections because, like the mucus, lipid is lost

KEY

ED, excretory duct
ID, intercalary duct
S, septa
SA, serous acini
SD, striated duct
arrows (Fig. 1), serous demilunes
arrows (Fig. 2, inset), lumens of serous acini

Fig. 1 (human sublingual gland), x 160; Fig. 2 (human parotid gland), x 160, (inset), x 640.

during preparation of the tissue. It should be noted that mucus is lost during the time that the tissue is in aqueous solutions, whereas lipid is lost during the time that the tissue is in the lipid solvents.

The submandibular, sublingual and parotid glands are sometimes designated as the major salivary glands. This distinguishes them from smaller glands, the minor salivary glands, which are located in the labial and buccal mucosa.

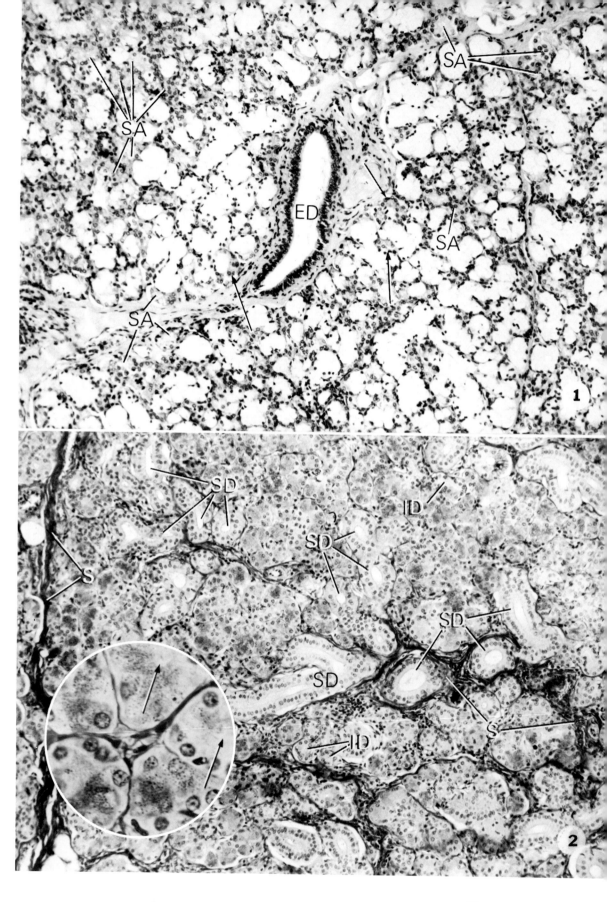

PLATE 10-5

Plate 10-6. Developing Tooth

During early fetal development, a plate of epithelium called the *dental lamina* grows into the underlying embryonic connective tissue (mesenchyme) from the oral epithelium. At regular intervals, where future teeth will be, the cells of the dental lamina proliferate and become the *enamel organs.*

The enamel organ (**EO**) appears as an expanded cell mass that has been invaginated by a connective tissue papilla, the *dental papilla* (**DP**) (Fig. 1). It is attached to the oral epithelium (**Ep**) by the dental lamina (**DL**). The junction between the enamel organ and the dental papilla assumes the shape of the future *dentino-enamel junction* before dentinogenesis or amelogenesis begins. The mesenchyme that surrounds the enamel organ and dental papilla forms a delicate fibrous sac called the *dental sac* (**DS**). This sac along with its contents is called the *tooth germ* (**TG**).

Figure 2 shows a tooth germ in which dentinogenesis and amelogenesis have just begun. The parts of the enamel organ are designated: the *inner enamel epithelium* (**A**) (these are called *ameloblasts* once they begin to form enamel), the *stratum intermedium* (**SI**), the *stellate reticulum* (**SR**), and the *outer enamel epithelium* (**OEE**). The dental papilla (**DP**) will become the future pulp cavity. At the periphery of the dental papilla are the columnar shaped *odontoblasts* (**O**) which produce *dentin* (**D**). The enamel (**E**) is deposited by ameloblasts on the surface of the previously formed dentin.

Figure 3 shows a tooth, stained with toluidine blue, at a later stage of development. The enamel (**E**) is unstained; however, the ameloblasts (**A**), dentin (**D**), and odontoblasts (**O**) stain intensely. The most recently formed enamel and dentin are at the bottom of the figure. A serial section of this region, stained with H & E, is examined at higher magnification in Figure 4. The sequence of events that are shown in Figure 4 (and in Fig. 2) are as follows: (**1**) cells of the enamel organ induce mesenchymal cells of the dental papilla to become odontoblasts; (**2**) the odontoblasts begin to produce dentin; (**3**) when the ameloblasts are confronted with the dentin, they deposit enamel on the outer dentinal surface.

In the formation of dentin, an organic

KEY

A, ameloblasts
D, dentin
DL, dental lamina
DP, dental papilla
DS, dental sac
E, enamel
EO, enamel organ
Ep, oral epithelium
O, odontoblasts
OEE, outer enamel epithelium
Pd, predentin
SI, stratum intermedium
SR, stellate reticulum
TG, tooth germ

Fig. 1 (pig), x 16; Fig. 2 (dog), x 40; Fig. 3 (rat), x 65, (inset), x 160; Fig. 4 (rat), x 160, (inset), x 640.

matrix containing collagenous fibers is produced by the odontoblasts. This calcifies to become dentin. The immediate product of the odontoblasts is called *predentin* (**Pd**). It stains less intensely than the dentin. The *odontoblastic process* (inset, Fig. 4) is contained in a *dental tubule* and both the process and its tubule extend through the entire thickness of the dentin.

In the early stages of amelogenesis, the ameloblasts secrete an organic matrix. Mineralization of this (as with the dentinal matrix) begins almost immediately. However, in teeth with a thin layer of enamel (e.g., rat), after the enamel reaches its full thickness it undergoes maturation. Organic material and water are removed, and the enamel continues to mineralize to a greater extent than occurs anywhere else in the body. During maturation the ameloblasts (inset, Fig. 3) acquire the characteristics of absorptive or transport cells. The maturation of enamel in human teeth (and in other teeth in which the enamel is thick) is more complex and not well understood.

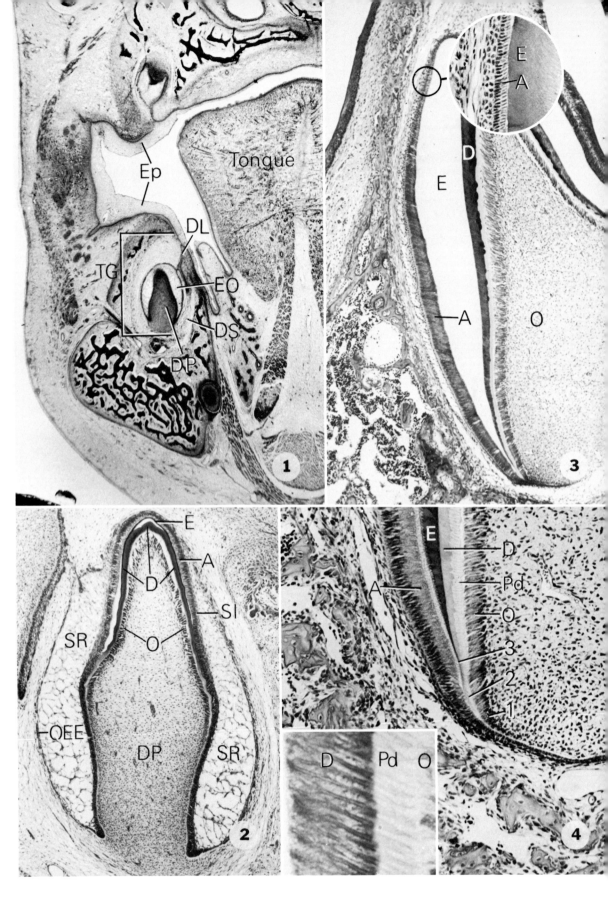

PLATE 10-6

Plate 10-7. ESOPHAGUS

The *esophagus* serves chiefly to convey food and other substances from the pharynx to the stomach. These materials are moved rapidly from the region where the respiratory system shares its passages with the alimentary structures. In this connection it should be noted that the oral cavity, pharynx, and the upper part of the esophagus contain striated muscle within their walls.

The wall of the esophagus is shown in Figure 1. The *mucosa* (**Muc**) consists of *stratified squamous epithelium* (**Ep**), a *lamina propria* (**LP**), and a *muscularis mucosae* (**MM**). The boundary between the epithelium and lamina propria is distinct, though somewhat uneven owing to the presence of numerous connective tissue papillae (**arrows**). The basal layer of the epithelium stains intensely and appears as a dark band, which is especially conspicuous at low magnifications. This is due in part to the cytoplasmic basophilia. The fact that the basal cells are small results in a high nuclear-cytoplasmic ratio which further intensifies the staining of this layer.

New cells are produced in the basal layer from which they migrate to the surface. During this migration, the shape and orientation of the cells change. This change in cell shape and orientation is also reflected in the appearance of the nuclei. In the deeper layers the nuclei are spherical; in the more superficial layers the nuclei are elongated and oriented parallel to the surface. The fact that nuclei can be seen throughout the epithelial layer as far as the surface indicates that this epithelium is not keratinized.

Whereas the boundary between the epithelium and lamina propria is striking, the boundary between the *mucosa* and *submucosa* (**Subm**) is less well marked but still readily discernible. The deepest part of the mucosa is the *muscularis mucosae* (**MM**) and this serves as the marker. The nuclei of the smooth muscle (**SM**) cells all appear spherical because the muscle cells have been cut in cross section (Fig. 2). The submucosa consists of irregular connective tissue with numerous blood vessels (**BV**). No glands are in the submucosa of Figure 1, but they are regularly present throughout this layer.

The *muscularis externa* (**ME**) in Figure 1 contains striated muscle (therefore the speci-

KEY

Adv, adventitia
BV, blood vessels
Ep, stratified squamous epithelium
LP, lamina propria
M(Sm), smooth muscle
M(St), striated muscle
ME, muscularis externa
MM, muscularis mucosae
Muc, mucosa
SM, smooth muscle
Subm, submucosa
arrows, connective tissue papillae

Fig. 1 (monkey), x 65, (inset), x 65; Fig. 2 (monkey), x 160; Fig. 3 (monkey), x 640.

men is from the upper part of the esophagus). Although the striations are not evident at this low magnification, reference to the inset and then to Figure 3 will substantiate this identification. The inset shows two kinds of longitudinally cut, oriented, fibrous type tissues. They stain differently, but of greater significance is the distribution and number of nuclei. In one case (Fig. 3), numerous elongated and oriented nuclei are scattered throughout; this is smooth muscle [**M(Sm)**]. In the other, fewer elongated nuclei are present; moreover, they are largely at the periphery of the bundles. This is striated muscle [**M(St)**]; the cross striations are clearly evident. Re-examination of Figure 1 shows that it consists of muscle bundles which resemble the striated muscle of Figure 3 in terms of nuclear number, orientation and location. The inset and Figure 3 are from the middle of the esophagus where both smooth and striated muscle are present. The distal third of the esophagus contains only smooth muscle.

External to the muscularis externa is the *adventitia* (**Adv**). (The term "adventitia" appeared earlier with respect to the walls of blood vessels. The term is also used in a more general way, in which case it refers to the outermost connective tissue layer of a structure which blends imperceptively with neighboring connective tissue.)

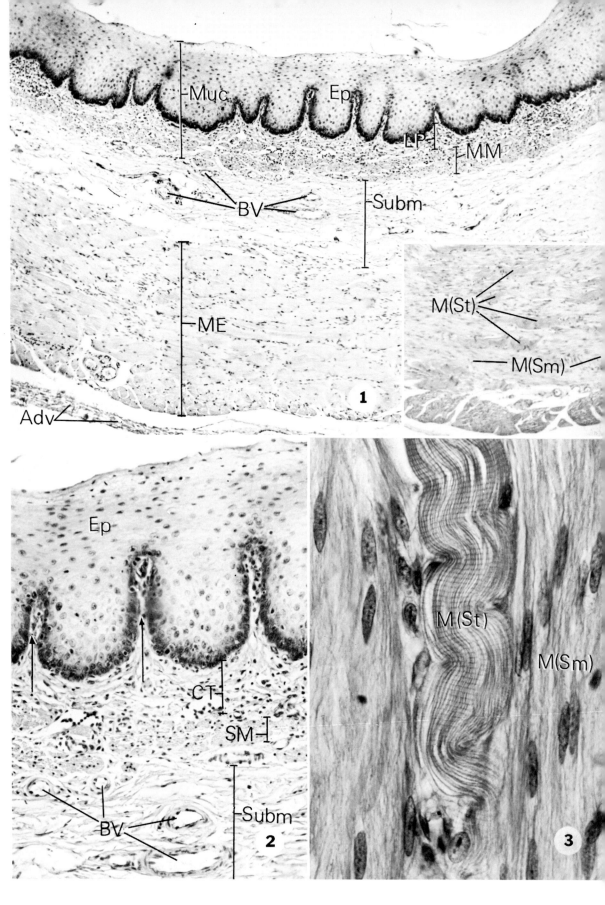

1 — Muc — Ep — LP — MM — Subm — BV — ME — Adv — M(St) — M(Sm)

2 — Ep — CT — SM — Subm — BV

3 — M(St) — M(Sm)

PLATE 10-7

Plate 10-8. ESOPHAGUS AND STOMACH, CARDIAC REGION

The surface of the stomach contains numerous and relatively deep depressions called *gastric pits* (**P**) or *foveolae*. Glands open into the bottom of the pits. The glands that are in the immediate vicinity of the cardiac orifice are called *cardiac glands*. (The entire gastric mucosa contains glands. These are of three types: fundic glands, cardiac glands, and pyloric glands. The location of cardiac glands has already been mentioned; pyloric glands are in the pyloric region; fundic glands are throughout the remainder of the stomach.)

The junction between the esophagus and the stomach is abrupt (Fig. 1). In the esophagus the epithelium (**Ep**) of the mucosa is stratified squamous and rests on a lamina propria that contains numerous papillae (**arrows**). In the stomach, the mucosa contains a surface of columnar epithelium (**Ep**) and numerous tubular glands (**Gl**) in addition to a highly cellular lamina propria (**LP**) (Fig. 2). Just beyond the junction in Figure 1, the gastric mucosa is folded and the glands are cut in cross section. At the actual junction, however, the glands are cut along a longitudinal axis. This region (**rectangle**) is examined at higher magnification in Figure 2.

The epithelium of the gastric surface and pits is columnar. However, it is a special type of epithelium in that each cell produces mucus. In other places where mucus is secreted onto a surface it is produced by goblet cells which share the surface with other cell types, or by mucous glands that are more deeply situated, or by a combination of these two arrangements. In the stomach, the cytoplasm of each surface and pit cell (Figs. 2 and 3) contains a mucous cup distal to the nucleus, so that the entire surface epithelium, and that of the pits, forms a mucous sheet comprised of *mucous surface cells* (**MSC**). The nucleus of each mucous surface cell is surrounded by non-mucous cytoplasmic material. In contrast, the nuclei of mucous gland cells (see below) appear to be in direct contact with the mucus.

The fundus of the gland (part furthest removed from the opening) also contains mucous cells (**MGC**) (Fig. 4), which discharge their product via a duct (**D**). The mucus appears to fill the entire cytoplasmic part of the cell, and the nucleus is pushed to the basal

KEY

AT, adipose tissue
D, duct
Ep, epithelium
Gl, glands
LN, lymph nodule
LP, lamina propria
MGC, mucous gland cells
MM, muscularis mucosae
MSC, mucous surface cells
P, gastric pits (foveolae)
arrowheads, chief cells of fundic glands
arrows, connective tissue papillae

Fig. 1 (monkey), x 40; Fig. 2 (monkey), x 160; Fig. 3 (monkey), x 640; Fig. 4 (monkey), x 640.

part, seemingly in direct contact with the mucous component of the cytoplasm. The mucus containing part of the cell appears clear because its content is lost during preparation of routine H & E sections. Cardiac glands are not very extensive; consequently, fundic glands are often included in specimens of the stomach cardia as they are in Figure 1. The **arrowheads** indicate where the darkly staining chief cells of fundic glands can be seen.

The round cells at the bottom of Figure 2, in the vicinity of the muscularis mucosae (**MM**), are mostly lymphocytes from the periphery of a lymph nodule (**LN**) that is just inside the stomach (Fig. 1). The light network in the submucosa is adipose tissue (**AT**).

Cardiac glands are easy to confuse with pyloric glands. For a consideration of this problem, see page 162.

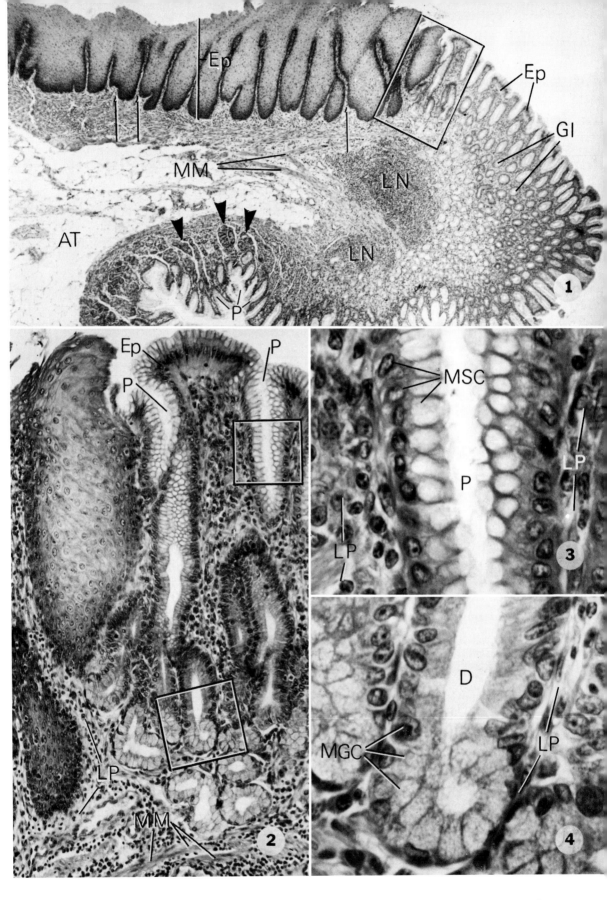

PLATE 10-8

Plate 10-9. STOMACH, FUNDIC REGION

The entire thickness of the stomach wall is shown in Figure 1. This is from the *fundic region* and is typical of the stomach except for the cardiac and pyloric regions. The *mucosa* (**Muc**), *submucosa* (**Subm**), *muscularis externa* (**ME**), and *serosa* (**S**) are indicated. The inner surface of the stomach is divided into areas that are designated mamillated areas. These areas are separated from neighboring mamillated areas by grooves (**asterisks**).

The surface of the gastric mucosa, including that of the *gastric pits* (**P**), is lined by a continuous sheet of mucous surface cells (Fig. 2). The *fundic glands* (**Gl**) extend from the bottom of the pits to the muscularis mucosae (**MM**). They are relatively straight tubular glands, except in the deep part of the mucosa where they become coiled. The glands are so numerous that they appear to make up almost the entire mucosa. In the mid-region of the mucosa the glands are tightly packed and the lamina propria (**LP**) appears as thin cellular strands that are squeezed between the glands. The lamina propria is more conspicuous under the surface and pit epithelium, and in the vicinity of the muscularis mucosae.

Several kinds of cells are present in the fundic glands. In the deep part of the gland (Fig. 3), the main cell type is the *chief cell* (**CC**). The nuclei of chief cells are characteristically in the basal part of the cell and surrounded by cytoplasm that stains with hematoxylin. Chief cells synthesize digestive enzymes. *Parietal cells* (**PC**) are also present in fundic glands. Their cytoplasm stains intensely with eosin. They are located among the chief cells, but are usually recessed from the lumen. Near the mid-portion of the gland the parietal cells become more numerous and their presence in larger numbers accounts for the marked eosin staining of this region. Parietal cells secrete hydrochloric acid. *Mucous neck cells* are near the opening of the glands into the pits. They are located between the parietal cells. These cells produce a mucous material that differs from that which is produced by the surface cells. *Argentaffin cells* are also present in the gastric glands, but special methods are required for their demonstration. Those argentaffin cells that fluoresce under UV light also exhibit a chromaffin reaction; these cells contain serotonin. Other

histochemically demonstrable cells, presumably within the argentaffin group, include specific cell types that secrete glucagon as well as those that secrete gastrin. Cytological differences among these various endocrine-secreting cells are more readily recognized in the electron microscope.

The submucosa consists of relatively dense connective tissue (Fig. 1). The muscularis externa (**ME**) is comprised of smooth muscle. It is described as being disposed into three layers: an inner oblique, a middle circular, and an outer longitudinal. However, these are difficult to discern. The serosa (**S**) consists of a layer of *mesothelium* resting on a small amount of connective tissue. A lymphatic vessel (**LV**) is in the serosa. The stomach wall contains nerve cells (**Gan C**) that are arranged in the same manner as in the intestinal canal (see page 170).

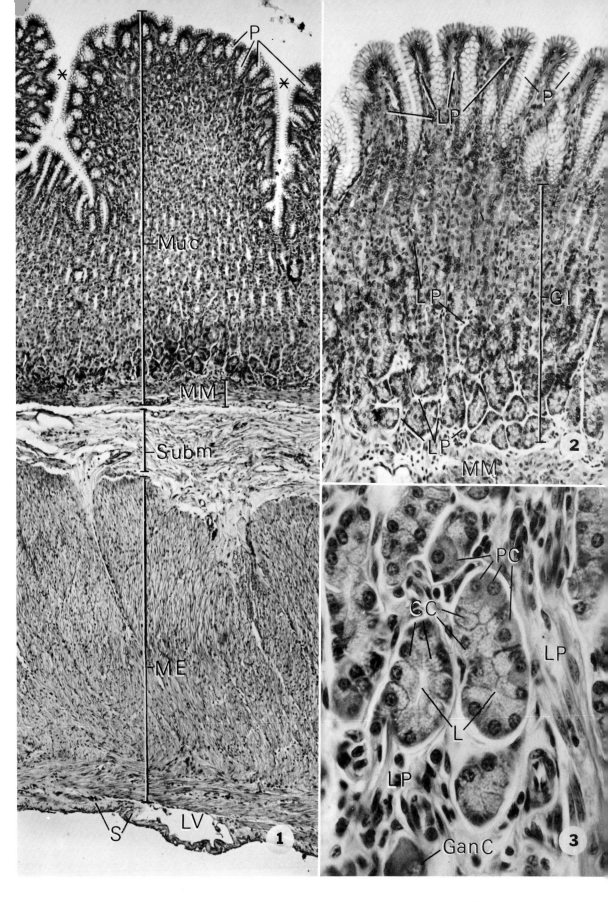

P

*

*

P

LP

P

Muc

LP

Gl

MM

LP

Subm

LP

MM

PC

CC

LP

ME

L

LP

S

LV

1

GanC

3

PLATE 10-9

Plate 10-10. STOMACH, PYLORIC REGION

The part of the stomach leading to the duodenum is called the *pyloric region*. The glands (**Gl**) in this region are shown in Figure 1. They are rather straight, and it is sometimes difficult to determine where the pits end and the glands begin. Glands are shown opening into gastric pits (**arrows**) in the upper part of Figure 1.

The fundic region of the pyloric glands (part farthest from the opening) is coiled and may appear oval or spherical when sectioned, even if the remainder of the gland has been cut longitudinally. Between the glands is the cellular lamina propria (**LP**). The deepest part of the mucosa is the muscularis mucosae (**MM**). Under this is the submucosa in which an artery (**A**) and vein (**V**) can be seen. The smooth muscle cells of the muscularis externa (**ME**) have been cut in cross section.

The **upper rectangle** of Figure 1 is examined at higher magnification in Figure 2. As was stated earlier (page 158), the columnar cells (**Ep**) that line the surface and pits of the stomach possess a mucous cup (**MC**) distal to the nucleus (**N**). The nucleus is surrounded by nonmucous cytoplasmic material (**BC**), and collectively the cells form a mucous sheet. A lymphocyte (**L**) has wandered into the epithelial layer from the lamina propria (**LP**).

The area within the **lower rectangle** is illustrated at higher magnification in Figure 3 and shows the fundic region of the pyloric glands. One gland has been cut in cross section (**asterisk**). The cells are polarized in the manner typical of cells that secrete onto a surface or into a lumen; that is, the nuclei are in the basal part of the cell, away from the lumen. These are *mucous gland cells*. They differ in appearance from the *mucous surface cells* in that the nuclei (of mucous gland cells) appear to be in direct contact with mucous material of the cytoplasm.

Pyloric and cardiac glands can be readily distinguished from fundic glands because fundic glands possess different cell types (chief and parietal) that are conspicuous in routine H & E sections. However, pyloric glands are difficult to distinguish from cardiac glands. Several pointers may be of assistance in distinguishing between these two. Obviously, if part of the esophagus is included in the specimen, the gastric component in its immediate

KEY

A, artery
BC, basal cytoplasm of mucous surface cells
Ep, epithelium
Gl, pyloric glands
L, lymphocyte
LP, lamina propria
MC, mucous cup
ME, muscularis externa
MM, muscularis mucosae
N, nuclei of mucous surface cells
V, vein
arrows, gastric pits

Fig. 1 (human), x 160; Figs. 2 and 3 (human), x 640.

vicinity is the cardiac region; if part of the duodenum is included in the specimen, the gastric component is the pyloric region. To some extent, distinguishing between pyloric and cardiac glands is based on familiarity and intangible impressions. The pyloric pits are usually described as being deeper than the cardiac pits; however, this difference may not always be evident. An additional feature that may be of use is: the cardiac glands appear to be more coiled and dilated in their fundic regions, whereas the pyloric glands appear to be less coiled and less dilated.

Although not specifically identifiable in routine H & E sections, argentaffin cells are also present among the epithelial cells of the pyloric mucosa. As was already noted, there are several types of argentaffin cells, and one of these, in the pyloric mucosa, has been shown to produce the hormone gastrin.

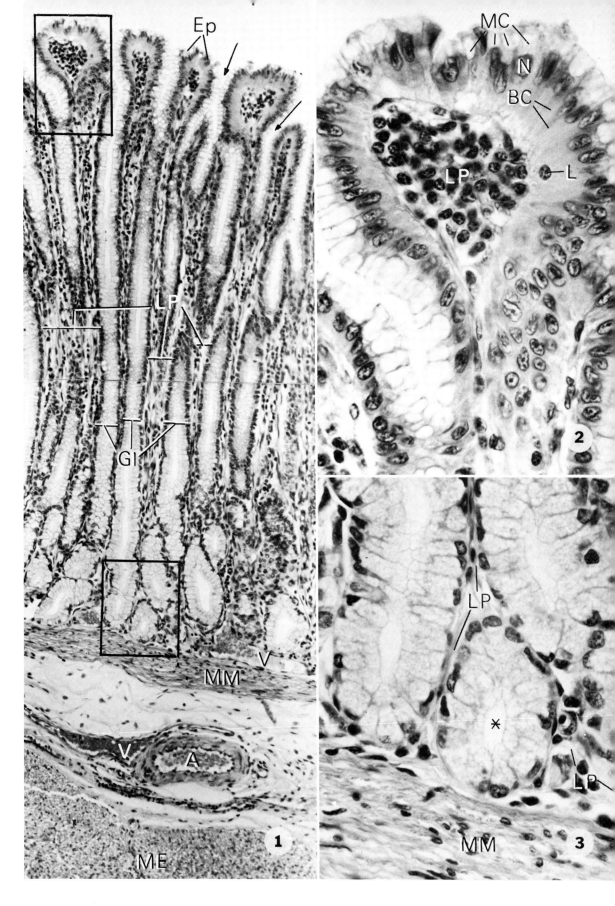

PLATE 10-10

DIGESTIVE SYSTEM

Plate 10-11. SMALL INTESTINE

The small intestine is a tube, about 20 feet long in man. It extends from the stomach to the large intestine and is divided into three parts: *duodenum, jejunum,* and *ileum.* There is, however, no sharp dividing line between these three regions. The duodenum can be distinguished from the jejunum and ileum because it contains glands in the submucosa. (They may not be present in the distal part of the duodenum.) The jejunum and ileum are not distinguished by any clear cut differences, but rather by relative differences.

The inner surface of the small intestine contains permanent circular folds (*plicae circulares, valvulae conniventes, valves of Kerckring*), which form ridges most of which are roughly at right angles to the long axis of the tube. Therefore, in a longitudinal section of the intestine (Fig. 1), these folds appear as a series of regular elevations (**PC**). However, some of these ridges branch and may travel in longitudinal directions for short distances; therefore, even in cross sections (Fig. 2) the plicae may resemble those that are seen in longitudinal sections. The plicae circulares begin in the duodenum; they are tallest and most numerous in the jejunum (Fig. 1) and become shorter and less numerous in the ileum.

Isolated nodules of lymphoid tissue are located in the proximal end of the intestinal canal. More distally they appear in increasingly larger aggregates, so that in the ileum (Fig. 2) aggregates of lymph nodules (**LN**), called *Peyer's patches,* are regularly found. These nodules are located opposite the mesenteric attachment. Note the interruption in the muscular layer (**arrowhead**) where blood vessels are traveling between the mesentery (**M**) and the submucosa.

Figure 3 shows an area comparable to that within the **rectangle** in Figure 1. It is, however, a cross section through the intestinal wall and shows a longitudinally oriented plica. In routine H & E sections the four layers of the intestinal wall are distinguished as follows: The *mucosa* (**Muc**) appears dark because of the large numbers of epithelial cells and the numerous cells in the lamina propria. It contains both *villi* (**V**) and *intestinal glands* (**IG**). The glands are also called *crypts of Lieberkühn.*

The submucosa (**Subm**) is the light-staining layer under the mucosa. It forms the core of the plica and contains large blood vessels (**BV**). The muscularis externa (**ME**) is external to the submucosa; it is disposed into two distinct layers: an inner circular and an outer longitudinal layer. The serosa (**S**) is the light-staining region external to the muscularis externa. Where the intestine has no serosa (visceral peritoneum), the layer external to the muscularis externa would be referred to as the adventitia. The duodenum is adherent to the posterior abdominal wall and therefore, much of the duodenal wall has an adventitia rather than a serosa.

The area within the **rectangle** in Figure 2 is examined at higher magnification in Figure 1 of Plate 10-14; a region comparable to that within the **large rectangle** (Fig. 3) is examined in Plate 10-12; a region comparable to the **small rectangle** (Fig. 3) is examined in Figure 3 of Plate 10-14.

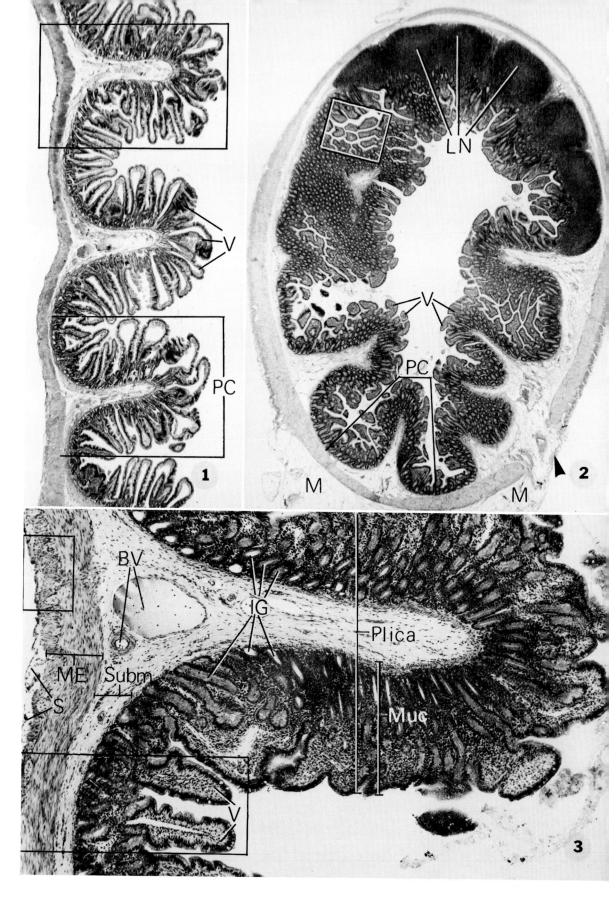

PLATE 10-11

Plate 10-12. DUODENUM

The *duodenum* is the shortest part of the small intestine, measuring about 10 to 12 inches in man. It is adherent to the posterior abdominal wall in the human and, therefore, nonmobile; it receives the secretions and other contents from the stomach, pancreas, liver, and gall bladder; and it contains glands in the submucosa.

Figure 1 shows a segment of the duodenal wall that is comparable to the **large rectangle** in Figure 3 of the preceding plate, i.e., a plica circulares is not included. The mucosa, submucosa (**Subm**) and muscularis externa (**ME**) are shown. The serosa (or adventitia) has been broken away. The mucosa occupies the upper part of the field. The villi project above the surface into the lumen of the duodenum; the glands "dip" into the supporting connective tissue. The **broken line** indicates the boundary between the villi and the glands.

Three kinds of cells are present on the surface of the villi (Fig. 2): columnar *absorptive cells* (**Ep**), *goblet cells* (**GC**), and argentaffin cells. The nuclei of the absorptive cells are elongate and located at the basal region of the cells. The absorptive cells of the small intestine possess a *striated border* (see Plate 10-13). The spherical nuclei (**arrows**) belong to lymphocytes which have migrated into the epithelial layer. The arrows point to cells which are clearly removed from the basement membrane. Argentaffin cells are in contact with the basement membrane, and as mentioned previously, argentaffin cells require special stains for their demonstration.

The lamina propria (**LP**) makes up the core of the villus. It contains large numbers of round cells. Most of these are lymphocytes. Plasma cells, eosinophils and macrophages are also present in smaller numbers. All of these cells are supported by a delicate stroma of reticular fibers (and cells) which resemble somewhat the stroma of lymphatic tissue. The lamina propria of the villus also contains smooth muscle cells (**SM**). Contraction of these cells accounts, in part, for the variation in height of neighboring villi. Villi also contain lacteals and blood vessels, but they are not evident in Figures 1 and 2.

The fundic regions of the intestinal glands (*crypts of Lieberkühn*) are shown in the upper part of Figure 3. These glands (**IG**) are rela-

KEY

BG, Brunner's glands
BV, blood vessels
D, duct
Ep, epithelium
GC, goblet cells
IG, intestinal glands
LP, lamina propria
ME, muscularis externa
MM, muscularis mucosae
SM, smooth muscle
Subm, submucosa
arrows, nuclei of lymphocytes
broken line, boundary between villi and glands

Fig. 1 (dog), x 65; Figs. 2 and 3 (dog), x 160.

tively straight. Note the highly cellular nature of the lamina propria (**LP**) which surrounds the glands. A more complete consideration of villi and intestinal glands can be found on pages 168 and 170.

The submucosa consists of irregular connective tissue. It differs from submucosa of other parts of the small intestine because it contains glands (Fig. 3), called *Brunner's glands* (**BG**). These are branched tubular or branched tubulo-alveolar glands whose secretory components consist of columnar epithelium. A duct (**D**) through which these glands open into the lumen of the duodenum is shown (Figs. 1 and 3) penetrating the *muscularis mucosae* (**MM**).

The two layers of the *muscularis externa* (**ME**) are shown in Figure 1. The inner circular layer is cut in cross section; the outer longitudinal layer is cut longitudinally. (Therefore, this is a longitudinal cut through the duodenum.)

The pancreatic duct and common bile duct enter the duodenum via a common opening called the *ampulla of Vater* (not shown). In some individuals there is an accessory pancreatic duct which also opens into the duodenum.

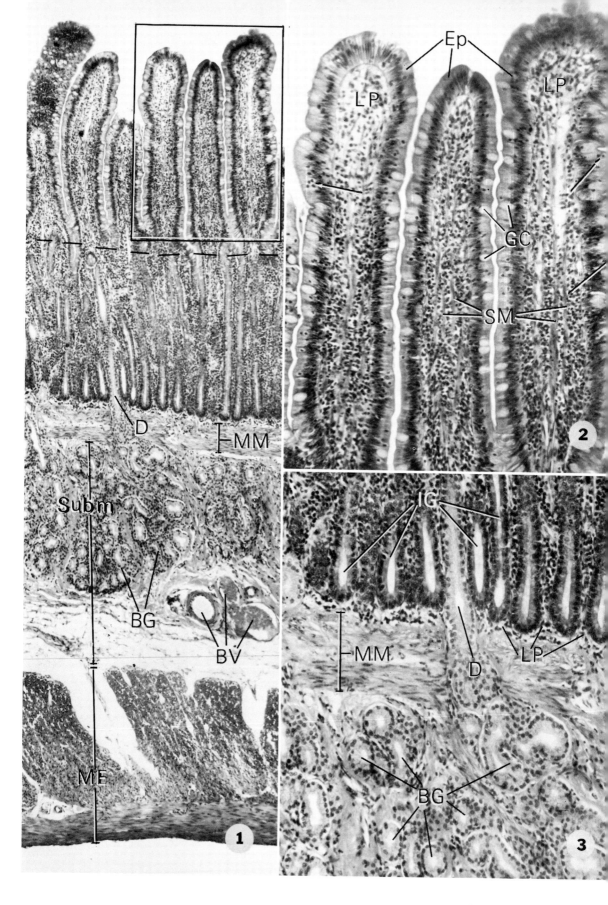

PLATE 10-12

Plate 10-13. VILLI

Villi are found only in the small intestine. They are fingerlike projections into the lumen, and are one of the modifications of the small intestine which serve to increase the amount of surface that is available for absorptive activity.

Whereas the plicae circulares have submucosa as their central core, the villi are mucosal projections (Fig. 1) and have lamina propria (**LP**) as their central core. The surface of the villus consists of columnar absorptive cells (**Ep**), goblet cells (**GC**) and argentaffine cells. Each villus contains a centrally located lacteal (**L**). This is a lymphatic capillary which begins in the villus. In this specimen, the lacteals are widely dilated. In addition to the lacteal, the lamina propria contains small blood vessels and smooth muscle cells.

The lacteals (**L**) are lined by extremely flat endothelial cells (Fig. 2). The nuclei of these cells appear as the elongated, dark-staining profiles [**E(N)**] directly at the surface. At each nuclear extremity, one can see the attenuated cytoplasm [**E(C)**] which constitutes most of the wall of the lacteal. The other elongated nucleus [**SM(N)**], close to the surface, does not belong to an endothelial cell since its cytoplasm [**SM(C)**] does not occupy a surface location. Its location and shape, in comparison to the other cells of the lamina propria, indicate that it is a smooth muscle cell. Nuclei of *plasma cells* (**PC**) can be seen. Other cells are difficult to identify, although some of those with pale staining nuclei are likely to be comparable to the reticular cells found in the stroma of lymphatic tissue.

The columnar absorptive cells contain a striated border (**SB**). Electron micrographs indicate that the striated border is due to the presence of closely packed, straight *microvilli* all of which are about the same height (see Plate 1-5). The cells rest on a basement membrane, which is not usually seen in H & E preparations. The cells are somewhat separated near the basement membrane and this enables one to identify the cell boundaries. However, the cell boundaries are also evident (**arrows**) near the surface where the cells are not separated. The nuclei of the absorptive cells all have essentially the same shape, orientation, and staining characteristics, and even if the cytoplasmic boundaries were not

KEY

E(C), cytoplasm of endothelial cell
E(N), nucleus of endothelial cell
Ep, epithelium
GC, goblet cells
L, lacteal
LP, lamina propria
Lym, lymphocytes
PC, plasma cells
SB, striated border
SM(C), smooth muscle cytoplasm
SM(N), smooth muscle nucleus
arrowheads, nuclei of goblet cell
arrows, boundaries of epithelial cells

Fig. 1 (monkey), x 160; Fig. 2 (monkey), x 640.

evident, the nuclei would be an indication of the shape and orientation of the cells.

A number of cells with round nuclei are scattered throughout different levels of the epithelial layer. Those which are close to and possibly in contact with the basement membrane may belong to argentaffine cells (or to lymphocytes). Other cells which are clearly removed from the basement membrane are lymphocytes (**Lym**). The remaining nuclei (**arrowheads**) belong to goblet cells (**GC**), which are located at different levels of the epithelial layer. The nucleus of the goblet cell is typically just basal to the mucous cup. The mucous cup of the goblet cells shows some pale staining material. Most, if not all, of the mucus is lost during preparation of routine sections. If mucus is retained, it stains intensely.

It should be noted that villi may differ in appearance according to plane of section, cellularity of lamina propria, degree of lacteal dilatation, etc.

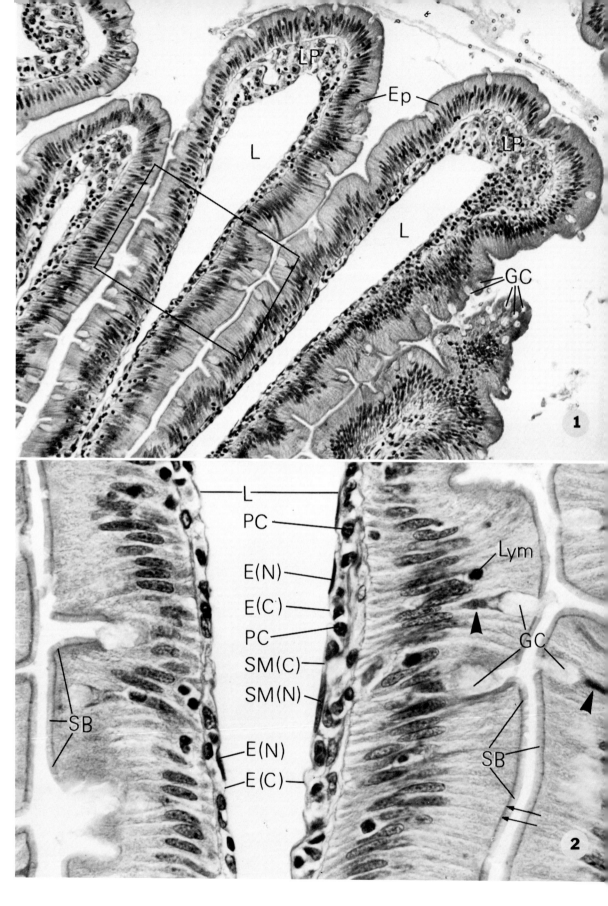

LP

Ep

L

LP

L

GC

1

L

PC

E(N)

E(C)

PC

SM(C)

SM(N)

Lym

GC

SB

E(N)

E(C)

SB

2

PLATE 10-13

Plate 10-14. INTESTINAL GLANDS AND MUSCULARIS EXTERNA

Figure 1 is a higher magnification of the area within the **rectangle** of Figure 2, Plate 10-11. *Villi* (**V**) and intestinal glands (**IG**) are shown; both have been cut in cross section. Since villi are finger-like projections into the lumen, they appear as islands of tissue surrounded by a space, the intestinal lumen. Each island has a central core of connective tissue, the lamina propria (**LP**), and an epithelial surface (**Ep**). Goblet cells (**GC**) appear as the light oval or spherical profiles in the epithelial layer. A lacteal (**L**) is evident in one of the villi.

The glands are invaginations into the underlying connective tissue. Because they are cut in cross section they exhibit a central lumen bounded by columnar cells. The glands are surrounded by the numerous connective tissue cells of the lamina propria. Since the intestinal glands are essentially straight tubular glands, they present similar profiles in any given plane of section.

The deeper regions of two intestinal glands are shown at greater magnification in Figure 2. As indicated above, each is surrounded by the cellular connective tissue (diffuse lymphatic tissue) that constitutes the lamina propria (**LP**) and each has a central lumen (**asterisk**). Examination of the gland cells shows that the cytoplasm contains large (eosinophilic) granules. The cells which contain these granules are called *Paneth cells* (**PC**). Originally it was thought that these granules are typical secretory granules, possibly containing intestinal enzymes. More recent data shows that the granules contain lysosomal enzymes and that the Paneth cells may have an antimicrobial function. The epithelium of the intestinal glands also contains *argentaffin cells.*

The muscularis externa and serosa (**S**) are illustrated in Figure 3. This region is comparable to the **small rectangle** in Figure 3, Plate 10-11. The inner circular layer [**SM(C)**] and the outer longitudinal layer [**SM(L)**] are separated by a parasympathetic ganglion. This is part of *Auerbach's plexus.* Several *ganglion cells* (**Gan C**) with large spherical nuclei are evident. Parasympathetic ganglion cells are also present in the submucosa as components of *Meissner's plexus.* However, these are less numerous, and therefore more difficult to find.

KEY

Ep, epithelium
GC, goblet cells
Gan C, ganglion cells
IG, intestinal glands
L, lacteal
LP, lamina propria
M, mesothelium
PC, Paneth cells
S, serosa
SM(C), circular layer of smooth muscle
SM(L), longitudinal layer of smooth muscle
V, villi
asterisk, lumen of intestinal glands

Fig. 1 (monkey) x 160; Fig. 2 (human), x 640; Fig. 3 (monkey) x 640.

The serosa (**S**) consists of simple squamous epithelium, mesothelium (**M**), which rests on delicate fibrous connective tissue.

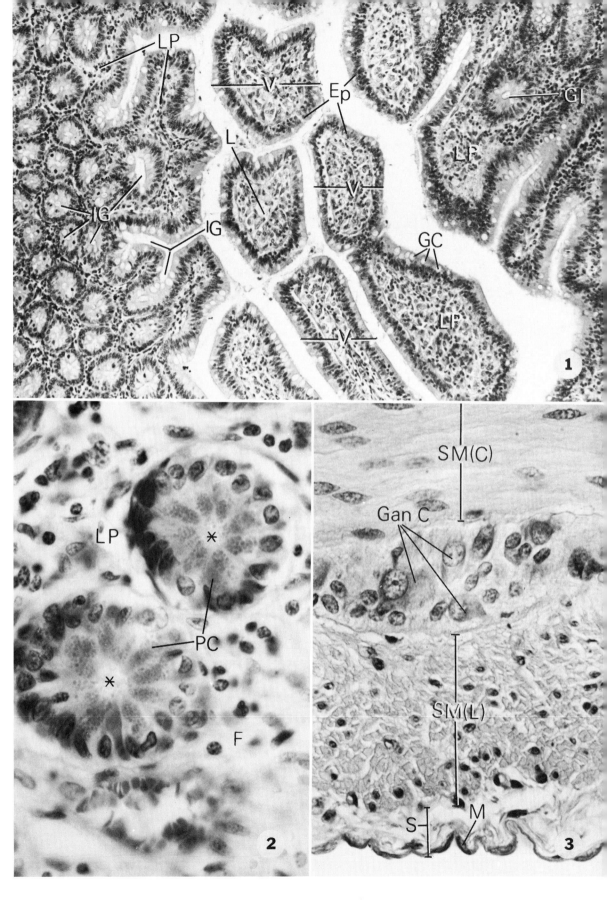

PLATE 10-14

Plate 10-15. APPENDIX AND LARGE INTESTINE

Appendix. The appendix is a finger-like process that is suspended from the cecum. Its wall is characterized by the presence of large numbers of lymphocytes which are organized as nodules. These are chiefly in the submucosa, but may extend into the mucosa. The appendix has no villi or plicae circulares.

The wall of the appendix is illustrated in Figure 1. The *lumen* (**L**), *mucosa* (**Muc**), *submucosa* (**Subm**), *muscularis externa* (**ME**) and *serosa* (**S**) are shown. The mucosa contains straight tubular glands (**Gl**) which extend as far as the muscularis mucosae (**MM**) (Fig. 2), and are surrounded by a highly cellular lamina propria (**LP**). Most of the cells of the lamina propria are lymphocytes; however, other cells characteristic of lymphoid tissue are also present. Lymphocytes (**Lym**) may be so numerous in the mucosa and submucosa that they obscure the muscularis mucosae. The glands *(crypts of Lieberkühn)* contain large numbers of goblet cells, and in their fundic region may contain *Paneth cells* and *argentaffin cells.*

The submucosa (**Subm**) consists of a rather dense irregular connective tissue. Some adipose tissue (**AT**) and two aggregations of lymphocytes (**Lym**) are shown in Figure 1. Although the fibrous nature of the submucosa is readily evident in Figure 1, in other specimens the amount of lymphatic tissue may be sufficiently great to obscure the fibrous material.

The muscularis externa (**ME**) is comprised of an inner circular layer and an outer longitudinal layer of smooth muscle. External to the muscularis externa is the serosa (**S**).

Large intestine. The wall of the large intestine (colon) contains the same layers that are found in the stomach and small intestine. However, the large intestine has no villi or plicae circulares. The mucosa (**Muc**) contains straight tubular glands (crypts of Lieberkühn) that extend throughout the entire thickness as far as the muscularis mucosae (see Plate 10-16). The glands, as in the appendix, contain large numbers of goblet cells. Argentaffin cells are present, however, Paneth cells are rarely found.

The submucosa (**Subm**) consists of a rather dense irregular connective tissue. Adipose tissue (**AT**) and blood vessels can be seen in

KEY

AP, Auerbach's plexus
AT, adipose tissue
Gl, glands
L, lumen
LP, lamina propria
LV, lymphatic vessel
Lym, lymphocytes
ME, muscularis externa
MM, muscularis mucosae
Muc, mucosa
S, serosa
SM(C), circular layer of smooth muscle
SM(L), longitudinal layer of smooth muscle
Subm, submucosa

Fig. 1 (human), x 40; Fig. 2 (human), x 160; Fig. 3 (monkey), x 65.

this layer. The muscularis externa (**ME**) consists of an inner circular layer [**SM**(C)] and an outer longitudinal layer [**SM**(L)]. The smooth muscle cells of the outer layer are grouped into three separate, longitudinal bundles (taenia coli), one of which is shown in Figure 3. The regular arrangement of muscle cells helps to distinguish the muscularis externa from the irregular arrangement of fibers that constitute the submucosa. The light areas between the two muscular layers contain components of Auerbach's plexus (**AP**).

The serosa (**S**) is similar to that of the small intestine. The space (**LV**) in the serosa is not an artifact; it is a lymphatic vessel. This cannot be established at the low magnification of Figure 3, but was determined by examination of this slide and its serial neighbors at higher magnification.

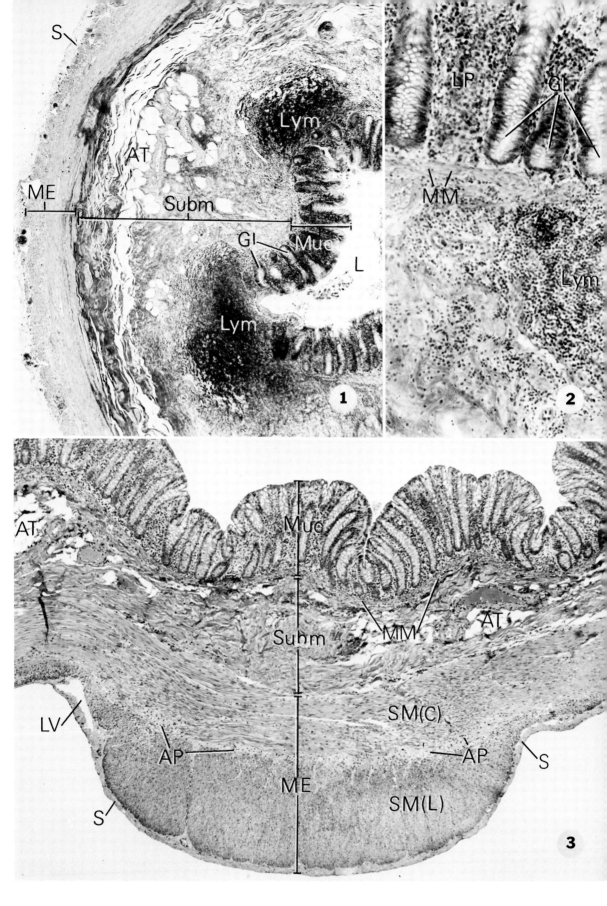

PLATE 10-15

Plate 10-16. Mucosa of Large Intestine

The mucosa (**Muc**) and part of the submucosa of the large intestine are shown in Figure 1. The junction between the two is indicated by the muscularis mucosae (**MM**). A large number of lymphocytes are in the submucosa of this specimen. They are so numerous that at one point (**asterisk**) they obscure the muscularis mucosae and become continuous with the diffuse lymphoid tissue which constitutes the lamina propria (**LP**) of the mucosa. These lymphocytes are at the periphery of a lymph nodule.

The mucosa of the large intestine contains straight tubular glands (crypts of Lieberkühn). These extend as far as the muscularis mucosae. When a gland is cut longitudinally (**arrow**) it appears as an invagination of the surface epithelium (**EP**). When the glands are cut in cross section (Fig. 2) they present circular profiles with a central lumen.

The glands of the large intestine can be readily recognized because their lumens are invariably patent, as is evident in Figures 1, 2, and 3.

The cross-sectioned glands in Figure 2 are surrounded by the highly cellular lamina propria (**LP**). Immediately surrounding the glands are elongated, flattened nuclei (**arrowheads**). Cytoplasmic material can be seen extending from the extremities of these nuclei. This cytoplasm is extremely attenuated; moreover, it is very close to the base of the epithelial cells (**EP**) and it could be confused with a basement membrane if it were not related to a nucleus. Electron micrographs of cells with elongated nuclei that are related to tubular glands in this fashion indicate that they are smooth muscle.

The surface cells of the mucosa are largely columnar absorbing cells. They possess a striated border which is less prominent than that of the small intestine, but nevertheless readily seen (**arrows**) in well-prepared specimens (**inset,** Fig. 1). Goblet cells (**GC**) are very numerous within the gland. Although the epithelial cells (**Ep**) in the fundic region of the glands (Fig. 3) do not appear very different from those that are closer to the surface, they are regarded as being less differentiated. They give rise to new cells which will migrate to the surface to replace those cells that are constantly being desquamated.

KEY

Ep, epithelium
GC, goblet cells
LP, lamina propria
MM, muscularis mucosae
Muc, mucosa
arrow, longitudinally cut intestinal gland
arrowheads, nuclei of peritubular smooth muscle cells
arrows (inset), striated border
asterisk, numerous lymphocytes obscuring the muscularis mucosae

Fig. 1 (human), x 160; Fig. 2 and 3 (monkey), x 640.

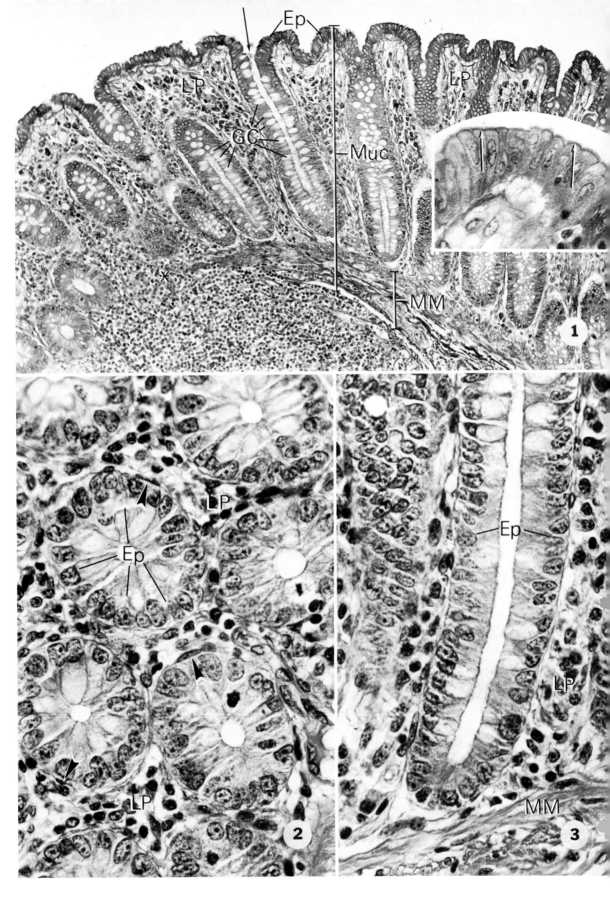

PLATE 10-16

Plate 10-17. LIVER I

The liver consists of large numbers of functional units called *lobules*. These are roughly cylindrical in shape with a venous channel, the *central vein*, traveling through the long axis. Irregular interconnecting sheets or plate-like arrangements of hepatic cells radiate outward from the central vein and constitute the parenchyma. Sinusoidal capillaries (*sinusoids*) separate the sheets of hepatic cells and empty into the central veins. In the human, the lobules are poorly delineated from their neighbors, and it is often difficult to determine where one lobule ends and the next begins.

In a low-power view of a liver section (Fig. 1), large numbers of hepatic cells appear to be uniformly disposed throughout the whole specimen. The plates of hepatic cells are one cell thick, but when sectioned, appear as interconnecting cords one or more cells thick according to the plane of section. The sinusoids appear as the light areas between the cords of cells. In addition to the sinusoids, three groups of blood vessels are present: (1) *central veins* (**CV**), (2) tributaries of hepatic veins (**HV**, Fig. 2), and (3) components of the *portal canal* (**PC**), namely, the branches of the *hepatic arteries* (**HA**) and *portal vein* (**PV**), which accompany the *hepatic ducts* (**HD**).

The central veins are larger than sinusoids. They are, in fact, the most distal radicles of the hepatic veins. Central veins travel alone, and have extremely thin walls. Several sinusoids can be seen emptying into the central veins of Figure 1 (**arrows**). Central veins empty into hepatic veins.

Figure 2 shows two hepatic veins (**HV**). The larger one is surrounded by a considerable amount of connective tissue. However, this connective tissue does not contain any other vessel of comparable size. This is a diagnostic characteristic of hepatic veins, i.e., a large vessel traveling alone. The smaller vein is surrounded by correspondingly less connective tissue.

A portal canal is examined at higher magnification in Figure 3. The hepatic artery, portal vein, and hepatic duct constitute a *portal triad*. The lumen of the portal vein (**PV**) is much larger than the lumen of the accompanying hepatic artery (**HA**), although the thickness of the walls is about the same.

KEY

CT, connective tissue
HA, branch of hepatic artery
HD, hepatic duct
HV, branch of hepatic veins
PC, portal canal
PV, branch of portal vein
arrows, sinusoids emptying into central vein
broken lines, boundary of liver lobule

Fig. 1 (human), x 65; Fig. 2 (monkey), x 65; Fig. 3 (monkey), x 160.

Both of these are readily distinguished from the hepatic duct (**HD**) which has a wall of columnar epithelium. Another portal canal is seen in Figure 1.

At this point it is well to re-examine Figure 1 in order to define the boundaries of a liver lobule. A lobule is readily identified when it is cut in cross section, and one has been delineated by the **broken lines**. The central vein, as its name implies, is centrally located. The hepatic cells and sinusoids appear to radiate outward from the central vein to the periphery of the lobule. Connective tissue and components of portal canals may be between adjacent lobules; however, very often, neighboring lobules are not separated by these structures and in these cases, the cords of hepatic cells seem to travel from one lobule to another.

The description of the liver lobule as presented above is the traditional version of liver organization. There is another interpretation of liver organization in which the portal canal is considered to be the center of the lobule. In either case, the identification of tissue elements (hepatic cells, sinusoids, "central" veins, hepatic veins and portal canals) is as given above.

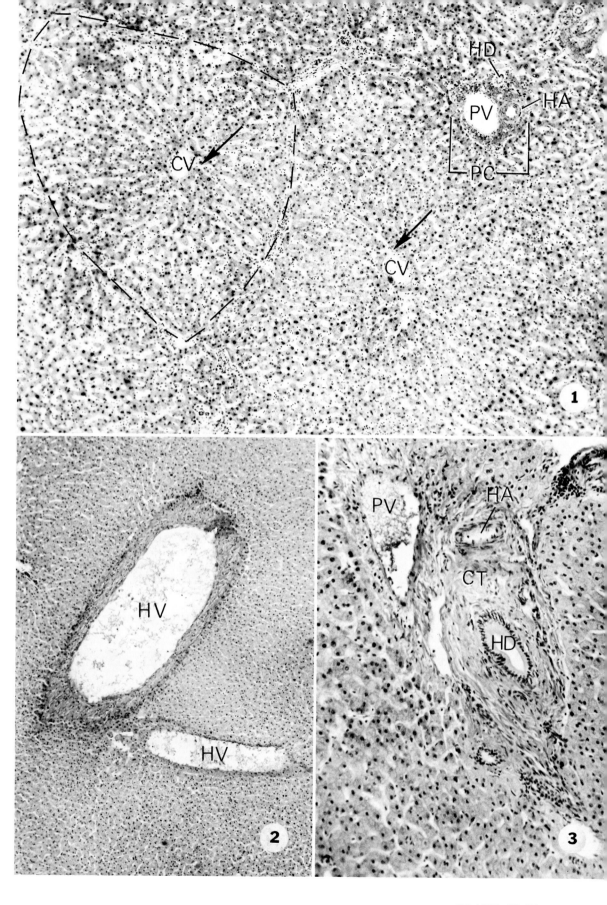

PLATE 10-17

Plate 10-18. Liver II

Hepatic cells are cuboidal cells that are arranged as interconnecting sheets one cell wide. In sections, these sheets or plates of cells appear as irregular interconnecting cords one or more cells wide according to the plane of section (Fig. 1). The nuclei of hepatic cells are characteristically large and spherical and they usually stain less intensely than the smaller nuclei of other cells in the liver. Not infrequently, two nuclei are found in the same cell (**asterisks**). The boundaries between adjacent cells are not always evident, although they can be seen in Figures 1 and 2.

The cytoplasm of hepatic cells is variable in appearance. For example, when a sufficient amount of glycogen is present in the cell, the cytoplasm has a flocculent appearance. In a fasted individual the cytoplasm is, in contrast, uniformly stained.

The area inside the rectangle in Figure 1 is shown at high magnification in Figure 2. Small, channel-like spaces called *bile canaliculi* are located between the cells. They appear as small oval structures between adjacent cells (**brackets**). Actually these are places where adjacent cell membranes are separated to form a conduit. Small hepatic ducts (**HD**) are also evident in Figures 1 and 2. They consist of cuboidal cells; the small lumen can be distinguished in Figure 2. The bile canaliculi collect bile from the hepatic cells and convey it to the hepatic ducts. The ducts enter the interlobular connective tissue where they accompany a hepatic artery and a portal vein as part of a portal triad. Whereas the hepatic artery and portal vein carry blood to the liver, the hepatic ducts carry bile away from the liver.

The sinusoids are lined by two types of cells, endothelial cells and Kupffer cells. The endothelial cells do not display the intimate cell to cell contact typical of endothelium in other blood vessels. Rather, it seems likely that small intercellular openings between endothelial cells may exist thereby providing for ready passage of plasma (but not blood cells) through the wall of the sinusoids. The Kupffer cells are phagocytic. When particulate material is injected into the bloodstream, Kupffer cells phagocytize this material and thereby remove it from the blood. Kupffer cells have irregularly shaped, often elongated

KEY

HD, hepatic duct
arrows, unstained nuclei of Kupffer cells
asterisks, binucleate cells
brackets, bile canaliculi

Fig. 1 (monkey), x 640; Fig. 2 (monkey), x 1240; Fig. 3 (rat), x 640.

nuclei and variable amounts of cytoplasm. The nuclei often appear to project into the lumen of the sinusoids. A small space, the *space of Disse*, is situated between the sinusoidal wall and the hepatic cells. This space is not usually seen in well-preserved specimens. A perisinusoidal cell capable of accumulating lipid is present within the space of Disse. This cell type is difficult to distinguish from cells which form the sinusoidal wall. In addition, with the electron microscope, occasional bundles of collagen fibers are observed in the space of Disse. These collagen fibers are regarded to be the basis for the reticulum which can be demonstrated with special silver staining procedures.

Figure 3 is an unstained section of a liver from an animal that was injected with trypan blue. The trypan blue was phagocytized by the Kupffer cells and can be seen as it fills the cytoplasm and partly surrounds the clear, unstained nuclei (**arrows**).

The blood of the portal vein comes from the alimentary canal, pancreas, and spleen; by this arrangement materials that are absorbed from the alimentary canal can be acted on by the liver before they enter the systemic circulation. The liver not only modifies and removes portal blood constituents, but it also participates in maintaining certain blood components of the systemic circulation at appropriate levels. Branches of the portal vein and hepatic artery both open into the sinusoids. Blood then enters the central veins and leaves the liver via the hepatic veins.

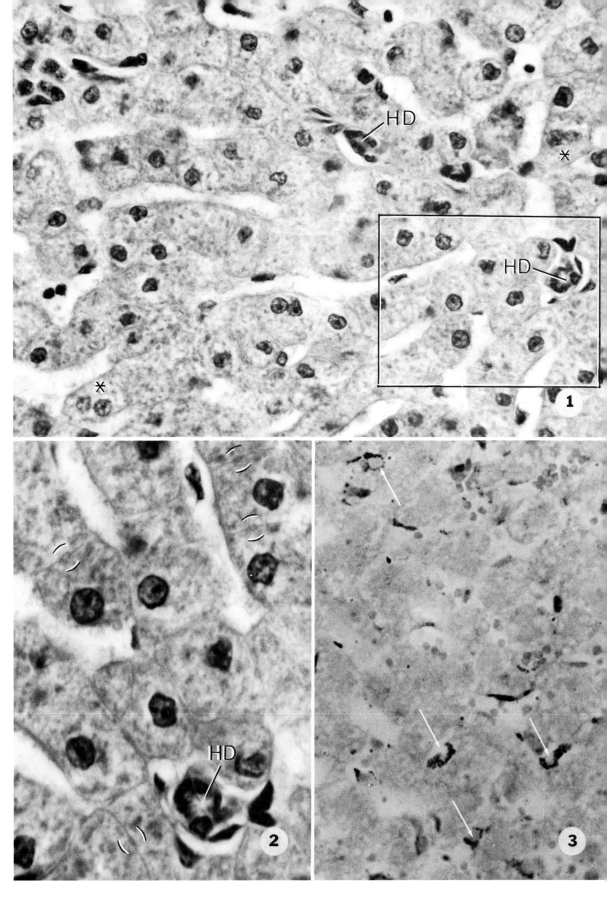

PLATE 10-18

Plate 10-19. GALL BLADDER

The gall bladder is a hollow, pear-shaped organ which concentrates and stores the bile. Its wall (Fig. 1) is comprised of a mucosa (**Muc**), *muscularis* (**Mus**), and an adventitia (**Adv**), or, on its free surface, a serosa. The mucosa (Fig. 2) consists of a simple columnar epithelium (**Ep**) resting on loose, irregular, connective tissue (**CT**); the muscularis consists of interlacing bundles of smooth muscle (**SM**); the adventitia (Fig. 1) consists of irregular connective tissue and contains a considerable amount of adipose tissue (**AT**) and blood vessels (**BV**).

The mucosa is thrown into numerous folds when the muscularis is contracted. This is the usual histological appearance of the gall bladder unless, of course, steps are taken to fix and preserve it in the distended state. Occasionally the section cuts through a recess in a fold and the recess may then resemble a gland (**X**). The mucosa however does not possess glands except in the neck.

The epithelial lining (**Ep**) of the gall bladder consists of absorptive cells. They have certain characteristics which may assist the student in identifying the gall bladder and distinguishing it from other organs. Only one cell type is present in the epithelial layer (Fig. 3). These are tall columnar cells; the nuclei are in the basal portion of the cell. The cells possess a delicate *striated border* (**arrows**). However, this is not always evident in routine H & E sections. The cytoplasm stains rather uniformly with eosin. This is related to its absorptive function and is in contrast to the staining of cells that are engaged in the production of proteinaceous material. Such cells possess basophilic material within their cytoplasm; moreover, the cytoplasm of protein-secreting cells may stain unevenly, owing to the presence of Golgi material and secretory granules.

The muscle cells can be recognized largely by their organization (Fig. 2). Note that groups of elongated nuclei are oriented in generally the same direction. In many places, the nuclei appear as slight thickenings in an eosinophilic fiber (the smooth muscle cytoplasm). This is a particularly strong diagnostic feature of smooth muscle. In this preparation the cytoplasm of the muscle cells stains a slightly

KEY

Adv, adventitia
AT, adipose tissue
BV, blood vessels
CT, connective tissue
Ep, epithelium
Muc, mucosa
Mus, muscularis
SM, smooth muscle
X, mucosal recess
arrows, striated border

Fig. 1 (monkey), x 75; Fig. 2 (monkey), x 185; Fig. 3 (monkey), x 720.

different hue from the connective tissue and further facilitates its recognition.

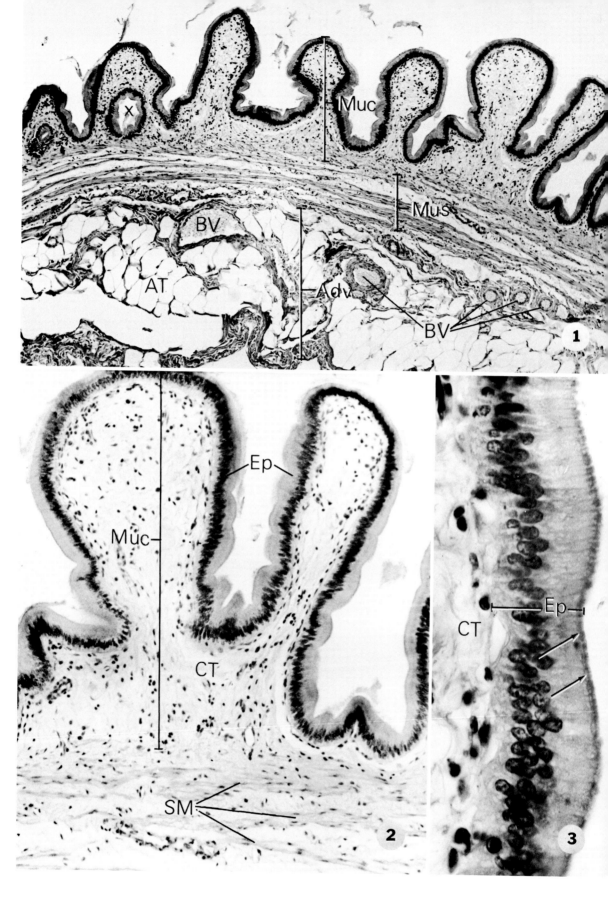

PLATE 10-19

Plate 10-20. PANCREAS

The *pancreas* is a compound tubulo-acinous gland. In addition to the exocrine component, it also contains *islets of Langerhans* which are endocrine components. A section through the pancreas is shown in Figure 1. It shows three islets of Langerhans (**IL**), a large duct (**D**), some smaller ducts (**arrows**), and, throughout most of the field, the acinous components (**A**). A ganglion cell (**arrowhead**) is in the lower left of the figure.

The acini consist of serous-type cells. Characteristically, the nuclei occupy a basal location within the cell. The cytoplasm in the basal part of the cell stains intensely with hematoxylin. The acini appear as spherical or elongated aggregates of cells. The islets of Langerhans, on the other hand, appear as larger aggregates of cells. The nuclei of the islet cells do not show any particular arrangement and the cytoplasm stains less intensely than the cytoplasm of the acinar components. Therefore, the islets usually appear as large islands of lightly stained cells among the darker acini.

The large duct (**D**) in the center of the field is surrounded by a moderately large amount of connective tissue (**CT**). It consists of columnar cells which surround a distinct lumen. The smaller ducts (**arrows**) can be recognized by the arrangement of the nuclei and the fact that the cytoplasm stains less intensely than the cytoplasm of the acinous cells. If the duct is collapsed or cut tangentially, it may simply appear as a row of nuclei.

Figure 2 shows an islet of Langerhans at higher magnification. Three types of cells can be demonstrated in special preparations, *A or alpha cells*, *B or beta cells*, and *D cells*. However, the different cell types cannot be distinguished with assurance in routine H & E sections. Insulin is produced by the beta cells; glucagon is produced by alpha cells; and gastrin is produced by D cells. In addition to the well-known A, B, and D cells, several other cell types have been described in the islets of various species. These include: EC cells (enterochromaffin cells), which secrete 5-hydroxytryptamine; D_1 cells, which are said to produce a vasoactive intestinal peptide; and possibly P and F cells, whose function is not known.

Surrounding the islets in Figure 2 are the

KEY

A, acini
CT, connective tissue
D, duct
IL, islets of Langerhans
arrowhead (Fig. 1), ganglion cell
arrowheads (Fig. 2), centro-acinous cells

Fig. 1 (monkey), x 160; Fig. 2 (monkey), x 640.

acini of the pancreas. The cells which make up the acini contain a large amount of basophilic cytoplasm. The acini also contain a small cell with pale-staining cytoplasm. These are the *centro-acinous cells* (**arrowheads**). They occupy a central position within the acinus and are the beginning of the duct. Although these cells occupy a central axial position in the acini, they frequently appear to have a peripheral position owing to the plane of section.

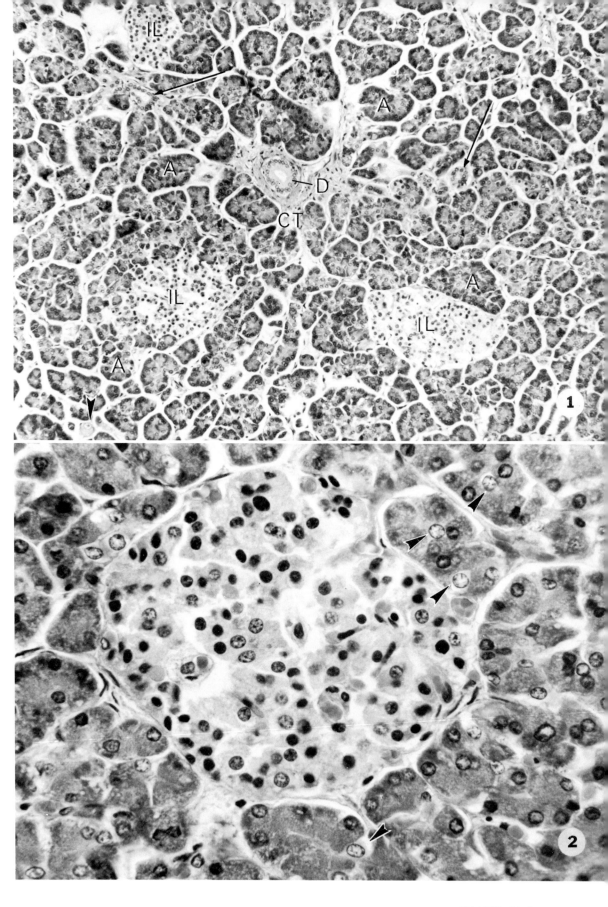

PLATE 10-20

11 RESPIRATORY SYSTEM

THE RESPIRATORY SYSTEM consists of the lungs and the respiratory passages that lead to and from the lungs. The respiratory passages include the nose (and, during forced breathing, mouth), naso- and oropharynx, larynx, trachea, and the two bronchi. Each bronchus enters a lung and continues to branch into smaller passages with increasingly thinner walls. These intrapulmonary branchings are called the bronchial tree. Blood vessels also enter the lungs with the bronchi; the blood vessels branch, and ultimately come into intimate contact with the terminal units of the bronchial tree, called the *alveoli*. This intimate relationship between pulmonary capillaries and alveolar air spaces is the structural basis for the main function of the respiratory system, namely, gas exchange within the lungs. This relationship is strikingly illustrated in the histological appearance of a lung section.

For most of its length, the respiratory passages are covered by a mucous film. This is produced by glands within the wall of the respiratory passages and by single-celled glands (*goblet cells*) within the surface epithelium. Although the mucus serves several functions, such as trapping inspired particulate matter, moistening the air, and keeping the underlying tissues moist, it must be regularly removed. For this purpose, cilia are present on the surface of most of the cells that line the respiratory passages and upper part of the bronchial tree. It should be noted that cilia extend more distally into the bronchial tree than the mucus-producing glands.

The main function of the respiratory passages is to serve as an air conduit, and the structure of the walls reflects this function. Cartilage is present within the walls of the respiratory passages and the proximal part of the bronchial tree. The cartilage is arranged so that the passageways remain patent.

Parts of the respiratory system also serve other functions. For example, the olfactory mucosa serves as a receptor for smell, and the larynx serves in phonation. In both of these, advantage is taken of the air movement that is a consequence of respiration.

Plate 11-1. Olfactory Mucosa

The *olfactory mucosa* is located in the roof and adjacent upper walls of the nasal cavity. It consists of a pseudostratified columnar epithelium which rests on a supporting connective tissue (Fig. 1).

The olfactory epithelium contains three cell types: *receptor cells, sustentacular cells,* and *basal cells.* The surface is modified by the presence of cilia and other specializations. It is not possible to identify the various cell types on the basis of cytologic characteristics in H & E preparations. However, on the basis of location of the nuclei, some estimate is possible. A "cytoplasmic zone" without nuclei immediately under the surface (Fig. 2) can be distinguished from a "nuclear zone." The nuclei of sustentacular cells (**Sus**) are located in the most superficial part of the nuclear zone, immediately adjacent to the cytoplasmic zone. The nuclei of the basal cells (**Bas**) are located in the deepest part of the nuclear zone, immediately adjacent to the connective tissue. The broadest part of the nuclear zone contains the nuclei of the receptor cells (**Rec**).

A *receptor cell* is a bipolar type of neuron which retains a surface location. It contains a distal process that extends from the perikaryon to the surface, and at the surface it possesses a bulbous expansion, called the *olfactory vesicle*. This structure contains numerous cilia. The olfactory vesicle is not always evident in H & E preparations and is not clear in Figure 2. The proximal part of the receptor cell extends toward the basal region of the olfactory layer. Here it continues as a slender axon which, along with the axons of other receptor cells, forms nonmyelinated nerve bundles (**N**) that proceed through the connective tissue, through the cribriform plate, and into the cranial cavity. The axons of the receptor cells are extremely slender and appear as dots in cross section through the nerve. Nuclei of supporting cells are also evident within the nerve bundles.

The *basal cells* have only a small amount of cytoplasm which is confined to the vicinity of the nucleus and does not reach the surface. The *sustentacular cells* extend through the entire thickness of the epithelium. These cells do not contain cilia.

The connective tissue of the olfactory mu-

cosa contains not only numerous bundles of the olfactory nerves, but also special glands called *Bowman's glands* (**Gl**). These glands contain a pigment that stains intensely with hematoxylin. Ducts from the glands carry secretions to the mucosal surface. A number of these are seen just as they are about to penetrate the epithelium. Numerous blood vessels are present in the connective tissue.

The empty vessels with a flat epithelial lining are lymphatic vessels (**Lym**). They can be distinguished from arteries (**A**) and veins (**V**) because their walls are extremely thin, and also because they contain no blood cells. Although the absence of blood cells does not justify an identification of lymphatic vessels, the absence of cells in extremely thin-walled vessels is diagnostic, especially if all of the other vessels contain blood cells.

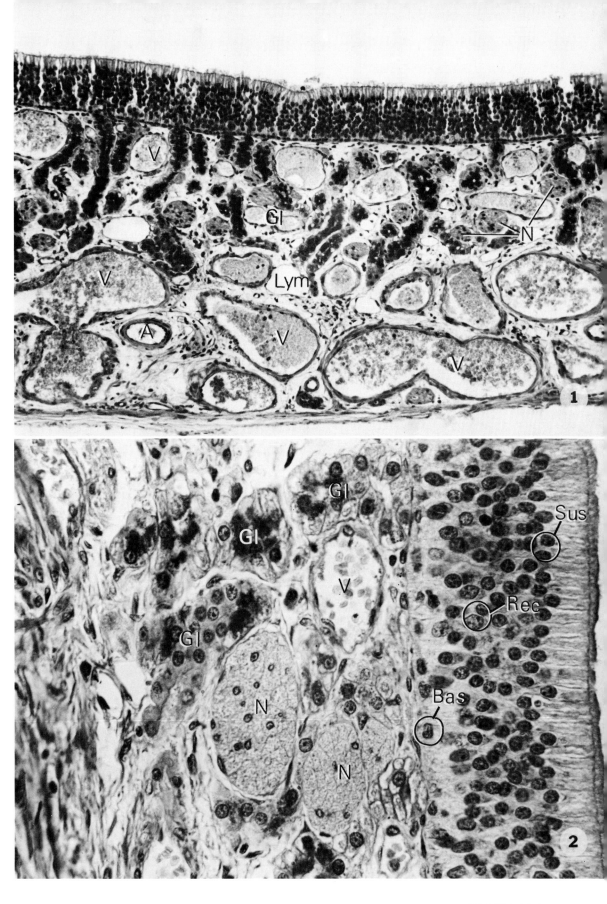

PLATE 11-1

Plate 11-2. THE LARYNX

The larynx is the part of the respiratory passage which functions in the production of sound. It consists of a cartilaginous framework to which muscles are attached and a mucosal surface which varies in character in different regions. The muscles move certain cartilages with respect to others; in doing so, they bring about a greater or lesser opening of the glottis and a greater or lesser tension on the vocal folds. In this way, vibrations of different wavelengths are generated by the passing air.

The *vocal folds* are ridge-like structures which are oriented in an anterior-posterior (ventral-dorsal) direction. In frontal sections (Fig. 1), the vocal folds (**VF**) are cross sectioned, giving the appearance seen in the illustration. The two vocal folds and the space between them constitute the *glottis*. Just above each vocal fold is an elongated recess called the *ventricle* (**V**), and above the ventricle is another ridge called the *ventricular fold* (**VnF**) (or sometimes, the false vocal fold). At the bottom of the figure are the cricoid (**CC**) and tracheal cartilages (**TC**). These cartilages are ring (cricoid) and C-shaped and appear paired in frontal sections. Examination of these at higher magnification would reveal typical lacunae separated by a matrix that stains intensely with hematoxylin, thus accounting for their dark appearance. Below and lateral to the vocal folds are the *vocalis muscles* (**VM**). At the top of Figure 1 is one of the laryngeal cartilages, the *epiglottis* (**E**), and above this, part of the tongue. The irregularly oval-shaped masses within the tongue are the *lingual tonsils* (**LT**).

A higher magnification of a vocal fold is shown in Figure 2. This figure includes the covering epithelium, the underlying connective tissue (**CT**), the vocalis muscle (**VM**), and some mucous glands (**Gl**). The connective tissue under the crest of the vocal fold contains a large amount of elastic material and is referred to as the vocal ligament (**VL**). Although the elastic material is not evident in H & E sections, the approximate location of the vocal ligament is indicated in Figure 2. The variations in the laryngeal epithelium can be seen in Figures 3 to 5. These figures are higher magnification of the three rectangles, from top to bottom, respectively, in Figure 2.

KEY

BM, basement membrane
CC, cricoid cartilage
CT, connective tissue
E, epiglottis
Gl, mucous glands
LT, lingual tonsils
PSE, pseudostratified columnar epithelium (ciliated)
SCE, stratified columnar epithelium
SSE, stratified squamous epithelium
TC, tracheal cartilage
V, ventricle
VF, vocal fold
VL, vocal ligament
VM, vocalis muscle
VnF, ventricular fold
arrows (**Fig. 2**), extent of stratified squamous epithelium

Fig. 1 (monkey), 4; Fig. 2 (human), x 40; Figs. 3–5 (human), x 640.

The surface of the vocal fold (Fig. 3) is comprised of stratified squamous epithelium (**SSE**). This is in contact with a thick homogeneous-appearing basement membrane (**BM**) which separates the epithelium from the underlying connective tissue. Stratified squamous epithelium constitutes only part of the epithelial lining of the larynx. It extends from the upper left portion of Figure 2 (**arrow**) to the lower right of the figure (**arrow**) and can be readily identified even at low magnification by virtue of the intense staining of the basal cell layer.

The lower part of the larynx is surfaced by ciliated pseudostratified columnar epithelium (Fig. 5). This epithelium (**PS**) consists of two cell types: basal cells and ciliated cells. A third type of epithelium, stratified columnar (**SCE**) is present on the laryngeal surface (Fig. 4). This epithelium forms a transition between the stratified squamous epithelium and the pseudostratified ciliated epithelium. Although it resembles the pseudostratified epithelium, the surface cells of stratified columnar epithelium do not touch the basement membrane.

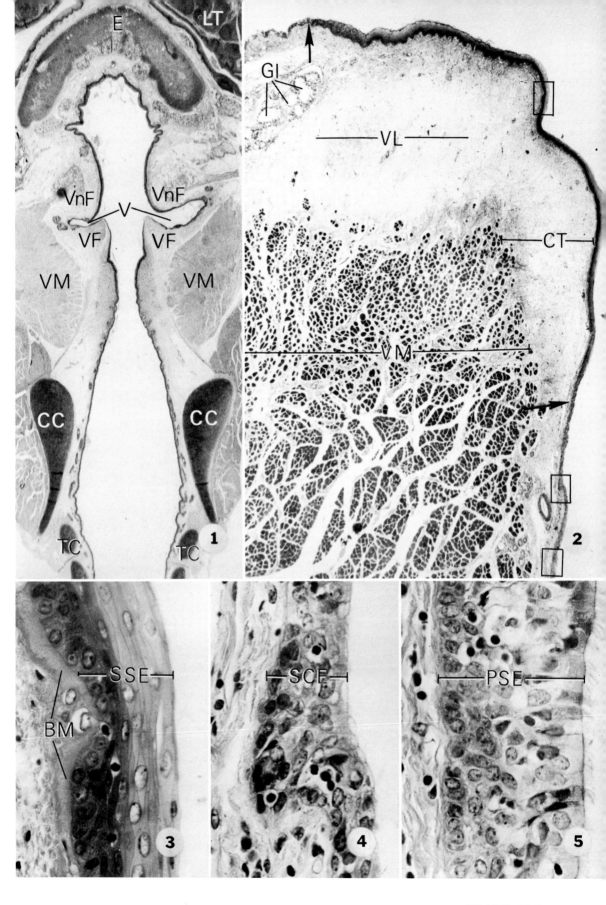

PLATE 11-2

Plate 11-3. Trachea and Bronchus

The trachea extends from the larynx to about the middle of the throat, where it divides into two bronchi. Its primary function is to serve as a conduit for air. The lumen of the trachea is held open by a series of C-shaped hyaline cartilages which form the framework of the wall. Posteriorly, cartilage is lacking whereas smooth muscle and fibroelastic tissue are present.

The wall of the trachea consists of the following layers (see Fig. 1): From the inside (luminal surface) there is a *mucosa* (**Muc**), *submucosa* (**Submuc**), *cartilaginous layer* (**Cart**), and an *adventitia* (**Adv**).

The **rectangle** in Figure 1 outlines the area shown in Figure 2 at higher magnification. The mucosa consists of ciliated pseudostratified columnar epithelium (**Ep**) resting on a highly elastic lamina propria (**LP**). A division between the mucosa and submucosa is not evident in H & E sections, but the boundary (**double-headed arrow**) is marked by the presence of an elastic layer that is revealed with special stains. Seromucous glands (**Gl**) and their ducts are present in the submucosa (Fig. 2). Glands are also present in the posterior part of the trachea where there is no cartilage; here they often extend through the muscle layer into the adventitia.

Three cell types are present in the tracheal epithelium: *basal cells, ciliated columnar cells,* and *goblet cells* (Fig. 3). Basal cells, at the base of the epithelial layer, can be recognized by their spherical, densely staining nuclei (**N Bas**), which are close to the basement membrane. These cells contain little cytoplasm.

The ciliated columnar cells extend from the basement membrane to the surface. The nuclei of these cells (**N Col**) are generally oval and tend to be located in the mid-region of the cell. Moreover, they are somewhat larger and paler staining than the basal cell nuclei. At their free surface they contain numerous cilia which, together, give the surface a brush-like appearance. At the base of the cilia one sees a dense line. This is due to the linear aggregation of structures referred to as *basal bodies* that are connected to the proximal end of each cilium.

Interspersed between the ciliated cells are mucus-secreting goblet cells (**GC**). They ap-

KEY

Adv, adventitia
Cart, cartilaginous layer
Ep, epithelium
Gl, glands
GC, goblet cell
LP, lamina propria
Muc, mucosa
N Bas, nuclei of basal cells
N Col, nuclei of columnar cells
SM, smooth muscle
Submuc, submucosa
arrows (Fig. **3**), nuclei of goblet cells
double-headed arrow (Fig. **2**), approximate boundary between mucosa and submucosa

Fig. 1 (dog), x 65; Fig. 2 (dog), x 160; Fig. 3 (monkey), x 640; Fig. 4 (dog), x 40.

pear empty because the mucus is lost during tissue preparation. Characteristically, the flattened nuclei are at the base of the mucous cup (**arrows**).

Although basement membranes are not ordinarily seen in H & E preparations, one is regularly seen under the epithelium in the human trachea. It is conspicuous because of its thickness.

The trachea divides into two *bronchi,* one of which goes into each lung. The bronchi branch several times, decrease somewhat in diameter, and undergo certain structural changes (Fig. 4). The large C-shaped cartilages are now replaced by smaller plates (**Cart**) which completely surround the bronchus. The connective tissue of the bronchus contains a large number of elastic fibers. However, the discrete elastic layer is replaced by smooth muscle (**SM**) which now appears at the boundary between the mucosa and submucosa. The mucosa remains essentially the same, except for the presence of smooth muscle. The description of ciliated pseudostratified columnar epithelium given above also applies to the epithelium of the bronchi.

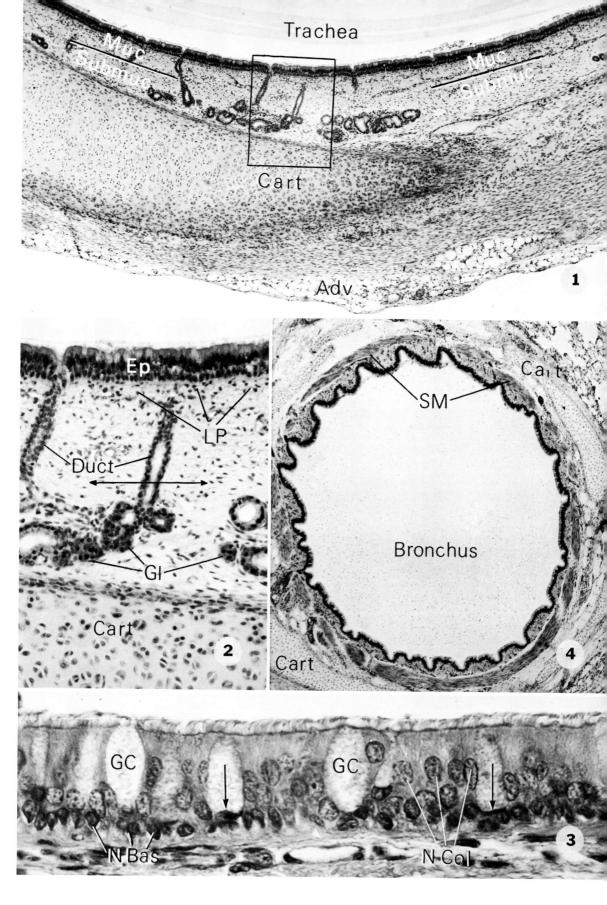

Trachea

Muc
Submuc

Muc
Submuc

Cart

Adv

1

Ep

LP

Duct

Gl

Cart

2

SM

Cart

Bronchus

Cart

4

GC

GC

N Bas

N Col

3

PLATE 11-3

Plate 11-4. BRONCHUS AND BRONCHIOLE

Each bronchus enters a lung at a site called the *hilus*. The hilus also serves as the portal for the pulmonary artery and veins, bronchial artery and veins, nerves, and lymphatic vessels. Sections that include the larger respiratory passages often show these structures.

Figure 1 is a segment of the wall of a *bronchus*. Its cartilage is not included in the illustration. The section shows the ciliated pseudostratified columnar epithelium (**Ep**) cut obliquely. The goblet cells appear as the clear spherical structures. Under the epithelium, in the lamina propria, are a number of round cells, mostly lymphocytes (**Lym**) comprising diffuse lymphatic tissue. In the bronchus, smooth muscle (**SM**) marks the boundary between the mucosa and submucosa, in contrast to the trachea where no boundary is evident. Below the smooth muscle is dense connective tissue (**CT**) and glands (**Gl**) of the submucosa. The submucosa also contains a collection of ganglion cells (**Gan C**). These are parasympathetic ganglia, and are recognized by their large cell bodies which contain an extremely large, spherical, pale-staining nucleus.

As the respiratory tube proceeds more distally, certain elements are lost and the tube is now called a bronchiole rather than a bronchus. In a *bronchiole* the cartilage is no longer present; the seromucous glands of the submucosa disappear; goblet cells are reduced in number or entirely missing; and the epithelium becomes simple columnar, but is still ciliated. On the other hand, the smooth muscle remains and forms a conspicuous component of the wall. Elastic tissue is also a conspicuous feature of the wall but, again, requires special elastic tissue stains for its demonstration.

It should be emphasized that the changes from bronchus to bronchiole are gradual and some elements remain longer than others; therefore, one may encounter a respiratory tube showing features of both, such as that shown in Figure 2. A small amount of cartilage (**Cart**) is still present in this instance. However, it should be noted that the glands have disappeared and the smooth muscle (**SM**) constitutes a major component of the wall.

The epithelium of a bronchiole is shown in Figure 3. This is simple columnar ciliated epi-

KEY

BV, blood vessel
Cart, cartilage
CT, connective tissue
Ep, epithelium
Gan C, ganglion cells
Gl, glands
Lym, lymphocytes
SM, smooth muscle
arrows, alveoli in wall of respiratory bronchiole

Fig. 1 (monkey), x 160; Fig. 2 (monkey), x 65; Fig. 3 (monkey), x 640; Fig. 4 (monkey), x 40.

thelium. At the base of the cilia are the basal bodies which appear as a dark line.

Figure 4 shows the alterations that occur as the respiratory tube is followed more distally. Evidently a branching has recently occurred; the larger part of the tube is on the left, whereas, on the right, the knife has cut the passage at two places. Above the respiratory passage is an accompanying blood vessel (**BV**) and a dense aggregation of lymphocytes (**Lym**) in the form of a nodule. Alveolar spaces are seen in the remainder of the section. The respiratory passage, moving across the field to the right, loses more and more of its elements until the wall loses its continuity and is partly made up of *alveoli* (**arrows**). At this point, the tube is called a *respiratory bronchiole* because gas exchange occurs through the alveolar part of the wall. Proximal to this point the bronchiole is called a *terminal bronchiole*. Air exchange does not occur through the wall of the terminal bronchiole or through the more proximal parts of the respiratory tree.

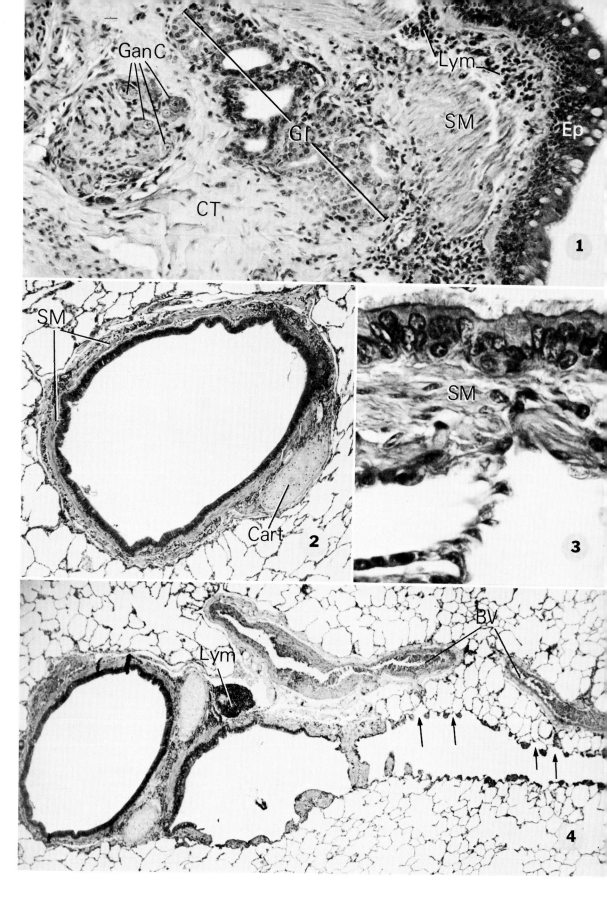

PLATE 11-4

Plate 11-5. Respiratory Bronchiole, Alveolar Duct, Alveolar Sac, and Alveolus

The illustrations on the accompanying plate show those parts of the bronchial tree through which air exchange occurs with the blood stream; namely, the *respiratory bronchiole, alveolar duct, alveolar sac,* and *alveolus.* "Alveolar air" is contained within these spaces.

The respiratory bronchiole (Fig. 1) retains some of the characteristics of a terminal bronchiole, since part of the wall, like that of the terminal bronchiole, is thick. However, as stated in the text on page 192, in addition to the thick segments which contain smooth muscle, alveolar sacs (**arrows**) also form part of the wall. Even at low power, the thick muscle-containing segments of the wall can easily be distinguished from the alveolar pockets. The muscle (**SM**) is easily recognized where it has been cut in a longitudinal fashion (Fig. 1). However, it is difficult to recognize when only small areas of the thick segments appear in the section. Surrounding the respiratory bronchiole in the remainder of the figure are the alveolar air spaces of the lung.

The area within the **rectangle** in Figure 1 is shown in Figure 2 at higher magnification. This permits a more detailed examination of the wall of the respiratory bronchiole. The surface of the respiratory bronchiole consists of cuboidal epithelium (**Ep**), and this rests on a very small amount of connective tissue. It should be noted that these epithelial cells are extremely small. The main component under the epithelial lining is the smooth muscle (**SM**). However, as indicated above, it is sometimes difficult to recognize.

When the respiratory bronchiole (**RB**) loses its thick components, it opens into the terminal part of the bronchial tree (Fig. 3), namely, the alveolar duct, alveolar sacs, and alveoli. The most distal component of the respiratory tube is the alveolus (**A**). Groups of alveoli clustered together and sharing a common opening are referred to as alveolar sacs (**AS**). Alveoli that form a tube are referred to as alveolar ducts (**AD**).

The alveolar wall consists of flattened epithelial cells in close contact with a capillary and a delicate connective tissue framework (Figs. 4 and 5). Actually, the epithelium of adjacent alveoli share capillaries and connective tissue so that the wall between neighboring alveoli consists of epithelium on each air surface, separated by a minute connective tissue compartment which contains the capillaries.

The alveolar epithelium contains two types of cells: squamous pulmonary epithelial cells (pneumocytes type I) and septal cells (pneumocytes type II, great alveolar cells). The squamous pulmonary epithelial cells are more numerous. They form a continuous lining of the alveolar wall except for occasional septal cells. The cytoplasm of the squamous cells is extremely attenuated and it is not possible to ascertain the limits of the cell in H & E sections. The septal cells have a rounded shape. They may bulge slightly into the alveolus and when this happens (arrow-heads, Figs. 4–5) the septal cell is easily identified. The septal cell in these illustrations display a nucleus and typically, a distinguishable amount of cytoplasm. Septal cells are thought to be active in the production of surfactant. The alveolar wall also contains macrophages which may contain phagocytized material and which are then called *dust cells.* Although it is difficult to distinguish squamous pulmonary epithelium, capillary endothelium, and connective tissue cells from one another, the capillary lumen can usually be identified by the presence of blood cells. Several red blood cells (**RBC**) and a white blood cell (**WBC**) can be recognized within the capillaries of the alveolar wall (Figs. 4–5).

KEY

A, alveolus
AD, alveolar duct
AS, alveolar sac
Ep, epithelium
RB, respiratory bronchiole
RBC, red blood cell
SM, smooth muscle
WBC, white blood cell
arrowheads, septal cells
arrows, alveolar sacs

Fig. 1 (monkey), x 65; Fig. 2 (monkey), x 160; Fig. 3 (monkey), x 65; Fig. 4 (monkey), x 640; Fig. 5 (monkey), x 960.

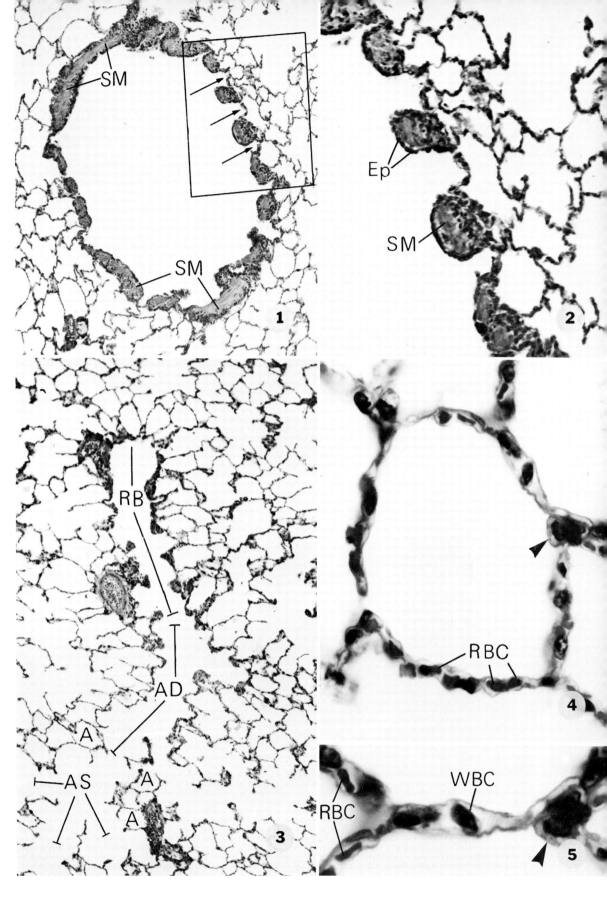

PLATE 11-5

12 URINARY SYSTEM

THE URINARY SYSTEM consists of the paired kidneys and ureters, the urinary bladder, and the urethra.

The functional unit of the kidney is the *nephron*. It consists of a tuft of capillaries, the *glomerulus,* and a *renal tubule.* The tubule begins as an expanded bulb, called the *renal capsule* or *Bowman's capsule.* This is in close association with the glomerulus and together, the glomerulus and the renal capsule form a filtering apparatus called the *Malpighian corpuscle.* The remaining parts of the renal tubule are designated, in order: the *proximal convoluted tubule, Henle's loop,* and the *distal convoluted tubule.* Henle's loop can be further subdivided into a proximal thick straight segment (or the thick descending limb), the thin segment which usually includes the loop itself, and the distal thick straight segment (or the thick ascending limb). The distal thick segment may form the loop instead of the thin segment. The distal convoluted tubule continues into the arched collecting tubule and then the arched collecting tubule enters a common *collecting* tubule that serves a number of nephrons.

Because of the way in which nephrons and collecting tubules are arranged, when a cut surface of the kidney is examined, the outer part of the kidney (the cortex) looks different from the inner part (the medulla). An entire nephron cannot be seen in a single section owing to its tortuosity. It is nevertheless well to know that parts of the nephron are in the cortex and parts are in the medulla. The medulla consists of conical shaped structures named the pyramids. The base of the pyramid faces the cortex and the apex faces toward the hilus of the kidney. The apex of the pyramid opens into a minor calyx, of which there are several, and the minor calyces join to form major calyces which finally open into the funnel shaped renal pelvis. The renal pelvis leads to the ureter. The apical portion of the pyramid which actually opens into the minor calyx is called the papilla.

The pyramid consists of collecting tubules, the loops of Henle (including their ascending and descending limbs) and blood vessels. These are relatively straight structures which, with the unaided eye, appear as radiations that extend from the apex to the base of the pyramid. The collecting tubules approach the apex of the pyramid ultimately to pour their product, the urine, into the minor calyx. However, shortly before the collecting tubules reach the apex, they join to form slightly larger tubular ducts called the papillary ducts of Bellini.

The cortex consists of the cortical labyrinth (Malpighian corpuscles, promimal and distal convoluted tubules, and arched collecting tubules) and the medullary rays (the proximal straight segment, the distal straight segment and the collecting tubules). The medullary rays appear to be radiating from the pyramids into the cortex. Cortical substance is also between the pyramids. A pyramid and its cortical cap are referred to as a renal lobe; a medullary ray and its contiguous cortical substance is referred to as a renal lobule.

Renal arteries branch within the kidneys, and the successive segments are called: the interlobar arteries (adjacent to the pyramids), arcuate arteries (at the cortico-medullary junction) and interlobular arteries (in the cortex). Interlobular arteries give rise to afferent arterioles which open into the glomerulus. From this point on, the arrangement of vessels in the kidney is unique. The capillaries that form the glomerulus receive an afferent arteriole (as already mentioned) and feed into an efferent arteriole which leaves the renal corpuscle. The efferent arterioles continue in one of three possible routes: 1) Efferent arterioles in the outer part of the cortex open into a second capillary network, the peritubular capillaries, which surround the convoluted tubules of the cortex; 2) Efferent arterioles in the inner part of the cortex continue as straight vessels (arteriolae rectae) into the medulla and then they open into the peritubular capillary network in the medulla; and 3) Efferent arterioles close to the base of the pyramid open directly into the peritubular capillary network in the medulla. In addition, the arteriolae rectae make a U-turn in the pyramid (much like the loop of Henle) and the ascending straight vascular limb (venulae rectae) returns to the base of the medulla to then empty into the arcuate vein. The descending and ascending straight vessels together with the loop of Henle and collecting ducts serve as the basis for the countercurrent exchange whereby urine is concentrated in the medulla.

The kidneys also serve in blood pressure regulation by the production of renin (a substance involved in activating angiotensinogen). Renin is produced by juxtaglomerular (JG) cells. These are modified smooth muscle cells in the wall of the afferent arteriole, just where the afferent arteriole enters the glomerulus. In addition, the distal convoluted tubule forms a specialization, the macula densa, which is adjacent to the JG cells. In some manner, not yet known, the macula densa is thought to be functionally associated with the JG cells.

Plate 12-1. KIDNEY I

The cortex of the kidney is shown at low power in Figure 1. The most striking feature of the kidney cortex is the presence of numerous *renal corpuscles* (**RC**). They appear as the spherical bodies surrounded by a small clear space. Surrounding the renal corpuscles are the *proximal* and *distal convoluted tubules*. These present a variety of profiles in sections, most of which appear oval or spherical. However, because of their convolutions, it is also possible to find some whose profile resembles a U, J, or even an S. The renal corpuscles (**RC**), convoluted tubules (unlabeled), and larger blood vessels (**BV**) make up the part of cortex that is referred to as the *cortical labyrinth* (**CL**).

In Figure 1, the cortical labyrinths are separated by groups of tubules oriented in the same direction. These tubules, collectively, are referred to as the medullary rays (**MR**). Each tubule within a medullary ray follows a rather straight course traveling to or from the medulla. When the medullary rays are cut longitudinally, the tubules present elongated profiles as they do in Figure 1.

The cortex of the kidney is also shown at low power in Figure 2, but the plane of section is at a right angle to that of Figure 1, and the medullary rays (**MR**) are thus cut in cross section. In this case, the tubules of the medullary rays appear oval or spherical, but the convoluted tubules and renal corpuscles of the cortical labyrinth appear as they do in Figure 1. A random gathering of yarn to form a ball, when sectioned, would present the same kind of profiles regardless of the plane of section; a package of cigarettes, on the other hand, will appear as circular profiles if cut in cross section, or as elongated profiles if cut longitudinally. For these reasons, the convoluted tubules present the same type of profiles in Figures 1 and 2, whereas the medullary rays present different profiles, depending on the plane of section. The appearance of the medullary rays can therefore give some indication regarding the plane of section. The closeness of the medullary rays and the large-sized blood vessels (**BV**) indicate that this section is close to the medulla. The arteries and veins in the cortex are interlobular arteries and veins.

Figure 2 is a silver preparation designed to

KEY

BV, blood vessel
CL, cortical labyrinth
MR, medullary ray
RC, renal corpuscle
arrow (inset), vascular pole

Fig. 1 (human), x 40; Fig. 2 (human), x 40; (inset), x 160.

illustrate the stroma of the kidney. The stroma appears as the black material that surrounds the tubules and the renal corpuscle (**RC**) (inset). The place where the blood vessels enter the renal corpuscle (the *vascular pole*) is indicated by an **arrow**. The very beginning of the proximal convoluted tubule is present on the opposite side of the renal corpuscle (the *urinary pole*); however it is not included in the illustration (see next plate).

With the electron microscope, small bundles of collagen fibrils are found within the interstitium, that is, the space between the tubules and the space between blood vessels and tubules. These collagen fibrils constitute the stroma of the kidney cortex and it is likely that they are blackened by the silver preparation. Traditionally these blackened fibers have been thought to be reticular fibers. The interstitium of the medulla is somewhat more extensive and in addition to small bundles of collagen fibrils, the medullary interstitium contains considerable amounts of basement membrane like material.

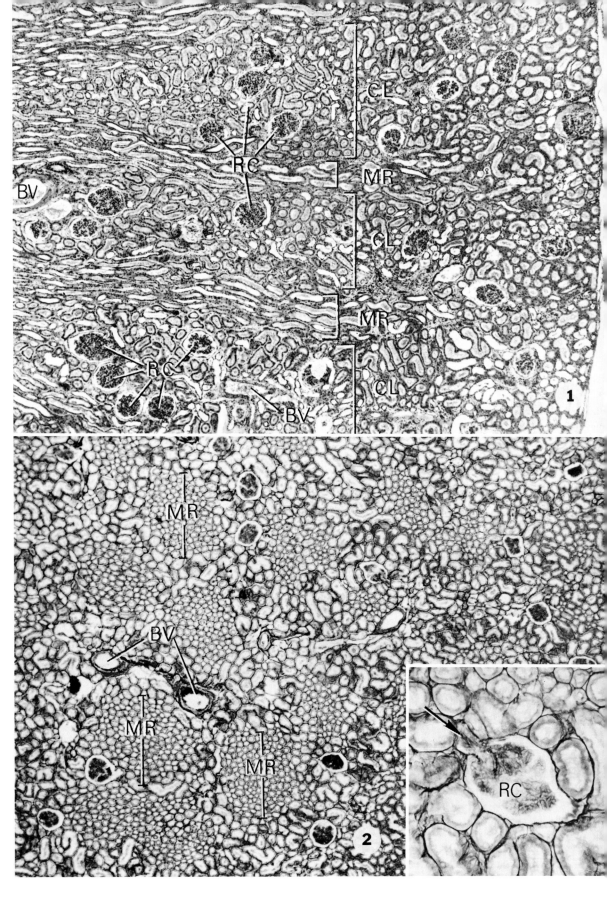

PLATE 12-1

Plate 12-2. KIDNEY II

The components of the cortical labyrinth are shown in Figure 1. A renal corpuscle is in the center of the field, and both the urinary and vascular poles are included in the section. The junction between the parietal layer of Bowman's capsule and the proximal convoluted tubule is clearly seen at the urinary pole (**arrowheads**); a distal convoluted tubule (**D′**) is adjacent to the blood vessels at the vascular pole. The side of this tubule that is in direct apposition to the blood vessels reveals a greater number of nuclei and is slightly thicker than the opposite side; this is the *macula densa* (**MD**). The macula densa is adjacent to the juxtaglomerular cells (**arrow**) of the afferent arteriole and the latter can usually be identified on this basis.

Proximal convoluted tubules are distinguished from distal convoluted tubules in a number of ways: (1) The proximal tubule is more than twice as long as the distal tubule; consequently, the majority of tubules in a given area will be proximal. (2) Proximal tubules have a slightly larger outside diameter than distal tubules, although the lumen may be smaller. (3) Proximal tubules have a distinct *brush border*, whereas the distal tubules have smaller surface projections and typically possess a cleaner, sharper luminal surface. (The brush border of the proximal tubules may be broken or even lost during preparation.) (4) The lumen of the proximal convoluted tubule is often star-shaped due to preparative procedures; this is less often the case with distal tubules. (5) Fewer nuclei appear in cross section of a proximal convoluted tubule than in distal tubules. (6) Both proximal and distal tubules possess *basal striations*, but they are less prominent in the distal.

Consider the two tubules marked **1** and **2** in Figure 1. In each, the luminal diameters are about the same. However, tubule **1** has a smaller outside diameter and shows about 16 nuclei; it is a distal tubule (**D**). Tubule **2** has a larger outside diameter and shows only about 12 nuclei; it is a proximal tubule (**P**). In Figure 2 notice the brush border (**arrows**) of the proximal tubules (**P**) and the relatively sharp surface of the distal convoluted tubule (**D**). Peritubular capillaries (**Cap**) can be seen between the tubules.

A precipitate is present in the lumen of the proximal convoluted tubules that are shown in Figure 1. While this may enable one to quickly recognize proximal tubules in this specimen, it should be pointed out and emphasized that this is not a regular feature and identification on this basis is tenuous.

Collecting tubules and arched collecting tubules (**C**) consist of cuboidal cells. A boundary can usually be seen between the cells, however, these boundaries are not always striking. Arched collecting tubule and collecting tubule cells do not possess basal striations. However, striations (**arrowheads,** Figs. 2 and 3) can be seen in the cytoplasm of the distal and proximal convoluted tubule cells.

A renal corpuscle and its vascular pole are shown at higher magnification in Figure 3. Surrounding the corpuscle is the parietal layer of Bowman's capsule (**BC**). It consists of flat, squamous cells. Some red blood cells can be seen within the capillaries (**arrows**) that make up the glomerulus. The visceral layer of Bowmans capsule is difficult to identify. These cells are highly specialized; they have interdigitating foot processes called pedicles; the cells themselves are called podocytes. The renal corpuscle also contains mesangial cells. These are chiefly at the vascular pole about the blood vessels, but they are also difficult to identify in routine H & E preparations.

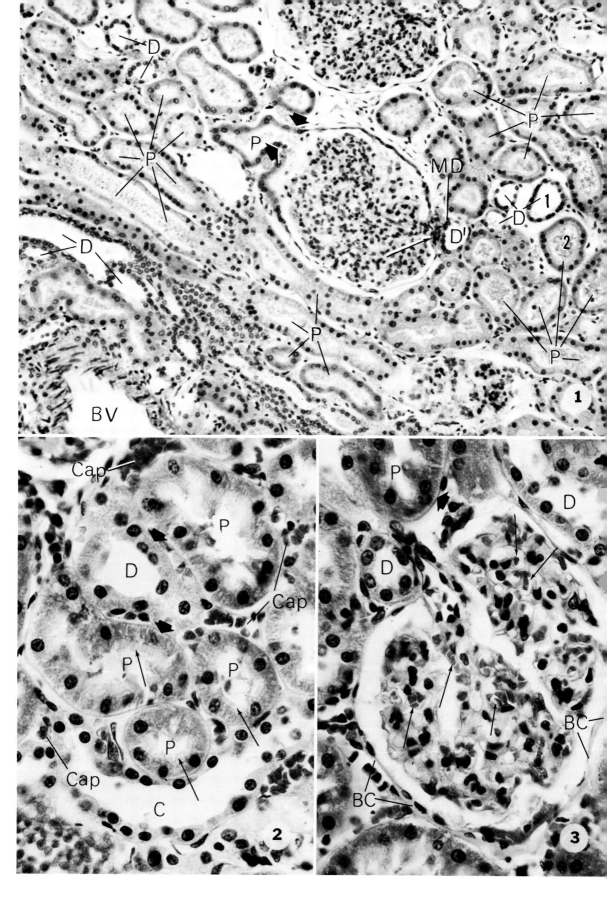

PLATE 12-2

Plate 12-3. KIDNEY III

The apex of a pyramid projecting into a *calyx* (**Ca**) is shown in Figure 1. Cortical substance is located on both sides of the illustration and can be recognized by the presence of renal corpuscles and the convoluted tubules. Adipose tissue (**AT**) surrounds the calyx, and in the adipose tissue are branches of the renal artery (**A**) and vein (**V**). The space occupied by the adipose tissue, the large blood vessels, and the calyces is referred to as the *renal sinus*. It is just inside the opening (hilus) on the medial side of the kidney.

The pyramid and calyx are shown in Figures 2 and 3 at higher magnification. Figure 2 shows the pyramid and wall of the calyx in cross section. Therefore, the collecting tubules (**C**) present circular profiles. They are comprised of cuboidal or columnar cells and characteristically exhibit prominent boundaries. It should be recalled that the boundaries between other cells of the kidney tubules are not distinct in H & E preparations. The smaller thin-walled tubules that are present in the pyramid in addition to the collecting tubules are either thin segments of Henle's loop or blood vessels (vasa recta). It is not always a simple matter to distinguish between these. As a general statement, cells that make up the thin segments have spherical nuclei which bulge into the lumen; endothelial nuclei, on the other hand, are flat. If the blood vessels contain red blood cells, the task of distinguishing between the two is simplified significantly.

The outer surface of the pyramid (**arrows**) is made up of a single layer of cuboidal or columnar cells which resemble the cells of collecting ducts, inasmuch as their cell boundaries are also evident.

Figure 3 shows essentially the same structures as shown in Figure 2, except that the collecting tubule (**C**) is cut longitudinally. Note the similarity between cells of the collecting tubule and cells that line the surface of the pyramid (**arrows**).

The surface of the calyx [**Ca(S)**] consists of *transitional epithelium* (**TE**) (Figs. 2 and 3). This epithelium is stratified and appears thicker than the simple epithelium on the surface of the pyramid. Transitional epithelium is presented in detail on pages 10 and 206.

KEY

A, renal artery
AT, adipose tissue
C, collecting tubule
Ca, calyx
Ca(S), surface of calyx
SM, smooth muscle
TE, transitional epithelium
V, renal vein
arrows, surface of pyramids

Fig. 1 (guinea pig), x 40; Fig. 2 (guinea pig), x 160; Fig. 3 (guinea pig), x 640.

Collagenous fibers are present in the connective tissue under the transitional epithelium of the calyx (Fig. 3). The wall of the calyces also contain smooth muscle. In Figure 1, near the bottom, the wall of the calyx has been cut tangentially. The lumen and epithelium have been missed, but the smooth muscle (**SM**) is included.

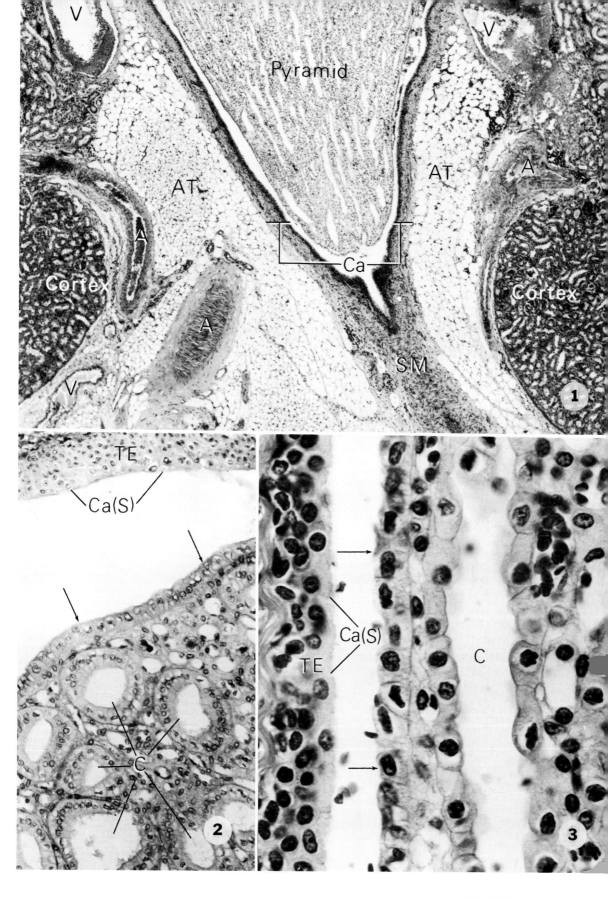

PLATE 12-3

Plate 12-4. Ureter

The ureters conduct urine from the kidneys to the urinary bladder. They not only serve as a route to the bladder but they contribute to the flow of urine by means of their regular peristaltic contractions. The wall of the ureters consists of a lining of transitional epithelium, smooth muscle, and supporting connective tissue. These components are organized as a *mucosa* (**Muc**), *muscularis* (**Mus**) and *adventitia* (**Adv**) and are illustrated in Figure 1. The lumen is characteristically star-shaped.

The wall of the ureter is examined at higher magnification in Figure 2. One can immediately recognize the lining of the inner surface which appears distinct and sharply delineated from the remainder of the wall. This inner, sharply delineated part, in direct contact with the lumen, is the transitional epithelium (**Ep**). The remainder of the wall is made up of connective tissue (**CT**) and smooth muscle. The latter can be recognized as the darker-staining layer with connective tissue on both sides. The section also shows some blood vessels (**A, V**) and adipose tissue (**AT**).

The transitional epithelium (**Ep**) and its supporting connective tissue (**CT**) constitute the mucosa (**Muc**). A distinct submucosa is not present, although the term is sometimes applied to the connective tissue that is closest to the muscle.

The muscularis (**Mus**) consists of smooth muscle. It is arranged as an inner longitudinal layer [**SM(L)**], a middle circular layer [**SM(C)**], and an outer longitudinal layer [**SM(L)**]. The outer longitudinal layer is present only at the lower end of the ureter. In a cross section through the ureter, the inner and outer smooth muscle layers are cut in cross section, whereas the circular middle layer of muscle cells is cut longitudinally. This is as they appear in Figure 2. The elongated and oriented nuclei of the middle layer are easy to recognize, but the inner and outer layers of muscle cells are more difficult to identify. The connective tissue external to the smooth muscle is referred to as the adventitia (**Adv**).

KEY

A, artery
Adv, adventitia
AT, adipose tissue
BV, blood vessels
CT, connective tissue
Ep, transitional epithelium
Muc, mucosa
Mus, muscularis
SM(C), circular layer of smooth muscle
SM(L), longitudinal layer of smooth muscle
V, vein

Fig. 1 (monkey), x 80; Fig. 2 (monkey), x 165.

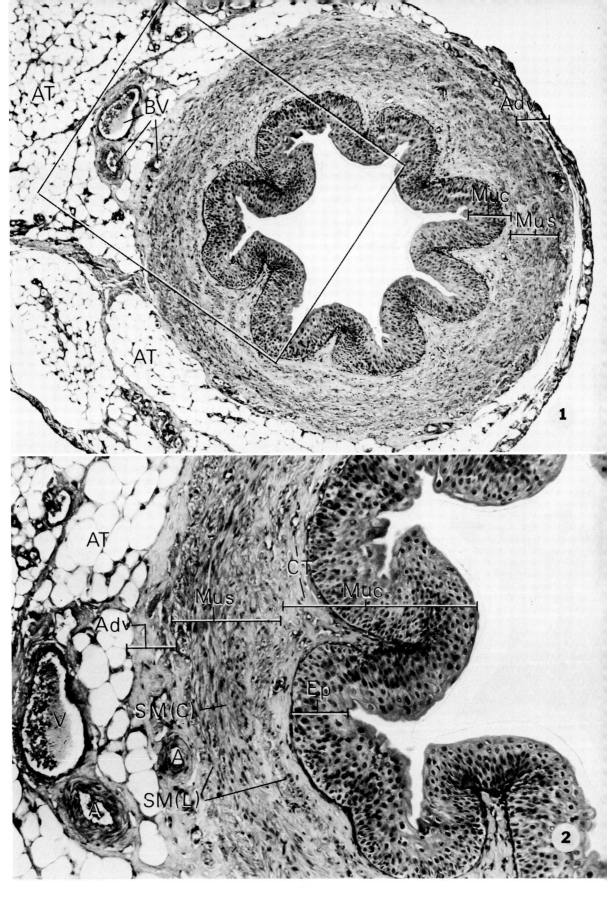

PLATE 12-4

Plate 12-5. URINARY BLADDER

The urinary bladder receives urine from the two ureters and stores it until it is discharged via the urethra. Its structure reflects these functions. It possesses a lining of transitional epithelium which adapts to changes in bladder volume, and the wall contains bundles of smooth muscle which function in discharging the urine.

The full thickness of the urinary bladder is illustrated in Figure 1. It shows the *mucosa* (**Muc**), the *muscularis* (**Mus**), and the *serosa* (**S**). The mucosa consists of transitional epithelium (**Ep**) and its supporting connective tissue (**CT**). A distinct submucosa is not present, although as with the ureter, the connective tissue closest to the muscle is sometimes referred to as a submucosa. The muscularis consists of smooth muscle which, like that of the ureter, is arranged in three layers: an inner longitudinal [**SM(L)**], middle circular [**SM(C)**], and outer longitudinal layer [**SM(L)**]. The smooth muscle in this preparation stains more intensely than the connective tissue. On the basis of organization, the bundles of smooth muscle cells can be recognized because they are surrounded by connective tissue (**CT**). This relationship is especially evident when the smooth muscle is cut obliquely or in cross section. When the smooth muscle is cut longitudinally, the relationship is less evident, but then the elongated profiles of the smooth muscle cell nuclei serve as a diagnostic feature. Morever, even at this low magnification, one can see some of the muscle cell nuclei in an intracellular location. Another extremely useful criterion for distinguishing smooth muscle from connective tissue in Figure 1 is that the number of nuclei in a given area of smooth muscle (**white circle**) is greater than the number of nuclei in a comparable area of connective tissue (**black circle**).

A serosa is present on the upper surface of the bladder; it consists of a layer of simple squamous epithelium (mesothelium) which rests on a small amount of supporting connective tissue. Elsewhere, the outer layer of the wall consists of a fibrous adventitia.

The **rectangles** in Figures 1 and 2 indicate areas that are examined at higher magnification in Figures 2 and 3, respectively, to show the transitional epithelium. In the contracted state the epithelium (**Ep**) is charac-

KEY

CT, connective tissue
Ep, epithelium
Lym, lymphocytes
Muc, mucosa
Mus, muscularis
S, serosa
SM(C), circular layer of smooth muscle
SM(L), longitudinal layer of smooth muscle
arrows, binucleate cells

Fig. 1 (monkey), x 65; Fig. 2 (monkey), x 160; Fig. 3 (monkey), x 640.

terized by the presence of dome-shaped cells at the free surface and large numbers of pear-shaped cells immediately under the surface cells. The cells at the surface are large and occasionally have two nuclei (**arrows**). Deeper cells, on the other hand, are smaller. Because of the absence of connective tissue papillae, the epithelial-connective tissue junction is rather even. An aggregation of lymphocytes (**Lym**) is immediately under the epithelial surface. This is not an unusual observation.

The thickness of the transitional epithelium depends on the degree of bladder (or ureteral) distention. In the empty ureter or bladder, it appears to be about five cells deep. However, when they are distended, it appears to have a thickness of only three cells, a basal layer, an intermediate cell layer, and a surface cell layer.

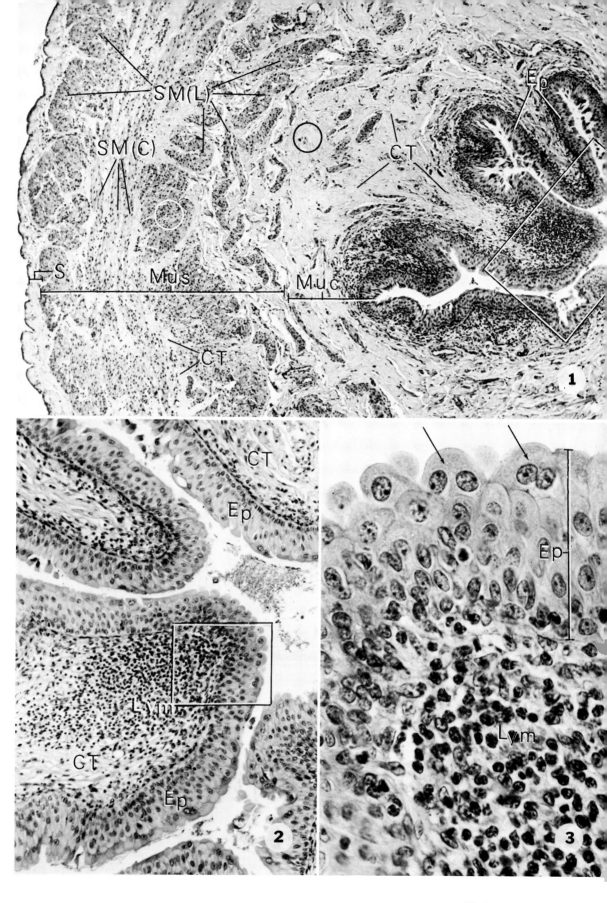

PLATE 12-5

13 MALE REPRODUCTIVE SYSTEM

THE MALE REPRODUCTIVE SYSTEM consists of two testes, the duct system leading from them, the penis, and the accessory glands. The testes produce both *sperm* and *hormones*. The sperm are produced by an extensively *coiled* system of tubules called the *seminiferous tubules*. In the human, spermatogenesis (the process of sperm formation) begins at about the time of puberty. Testosterone, the principal male hormone, is produced by cells called *interstitial cells of Leydig*. These cells are located in the interstices between the seminiferous tubules.

The seminiferous epithelium contains two distinctive cell types: supporting cells and spermatogenic cells. There is only one kind of supporting cell, designated the Sertoli cell. Sertoli cells do not divide. They provide mechanical, and possibly nutritional, support for the cells of the spermatogenic series, and they play a role in the maturation and release of the mature sperm. In addition, the Sertoli cells, by means of specialized junctions, form a barrier (the blood-testicular barrier) which divides the epithelium into a basal and adluminal compartment. This unique compartmentalization of the seminiferous epithelium, through which the germ cells must pass during their development, is concerned with the immunological isolation of the developing sperm once they are beyond the very early spermatocyte stage.

The spermatogenic cells are of several types, each of which represents a successive stage in the process of spermatogenesis. In the mature testis, spermatogenic cells undergo cyclical activity and at the end of each cycle of activity, sperm are produced. Sertoli cells also undergo changes which parallel in time those of the spermatogenic cells. In order to understand the histological appearance of the testis, it is well to comment on the place of cell division and cell associations as they related to the cycle of the seminiferous epithelium. For purposes of comparison and perspective, recall that elsewhere in the body, in the maintenance of stratified squamous epithelium, new cells are generated in the basal, or germinative, layer. As the cells differentiate, they approach the surface; however, during the differentiation and movement toward the surface, no further cell division occurs. In spermatogenesis, the spermatogonia also serve as a source of new cells and in this sense they constitute a germinative layer. However, as the cells differentiate and move toward the lumen, upon reaching a specific stage of development (now further removed from the basal layer), further cell divisions occur. Moreover, included in the divisions are two meiotic divisions which result in the reduction of the chromosome number. The production of new generations of cells in the basal layer occurs concurrently in the same region of the tubule with the production of more differentiated generations closer to the lumen. The process, however, is not random, and specific cell associations can be identified. (Thus, spermatids at a specific stage of development will always be associated with spermatocytes and spermatogonia at a specific stage of their development.) The number of recognizable cellular associations varies among mammals: in mice and rats there are 12 cellular associations; in the human there are six cellular associations. Whereas in most animals a given cellular association will occupy a variable length of a tubule, in the human the cellular associations constitute irregular, patch-like areas of the tubule. Thus, unlike other mammals, more than one cellular association may be observed in a single cross-sectional profile of a tubule. For this reason, the cellular associations are more difficult to identify in man, mainly because of the irregular and confusing boundaries that occur between adjacent cellular associations.

The duct system includes: the *straight tubules*, or *tubuli recti*, and *rete testes*, which are within the testes; the *efferent ductules*, which leave the testes; the *ductus epididymis*, a long, coiled tubule within the epididymis; the *ductus deferens*, which leaves the scrotal sac, enters the body cavity through the inguinal canal, and continues into the pelvis; the *ejaculatory duct*, which pierces the prostate gland; and the *urethra*, which finally courses through the penis. The urethra serves both the urinary system and the reproductive system as a terminal duct.

The accessory glands are the *seminal vesicles*, the *prostate gland*, and the two small *bulbourethral glands*. The seminal vesicles empty into the ductus deferens where it becomes the ejaculatory duct. The prostate gland surrounds the first part of the urethra and opens into it; the bulbourethral glands empty into the cavernous part of the urethra. All of these glands add their secretions to those of the seminiferous tubules, and the total mixture, containing spermatozoa, is referred to as *semen*.

The manner whereby spermatoza and fluid secretions are moved through the above-mentioned tubule and duct systems is not entirely clear. In some places, a thick layer of smooth muscle within the wall is obviously implicated. However, it should be noted that the amount of smooth muscle within the walls varies, and parts of the duct system (straight tubules and rete testes) have no muscle whatsoever.

Plate 13-1. Testis I

The *seminiferous tubules* are highly convoluted and in a section they present a variety of profiles (Fig. 1). Circular and oval profiles are the predominant forms. The lumens (L) of the tubules in a mature testis are conspicuous.

The framework of the testis consists of a capsule, called the tunica albuginea (TA), and septa (S), which divide the testis into compartments. Within each compartment are several seminiferous tubules. The tubules are surrounded by cells that display myoid features in the electron microscope. The contraction of the myoid cells is the basis for the slow peristaltic movement characteristic of the seminiferous tubules. Small blood vessels (BV), as seen in Figure 3, pass between the tubules. Broad lymphatic vessels also occupy an extensive space between the tubules. However, in routinely prepared specimens the lymphatic channels are collapsed and are usually not identifiable. Furthermore, the lymphatic endothelial cell nuclei and myoid cell nuclei are indistinguishable from one another (arrows, Fig. 3). Not infrequently, clusters of cells without a lumen (X), which represent tangential sections through a seminiferous tubule, are seen (Fig. 2). These should not be confused with Leydig cells (see Plate 13-2).

Note that in a particular section, the tubule walls do not all have the same appearance (Fig. 2). This is due to the groupings, or cell associations, that are characteristic of seminiferous epithelium (see chapter introduction).

Two distinctly different kinds of cells are present in the wall of the tubule (Fig. 3), cells of the spermatogenic series and *Sertoli cells*. The Sertoli cells differ from cells of the spermatogenic series in appearance and are considerably fewer in number. Whereas the cells of the spermatogenic series, excluding the spermatids in the later stages of development, have spherical nuclei, the nuclei of Sertoli cells (SC) are usually ovoid and often exhibit cleft-like indentations. Moreover, they are pale staining and radially oriented. The cytoplasm of Sertoli cells extends from the periphery of the tubule to the lumen, but the full extent cannot be seen in H & E sections.

The rectangle in Figure 2 marks an area which is depicted at higher magnification in Figure 3. Although it is from monkey, it corresponds rather closely to the epithelial grouping designated as stage II in man, and

KEY

BV, blood vessel
L, lumen of seminiferous tubule
PS, primary spermatocytes
S, connective tissue septum
SC, Sertoli cell nuclei
Sg, spermatogonia
St, spermatids
St°, late spermatids
TA, tunica albuginea
arrow, myoid and lymphatic endothelial cell nuclei

Fig. 1 (monkey), x 65; Fig. 2 (monkey), x 160; Fig. 3 (monkey), x 640.

it shows the cell types involved in spermatogenesis. At the periphery of the tubule are the *spermatogonia* (Sg), or primitive germ cells, about 12 μ in diameter. These differentiate into *primary spermatocytes*. Primary spermatocytes (PS) are about 17-19 μ in diameter, and lie next to spermatogonia, on the luminal side. The nuclei typically show chromatin that is in the process of organizing into chromosomal forms. Primary spermatocytes divide and form *secondary spermatocytes;* the latter are smaller than primary spermatocytes. Secondary spermatocytes divide into *spermatids* (St). Since the secondary spermatocytes are present for a very short duration, they are infrequently observed. Spermatids are about 9 μ in diameter, and are found in groups near the lumen of the tubule. Spermatids undergo differentiation and maturational changes to form sperm, which are released into the lumen. Late spermatids and sperm have small, dark staining heads. The heads shown in Figure 3 (St°) belong to late spermatids and, as such, still remain attached to the Sertoli cells. The tails, which are faintly evident, extend into the lumen.

In establishing a blood-testis barrier, Sertoli cells make intimate contact (occluding junctions) with neighboring Sertoli cells. The contact is made at a level which separates the spermatogonia from other cells of the spermatogenic series. Thus, by virtue of the occluding junctions between Sertoli cells, the seminiferous epithelium is divided into a basal compartment, containing the spermatogonia and very early primary spermatocytes, and an adluminal compartment containing the other cells of the spermatogenic cell series.

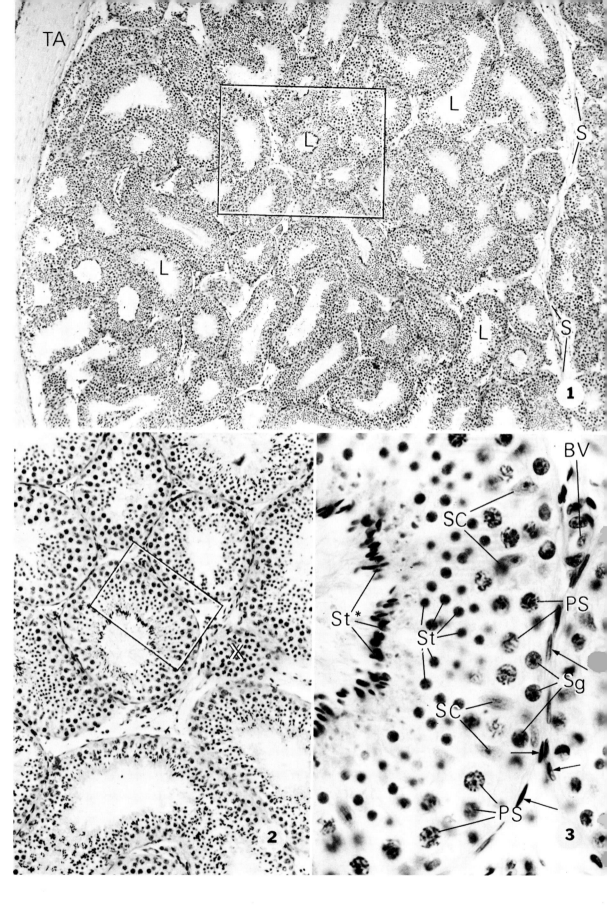

PLATE 13-1

Plate 13-2. Testis II

The variety of cell types that are indicative of spermatogenesis in the mature seminiferous tubules are not present in the testes before puberty (Fig. 1) or in the undescended testis. In fact, the "tubules" are actually solid cords of cells. In these cords, a cell which resembles Sertoli cells predominates. These are the future Sertoli cells. The cords also contain a second cell type, the gonocytes. These cells have a centrally placed, spherical nucleus. The cytoplasm takes little stain and appears as light ring around the nucleus. This gives the cell a distinctive appearance in histological sections (**arrows**, Figs. 1 and 2). Generally, these cells are found at the periphery of the cord, although some may be more centrally placed.

Interstitial cells of Leydig (**L**) are conspicuous in the newborn, a reflection of the residual effects of maternal hormones. However, the Leydig cells regress and do not become conspicuous again until puberty. In this preparation, the Leydig cells can be seen between the cords even at low magnification (Fig. 1). Leydig cells are ovoid or polygonal in shape (Fig. 2), and usually closely grouped so that adjacent cells are in contact with each other. The nucleus of the Leydig cell is spherical; the cytoplasm may appear vacuolated and empty due to the large amount of lipid which is lost during the tissue preparation. In the adult human, rod-shaped crystalloids may be seen within the cytoplasm. Despite the fact that these cells are mesodermal in origin and lie in a connective tissue stroma, they possess certain epithelial characteristics. They have large spherical nuclei; they have a relatively large amount of cytoplasm, the boundaries of which are readily seen in histological sections; and some of the cells contact each other without intervening fibrous material. For these reasons, these cells are referred to as epithelial-like, or epithelioid. Leydig cells produce testosterone and other steroid hormones.

In addition to the Leydig cells, the space between the cords contains a delicate connective tissue stroma and connective tissue cells (**CT**). Some blood vessels (**BV**) may be seen within this stroma; lymphatic vessels are also present, but, characteristically, they are empty and collapsed in routine H & E preparations

KEY

BV, blood vessels
CT, connective tissue
Ep, epithelium
L, Leydig cells
RT, rete testis
S, connective tissue septum
arrows (Figs. 1 and 2), gonocytes

Fig. 1 (monkey), x 160; Fig. 2 (monkey), x 640; Fig. 3 (human), x 40; (inset), x 640.

and are thus not evident. A delicate connective tissue septum (**S**) is also shown (Fig. 1), and typically the larger blood vessels are associated with septum.

Straight tubules and rete testes. In the posterior of the testis, the connective tissue of the tunica albuginea extends more deeply into the organ (Fig. 3). This inward extension of connective tissue is called the *mediastinum testis*. It contains a network of anastomosing channels called the *rete testis* (**RT**). The epithelium (**Ep, inset**) that lines these channels is generally cuboidal. However, there is some degree of variation and not infrequently, in some areas, the lining cells may be columnar or they may even be squamous. The epithelial cells possess a single cilium; however, this is difficult to see in routine H & E sections. The seminiferous tubules open into the rete testis by way of the *straight tubules*, or *tubuli recti*. The straight tubules are very short and are lined by Sertoli-like cells; no germ cell component is present. Both straight tubules and rete testes are in fact epithelial-lined, interconnective spaces in connective tissue. No special organization of the connective tissue can be seen, nor is smooth muscle present.

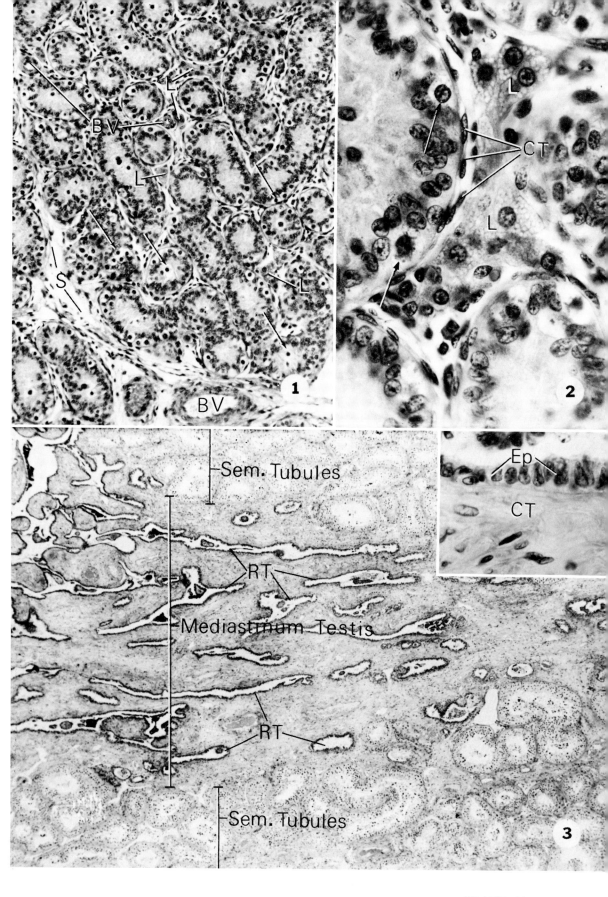

PLATE 13-2

Plate 13-3. EFFERENT DUCTULES AND EPIDIDYMIS

Efferent ductules. About eight to twelve efferent ductules leave the testis and serve as channels from the rete testis to the epididymis. The epithelium (**Ep**) that lines the efferent ductules is pseudostratified columnar. It is distinctive in that groups of tall columnar cells alternate with groups of cuboidal cells, giving the lumenal surface a more uneven or wavy appearance than the basal surface (Fig. 1). Some of the cells possess cilia. In addition to the columnar and cuboidal cells, basal cells are present, and for this reason the epithelium is designated pseudostratified columnar.

The efferent ductules are surrounded by a thin layer of circularly arranged smooth muscle cells (**SM**). The muscle is close to the epithelial surface, being separated from it by only a small amount of connective tissue. Some small blood vessels (**BV**) are shown in the wall of the efferent ductules and also in the surrounding connective tissue (**CT**).

Epididymis. The epididymis, by virtue of its shape, is divided into a *head, body,* and *tail.* It contains a convoluted tube called the *ductus epididymis,* into which the efferent ductules open.

A section through the epididymis cuts the duct in a number of places. The epithelium (**Ep**) which lines the duct contains two types of cells, principal cells and basal cells (**inset**). Because of this, the epithelium is designated pseudostratified columnar. The principal cells are tall columnar; those in the head and body are taller than those in the tail. The free surface of the principal cell contains *stereocilia* (**arrows**) which can be seen even with low magnification. These are extremely long, branching microvilli. They evidently adhere to each other during the preparation of the tissue to form the long tapering structures that are characteristically seen with the light microscope.

The duct of the epididymis is readily distinguished from the efferent ductules because the lumenal surface of the epithelium is more even than the luminal surface of the efferent ductule, and for many stretches, the luminal surface and the basal surface of the epithelial cells are parallel. In the epididymis, the nuclei of the columnar cells are typically elongated and located in the basal part of the cell. They are readily distinguished from the

KEY

BV, blood vessel
CT, connective tissue
Ep, epithelium
SM, smooth muscle
arrows, stereocilia

Fig. 1 (human), x 160; Fig. 2 (human), x 78; (inset), x 640.

spherical nuclei of the basal cells. In the efferent ductules the nuclei of the different cell types are not always easily distinguished from one another.

The duct contains circularly arranged smooth muscle (**SM**) cells which can be recognized by their elongated and oriented nuclei. The difference in staining between muscle and connective tissue also aids in distinguishing one from the other. The connective tissue (**CT**) has no special organization.

The smooth muscle cells within the duct in the head and body of the epididymis undergo rhythmic contractions which move the sperm toward the tail. These muscular contractions are not dependent on nervous stimulation. Maturation of sperm continues during the passage through the head and body of the epididymis. The smooth muscle cells within the duct in the tail responds to nerve stimulation and serves to discharge the sperm in the ejaculatory reflex.

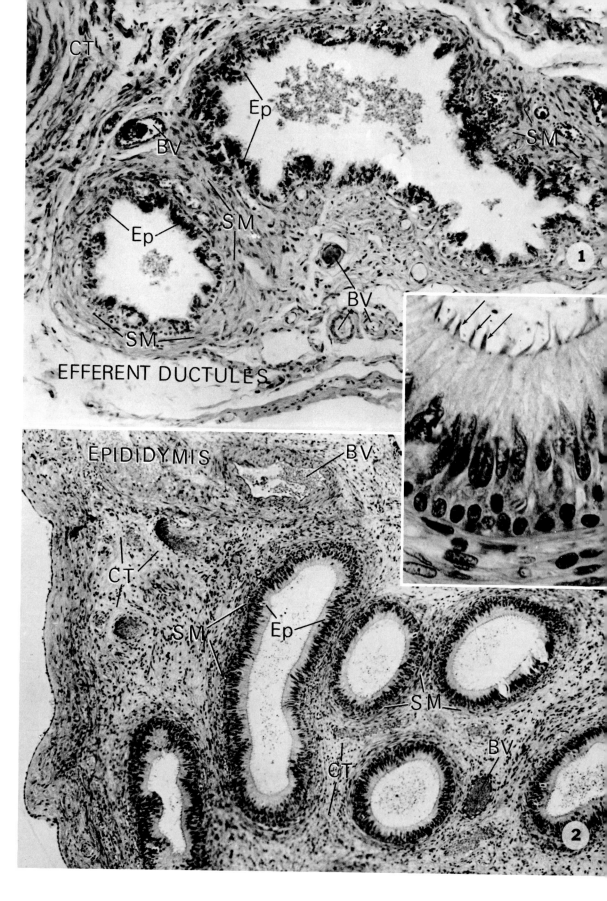

CT

Ep

BV

SM

Ep

SM

BV

SM

BV

EFFERENT DUCTULES

EPIDIDYMIS

BV

CT

SM

Ep

SM

CT

BV

1

2

PLATE 13-3

Plate 13-4. DUCTUS DEFERENS AND SEMINAL VESICLE

Ductus deferens. The ductus deferens continues from the duct of the epididymis. It leaves the scrotum and passes through the inguinal canal as a component of the spermatic cord. At the deep inguinal ring it continues into the pelvis, and behind the urinary bladder it joins with the seminal vesicle to form the ejaculatory duct. The ejaculatory duct then pierces the prostate gland and opens into the urethra.

A cross section through the ductus deferens is shown in Figure 1. The wall is extremely thick, owing mostly to the presence of a large amount of smooth muscle. The muscle contracts when the tissue is removed, causing longitudinal folds of the mucosa to form. For this reason, the lumen usually appears somewhat star-shaped in cross section.

The epithelial lining (**Ep**) of the ductus deferens consists of pseudostratified columnar epithelium which may contain stereocilia (Fig. 2). It resembles the epithelium of the epididymis. The elongated nuclei of the columnar cells are readily distinguished from the spherical nuclei (**arrow**) of the basal cells. (Spherical nuclei are easy to recognize if they are sufficiently numerous in an epithelial layer; they always appear spherical regardless of the plane of section. Elongated nuclei have variable appearances according to the plane of section.) The epithelium rests on a loose connective tissue (**CT**) which extends as far as the smooth muscle, and no submucosa is described.

The smooth muscle of the ductus deferens (Figs. 1 and 2) is arranged as a thick outer longitudinal layer [**SM(L)**], a thick middle circular layer [**SM(C)**], and a thinner inner longitudinal layer [**SM(L)**]. Blood vessels (**BV**) and nerves are in the connective tissue that surrounds the ductus deferens. A nerve bundle (**N**) is present just below the ductus deferens.

Seminal vesicle. The seminal vesicles are small elongated sacs that are folded upon themselves. Consequently, in a section, the lumen may be cut in several places (Fig. 3).

The *mucosa* of the seminal vesicles is characterized by being extensively folded or ridged. The ridges vary in size, and typically branch and interconnect with one another. The larger ridges may form recesses which contain smaller ridges, and when these are cut

KEY

BV, blood vessels
CT, connective tissue
Ep, epithelium
N, nerve
SM, smooth muscle
SM(C), circular layer of smooth muscle
SM(L), longitudinal layer of smooth muscle
arrow (Fig. 2), basal cell nucleus
arrowheads, villus-like appearance of mucosal folds
arrows (Fig. 3), arches formed by large mucosal folds

Fig. 1 (human), x 42; Fig. 2 (human), x 160; Fig. 3 (human), x 16; Fig. 4 (human), x 160.

obliquely, they appear as mucosal arches which enclose the smaller folds (**arrows**). When the plane of section is normal to the surface, the mucosal ridges appear as villi (**arrowheads**). The lower part of Figure 3 shows where the mucosa was cut tangential to the surface, but close to the base of the mucosal folds. Note how interconnecting folds appear as alveoli when cut in this manner.

The mucosa consists of a layer of pseudostratified columnar epithelium resting on a sparse but cellular connective tissue (**CT**) (Fig. 4). The basal cells are not particularly numerous and are difficult to identify.

The mucosa rests on a thick layer of smooth muscle (**SM**). The smooth muscle is described as consisting of an inner circular layer and an outer longitudinal layer, but these are difficult to distinguish. However, the difference in staining between the smooth muscle and connective tissue in this preparation makes it easy to distinguish these two components.

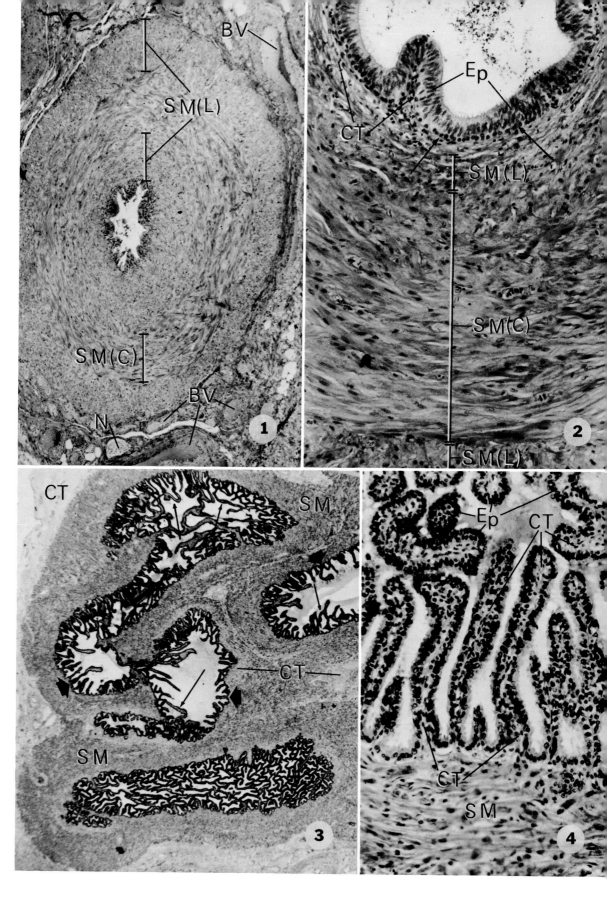

PLATE 13-4

Plate 13-5. PROSTATE GLAND

The *prostate gland* surrounds the first part of the urethra. It consists of about 40 tubulo-alveolar glands that are contained in a fibro-elastic stroma. The stroma is characterized by the presence of numerous small bundles of smooth muscle so that it can also be described as a fibromuscular stroma. Surrounding the gland is a fibroelastic capsule which also contains small bundles of smooth muscle. Ducts from the gland empty into the urethra.

A section of the prostate gland is shown in Figure 1. The capsule (**Cap**) is in the upper part of the figure; the glandular components in the lower part. The tube-alveoli of the gland vary greatly in form as evident from the illustration. They may appear as alveoli, as alveoli with branches, or as tubules with branches. They may appear open or they may be collapsed. Frequently, in older individuals, precipitates (*prostatic concretions*) (**PC**) are present in the lumen. These stain with eosin and may have a concentric lamellar appearance. With time, they may become impregnated with calcium salts.

The area enclosed within the **large rectangle** (Fig. 1), is shown at higher magnification in Figure 2, and shows some characteristic features of the tube-alveoli. In many places the epithelium bulges into the lumen; and sometimes the top of an epithelial fold is cut to give the impression of an island of cells in a lumen (**arrows**). Large numbers of closely packed nuclei are seen when a fold is cut obliquely or crosswise (**arrowheads**). This is one of the characteristic features of the prostate gland epithelium.

Figure 3 shows the epithelial cells at higher magnification. The epithelium consists mainly of columnar cells, although basal cells are also present. For this reason, the epithelium is classified as pseudostratified columnar. The columnar cells are described as containing secretion granules and lipid droplets, but these are not always evident. Many cells possess apical cytoplasmic protrusions (**arrows**) which seemingly break off into the lumen.

The various tube-alveoli are surrounded by a fibroelastic stroma containing smooth muscle (fibromuscular stroma). The smooth muscle is not organized in a way which sug-

KEY

BV, blood vessels
Cap, capsule
N, nerve bundle
PC, prostatic concretion
SM, smooth muscle
SM(L), smooth muscle, longitudinal section
SM(X), smooth muscle, cross section
arrowheads, nuclear clusters
arrows (Fig. 2), epithelial "islands"
arrows (Fig. 3), apical cytoplasmic protrusions

Fig. 1 (human), x 40; Fig. 2 (human), x 145; Fig. 3 (human), x 640; Fig. 4 (human), x 160.

gests that it belongs to any single tube or alveolus, as in the epididymis, but rather appears to be randomly dispersed in the stroma. In Figure 1, the staining of the muscle differs from the staining of the connective tissue. The muscle appears as the elongated dark fibers or as dark oval bodies (**SM**), in either case surrounded by a more extensive continuous phase of lighter-staining connective tissue. Some bundles of smooth muscle are also to be seen in the capsule. The **upper rectangle** in Figure 1 is examined at higher magnification in Figure 4. This shows the smooth muscle cut in longitudinal [**SM(L)**] and cross section [**SM(X)**], and also reveals the presence of a nerve bundle (**N**). The nerve stains very much like the connective tissue, but can be recognized by virtue of its organization and the presence of a perineurial sheath. These features would be more evident at higher magnifications.

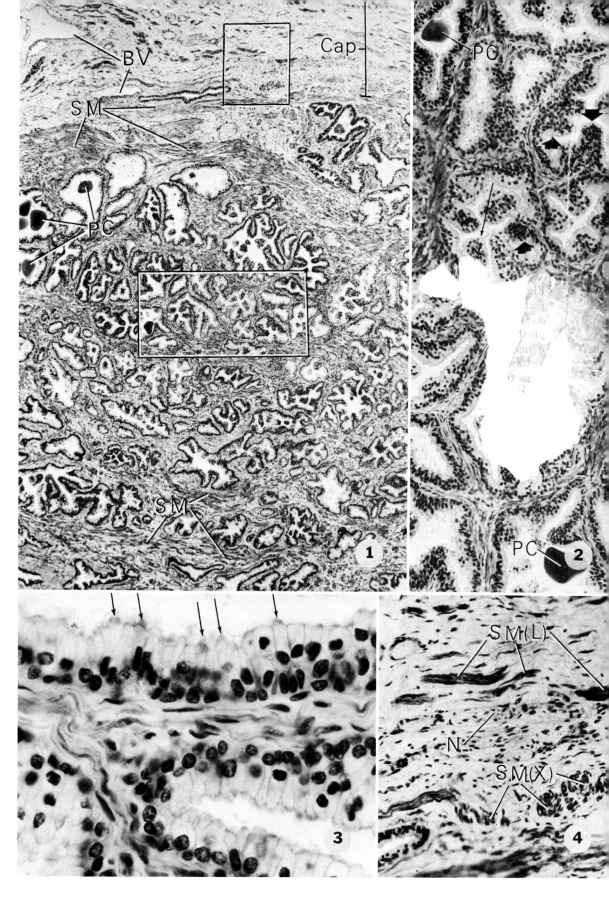

PLATE 13-5

14 FEMALE REPRODUCTIVE SYSTEM

THE FEMALE REPRODUCTIVE SYSTEM consists of the ovaries and a system of related ducts, the external genitalia, and the mammary glands. Under the influence of the pituitary gland the ovaries undergo cycles of activity. Like the testes, the ovaries are cytogenic glands inasmuch as they produce the ova; they are also endocrine glands since they produce estrogen and progesterone.

The ovarian hormones have very profound and widespread effects throughout the body at the time of puberty. They bring about the development of the female secondary sex characteristics and the full development of the reproductive ducts and genitalia. In the mature female, ovarian hormones bring about marked cyclical changes in the female duct system, especially in the uterus. Ovarian hormones are also involved in bringing about alterations in the mammary gland that lead to its becoming a lactating organ.

Although the *uterus* does serve certain duct functions, it is especially adapted to serve as the organ in which the fetus develops. During pregnancy the uterus participates with the embryonic tissue in forming the *placenta*. One of the chief functions of the placenta is to provide for the exchange of substances between the maternal and fetal circulations. At the end of gestation, the uterus undergoes contractions which expel the fetus, placenta, and contiguous membranes. The placenta also produces two protein hormones, chorionic gonadotropin and somatomammotropin and two steroid hormones, estrogen and progesterone. The placenta lacks certain enzymes for the complete synthesis of estrogen. In order to synthesize estrogen, the placenta requires a steroid precursor from the fetal adrenal gland.

Plate 14-1. OVARY I

The outer part (cortex) of a young, but sexually mature, ovary is shown in Figure 1 at low power. The surface consists of a single layer of epithelial cells. A higher magnification is required for their identification. Immediately under the surface epithelium is a layer of rather uniform thickness called the *tunica albuginea* (**TA**). Deep to the tunica albuginea and surrounded by a highly cellular connective tissue stroma are numerous spherical structures of uniform size, called the primordial (unilaminar) *follicles*.

At regular intervals, under the influence of pituitary hormones, some of the primordial follicles begin to undergo changes that lead to the development of a mature ovum. These changes include a proliferation of cells and total enlargement of the follicle up to the point where one follicle becomes mature. The ovum in the mature follicle is then released by a process called ovulation. The other follicles which began to proliferate at the same time degenerate. Therefore, it is not uncommon to see follicles in various stages of development or regression in the ovary. At least two developing follicles (**arrows**) and two regressing (*atretic*) follicles (**arrowheads**) are present in Fig. 1. The **large rectangle,** which includes one of each kind of follicle, is illustrated at higher magnification in Plate 14-2.

The surface of the ovary is shown in Figure 2. It consists of simple cuboidal epithelium and is referred to as *germinal epithelium* (**GE**). This epithelium has no striking surface specializations or cytoplasmic constituents that can be seen in routine sections. It is continuous with the *peritoneum* at the *mesovarium*. Whereas the peritoneum with its surface of squamous cells has a slick glistening appearance, the ovary with its surface of cuboidal cells has a dull appearance. The term germinal epithelium persists from the time when it was erroneously thought that the surface epithelium gave rise to the primordial follicles.

Figure 2 also shows the connective tissue which constitutes the tunica albuginea (**TA**). This connective tissue is continuous with the stroma of the ovary. Although it contains a large number of cells it is less cellular than the stroma.

KEY

FC, follicle cells
GE, germinal epithelium
N, oocyte nuclei
TA, tunica albuginea
X, oocyte with nucleus not shown
arrowheads, atretic follicles
arrows, developing follicles

Fig. 1 (monkey), x 65; Fig. 2 and 3 (monkey), x 640.

The unilaminar follicles within the **small rectangle** of Figure 1 are shown in Figure 3 at higher magnification. Each unilaminar follicle consists of a large *oocyte* which is completely surrounded by a single layer of flattened *follicle cells* (**FC**). The nucleus (**N**) of the oocyte is large and usually in an eccentric position. Because of its eccentric position it may not be included in the plane of section. Some oocytes (**X**) will therefore appear to be without a nucleus. Figure 3 also shows some characteristics of the cellular stroma. The stromal cell nuclei are spindle shaped and the cells appear to be arranged in bundles.

At the time of birth, all of the primordial follicles that will be available to the individual are already present in the cortex of the ovary. Moreover, in the newborn ovary, some of the follicles may show signs of development owing to the influence of maternal hormones which may pass through the placenta. Therefore, the ovary of a newborn may resemble the young mature ovary that is illustrated in Figure 1.

The inner part of the ovary, the medulla is continuous with the hilus. The medulla contains the larger blood and lymphatic vessels, smooth muscle cells and interstitial cells. The latter are clusters, or cords, of epitheloid cells which resemble endocrine glands in their cytological structure and in their relationship to blood vessels. Interstitial cells are present periodically in the mature ovary and they are thought to derive from the theca interna of degenerating secondary follicles (see Plate 14-2). In the human, interstitial cells are implicated in the synthesis of estrogens.

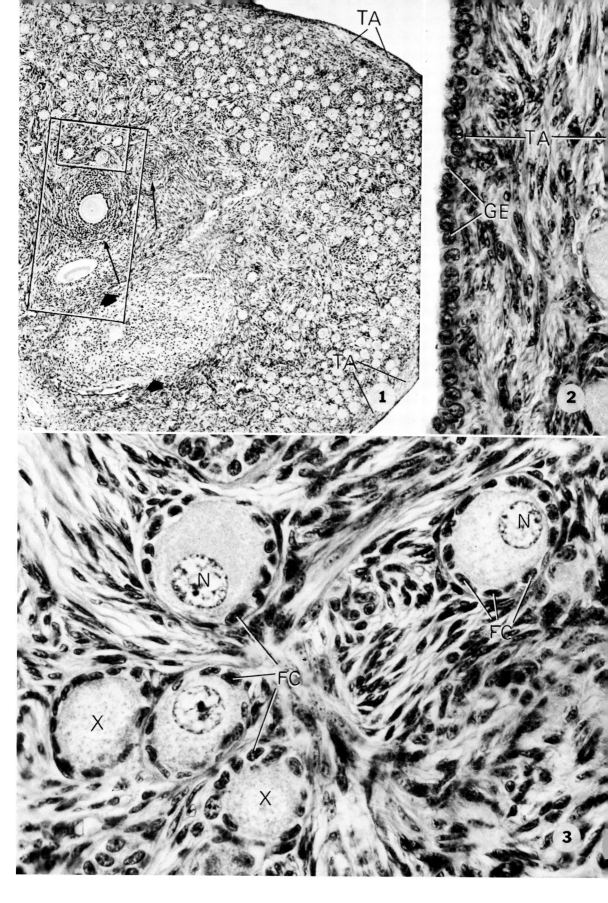

PLATE 14-1

Plate 14-2. Ovary II

At the onset of sexual maturity in the female the pituitary gland elaborates a hormone (*follicle-stimulating hormone, FSH*) which stimulates the development of primordial follicles into mature follicles. Under the influence of FSH, the single layer of investing follicle cells proliferates and becomes multilayered. The oocyte and its nucleus also enlarge, and a homogeneous appearing component, called the *zona pellucida* (**ZP**), forms between the oocyte and the follicle cells. A follicle undergoing these changes is called a primary follicle and is shown in Figure 1. This figure shows the area within the larger **rectangle** in Figure 1 of Plate 14-1 at higher magnification. Note the large number of follicle cells (**FC**) which now surround the enlarged oocyte. These cells developed from an original single layer of flattened cells.

The follicle cells continue to proliferate and form a rather large ovoid cellular mass with the ovum on one side. Small fluid-filled spaces appear between the follicle cells; these ultimately become an extremely large single cavity called the *antrum* or *follicular cavity*. A growing follicle in which these changes are occurring is called an antral, or a secondary follicle. A well-developed secondary follicle is shown in Figure 2. The ovum is located at one end in a mound of follicle cells called the *cumulus oophorus* (**CO**). The remaining follicle cells that surround the cavity (**Cav**) are now referred to as the *membrana granulosa* (**MG**) or as *granulosa cells*. A precipitate of the follicular fluid is within the cavity.

A higher magnification of the cumulus oophorus (Fig. 3) shows that the cells immediately in contact with the oocyte have a columnar shape. The apical cytoplasm of these columnar cells is just discernible (**arrow**). They are in correct relation to the oocyte only at the top; the space immediately below and to the left of the ovum is an artefact. A distinct zona pellucida (**ZP**) can be seen around the ovum. When the ovum is discharged, the columnar and other cumulus cells remain adherent to the oocyte. This surrounding ring of cells is referred to as the *corona radiata*.

The connective tissue around the secondary follicle also undergoes changes and it is subsequently referred to as the *theca*. Numerous

KEY

AF, atretic follicle
Cav, follicular cavity
CO, cumulus oophorus
FC, follicle cells
MG, membrana granulosa (stratum granulosum)
TE, theca externa
TI, theca interna
ZP, zona pellucida
arrow, apical cytoplasm of cells surrounding oocyte

Fig. 1 (monkey), x 640; Fig. 2 (monkey), x 65; Fig. 3 (monkey), x 160.

small blood vessels are present in the part of the theca, the *theca interna* (**TI**), immediately adjacent to the follicle cells. Some of the cells in this layer have round nuclei, are close to their neighbors, and may be described as being epithelioid. With the electron microscope these cells display the characteristics of endocrine cells; they produce estrogens. The outer part of the theca is more fibrous and is called the *theca externa* (**TE**). In contrast to the theca interna, the cells of the theca externa are more flattened. The boundary between the theca interna and theca externa is not sharply delineated.

Although a number of follicles begin the above-mentioned series of developmental changes, usually only one, the *Graafian follicle*, reaches maturity and will discharge an ovum. The others undergo regressive changes and degenerate. Therefore, a section of an ovary typically includes a number of regressing or *atretic follicles* (**AF**) (Figs. 1 and 2). In a regressing follicle, the oocyte degenerates. In addition, the theca cells proliferate and invade the granulosa cells so that, in some respects, a regressing follicle resembles a developing corpus luteum. However, the zona pellucida persists for some time in the atretic follicle, and when included in the section (**ZP**, Fig. 1), enables one to distinguish it from a corpus luteum. In these cases, the remains of the zona pellucida appears as an irregular homogeneous crescent or ring in a clear space that was formerly occupied by the degenerated oocyte. Ultimately, stromal elements replace the cellular elements.

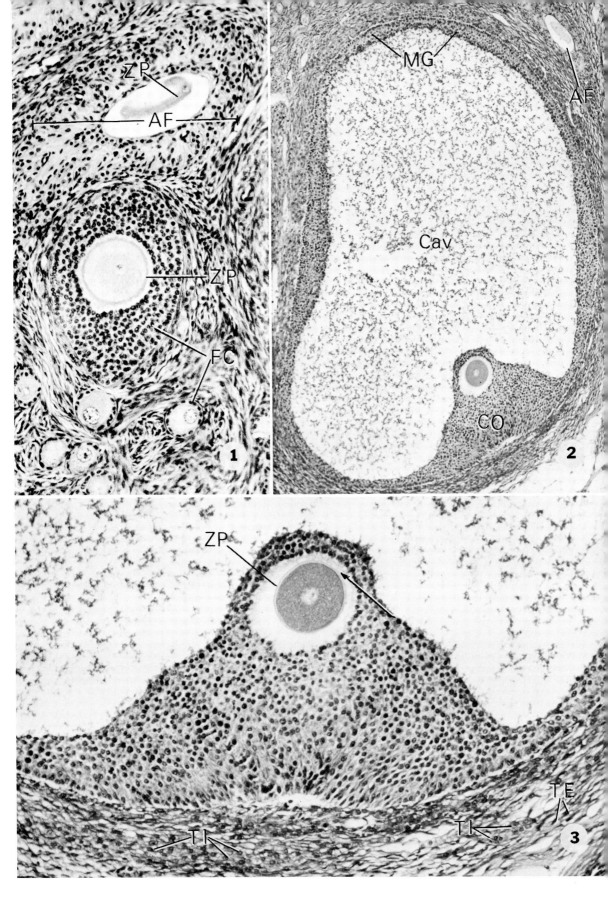

PLATE 14-2

Plate 14.3. CORPUS LUTEUM

After the oocyte and the surrounding cumulus cells are discharged from the mature ovarian follicle (ovulation), the remaining follicle cells (membrana granulosa) and the adjacent connective tissue (theca interna) undergo changes that result in the formation of a new functional unit, the *corpus luteum.*

The cells that previously constituted the membrana granulosa of the follicle undergo considerable enlargement and are then called *granulosa lutein cells* (**GLC**). They form an extremely thick and folded layer that surrounds the remains of the former follicular cavity (**Cav**) (Fig. 1). The cavity appears stellate because of the folded nature of the granulosa layer. The cavity usually contains serous material and variable amounts of fibrin. Immediately after the rupture of the follicle, however, it may also contain some blood. Subsequently, the cavity is invaded by connective tissue. Some connective tissue (**CT**) can already be seen at the periphery of the cavity shown in Figure 1.

At about the same time, the theca interna also undergoes changes. The cells of this layer become enlarged. They come to occupy the outer depressions (**arrows**) that are formed by the folded layer of granulosa lutein cells. These epithelioid cells having developed from the theca interna are now called *theca lutein cells* (**TLC**) and are an integral part of the corpus luteum (Fig. 2). Blood vessels (**BV**) accompany the theca lutein cells into the outer folds of the granulosa layer.

It should be noted that one can readily identify and distinguish between theca lutein cells (**TLC**) and granulosa lutein (**GLC**) cells on the basis of location. The granulosa lutein cells are related predominantly to the stellate-shaped former cavity, whereas the theca lutein cells are related predominantly to the outer connective tissue (**CT**) that surrounds the total structure.

When examined at higher magnification (Fig. 3), the granulosa lutein cells (**GLC**) can be seen to contain a large spherical nucleus and a large amount of cytoplasm. The cytoplasm contains lipid and pigment, therefore the name, corpus luteum. However, neither pigment nor lipid are evident in routine H & E sections because they are lost during tissue preparation. Theca lutein cells (**TLC**) also

KEY

BV, blood vessels
Cav, former follicular cavity
CT, connective tissue
GLC, granulosa lutein cells
TLC, theca lutein cells
arrows (Fig. 1), theca lutein cells
arrows (Fig. 3), nuclei of connective tissue and
  vascular cells

Fig. 1 (human), x 16; Fig. 2 (human), x 65; Fig. 3 (human), x 160.

possess spherical nuclei, but they are smaller than those of the granulosa lutein cells. Because of the difference in cell size, the nuclei of theca lutein cells are closer to each other than nuclei of granulosa lutein cells. Moreover, because of the smaller size, the theca lutein nuclei stain more intensely.

Connective tissue cells and small blood vessels from the theca externa ultimately come to invade the layer of granulosa lutein cells. The nuclei of the invading connective tissue and vascular cells appear flattened and elongated (**arrows**) in contrast to the round nuclei of the theca and granulosa lutein cells.

The changes whereby the ruptured ovarian follicle is transformed into a corpus luteum occur under the stimulus of a pituitary hormone (luteinizing hormone). The corpus luteum in turn elaborates another hormone, progesterone, which has a profound effect on the estrogen-primed uterus. If pregnancy occurs, the corpus luteum remains functional. However, if the ovum is not fertilized, the corpus luteum regresses after having reached a point of peak development, roughly two weeks after ovulation. The regressing cellular components of the corpus luteum are replaced by fibrous tissue and the structure is then called a *corpus albicans.*

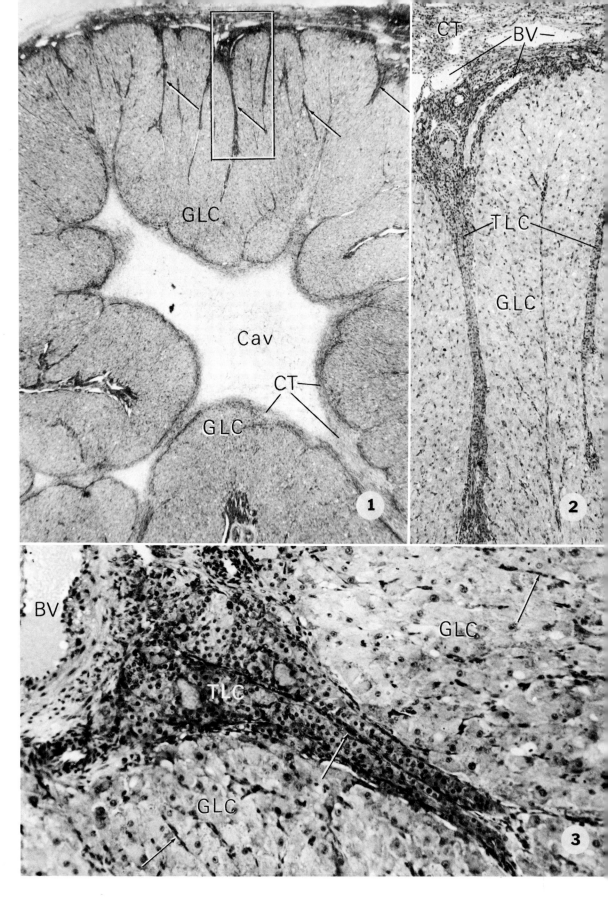

PLATE 14-3

Plate 14-4. Uterine Tube

The *uterine tubes (oviducts)* are joined to the uterus and extend to the ovaries where they present an open flared end for entry of the ovum. Fertilization of the ovum usually occurs in the uterine tube, and for the first several days, the developing embryonic cells are contained in the tube as they travel to the uterus. The tube undergoes cyclical changes along with those of the uterus but they are not nearly as pronounced. The tubal changes primarily involve the epithelial cells. They increase in height during the middle of the cycle, just about the time the ovum will be passing through the tube, but they become reduced during the premenstrual period. Some of the epithelial cells are ciliated; the number of ciliated cells increases during the follicular phase of the ovarian cycle.

The uterine tube varies in size and degree of mucosal folding along its length. The mucosal folds are more numerous near the open end and less numerous near the uterus. Near the uterus the tube is narrow and referred to as the *isthmus.* Then for about two thirds of its length it is in an expanded form and is referred to as the *ampulla.* Near the opening the tube flares outward and is called the *infundibulum.* It has fringed folded edges that are called *fimbria.*

A cross section through the ampulla of the tube is shown in the **inset** (middle of page). Many mucosal folds project into the lumen, and the complicated nature of the folds is evident by the variety of profiles that are seen. The remainder of the wall consists of smooth muscle and connective tissue.

The wall of the uterine tube is shown at higher magnification in Figure 1. It is described as consisting of a *mucosa* (**Muc**), a *muscularis* (**Mus**), and a *serosa* (not shown). The mucosa has a surface of simple columnar epithelium. Two kinds of cells are present (Fig. 2), nonciliated cells and ciliated cells (**Cil**). The ciliated cells have a round nucleus and a relatively clear cytoplasm. The cilia are clearly seen in Figure 2. The aggregation of basal bodies appears as the dense band at the base of the cilia. The nonciliated cells are also called *peg cells.* They have elongated nuclei and sometimes appear to be squeezed between the ciliated cells (**arrows,** Fig. 1). It may be that the ciliated and non-ciliated cells

KEY

BV, blood vessels
CT, connective tissue
Cil, ciliated cells
Muc, mucosa
Mus, muscularis
arrowheads, longitudinally sectioned smooth muscle
arrows, isolated peg cells

Fig. 1 (human), x 160; inset (human), x 16; Fig. 2 (human), x 640.

represent different functional states of the same cell type.

The connective tissue (**CT**) contains cells whose nuclei are arranged in a typically random manner. They vary in shape, being elongated, oval, or round. Their cytoplasm cannot be distinguished from the intercellular material (Fig. 2). Numerous lymphatic channels are in the mucosa of the oviduct but they are difficult to identify in routine H & E sections. The character of the connective tissue is essentially the same from the epithelium to the muscularis, and for this reason, no submucosa is described.

The muscularis (**Mus**) consists of smooth muscle which forms a relatively thick layer of circular fibers (Fig. 1) and a thinner outer layer of longitudinal fibers. The layers are not clearly delineated and no sharp boundary separates the two. In comparing the muscle and connective tissue the following points should be noted: the connective tissue is immediately under the epithelial surface and contains cells whose nuclei appear randomly arranged; in contrast, the smooth muscle is removed from the epithelium and the nuclei of the cells are oriented with respect to each other. When cut longitudinally the nuclei of muscle cells appear elongated, about the same size and roughly parallel (**arrowheads**). When cut in cross section the nuclei appear spherical. Some blood vessels (**BV**) are seen in the muscularis.

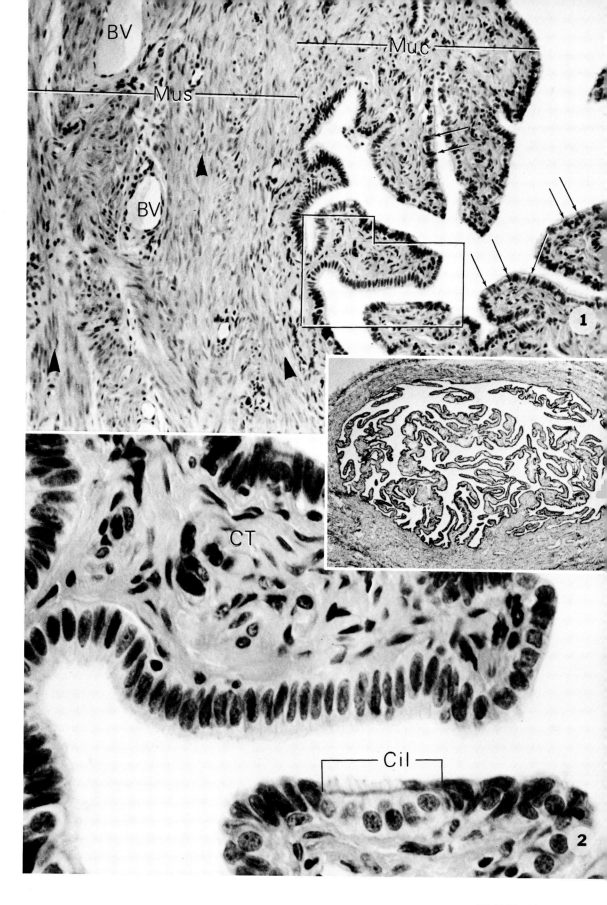

BV

Muc

Mus

BV

CT

Cil

1

2

PLATE 14-4

Plate 14-5. UTERUS

The mucous membrane of the uterus is called the *endometrium*. It is comprised of simple columnar epithelium and an extremely cellular connective tissue. Some of the epithelial cells are ciliated. Large numbers of tubular glands extend from the surface epithelium into the underlying connective tissue and the extent of the glands corresponds to the thickness of the endometrium. Deep to the endometrium is a thick layer of smooth muscle and connective tissue which constitutes the *myometrium*. The muscle cells are organized as interlacing bundles, separated by the connective tissue. External to the myometrium is either connective tissue or, over much of the uterine surface, a serosal cover, namely, the *visceral peritoneum*.

The uterus undergoes cyclical changes, during part of which implantation is possible. If implantation does not occur, the state of readiness is not maintained and much of the endometrium is sloughed off, constituting the menstrual flow. The part of the endometrium that is lost is referred to as the stratum *funtionalis*. The part that is retained is called the stratum *basalis*. The stratum basalis is the deepest part, and is close to the myometrium.

After the stratum functionalis is sloughed off, resurfacing of the raw tissue occurs. The epithelium (**Ep**) for this come from the glands (**Gl**) that are left in the stratum basalis (**SB**). Figure 1 shows the endometrium as it appears when resurfacing is almost complete. The endometrium is relatively thin at this time and over half of it consists of the stratum basalis. Below the endometrium is the myometrium (**M**) in which are a large number of blood vessels (**BV**).

Under the influence of estrogen, the various components of the endometrium proliferate (*proliferative stage*) so that the total thickness of the endometrium is increased (Fig. 2). The glands (**Gl**) are rather long and fairly straight within the stratum functionalis (**SF**). The connection of some glands to the surface epithelium (**Ep**) is shown (**arrows**). The stratum basalis (**SB**) remains essentially unaffected by the estrogen and appears much the same as in Figure 1. The stratum functionalis (**SF**), on the other hand, increases in thickness and comes to constitute about 4/5 of the endometrial thickness as shown in Figure 2.

KEY

BV, blood vessels
CT, connective tissue
SB, stratum basalis
Ep, epithelium
Gl, glands
M, myometrium
SB, stratum basalis
SF, stratum functionalis
arrows, junction of gland and surface epithelium

Fig. 1 (human), 40; Fig. 2 (monkey), x 16; Fig. 3 (human), x 65; Fig. 4 (human), x 160.

After estrogen acts on the endometrium to bring about the above changes, progesterone brings about additional changes (*secretory stage*). The endometrial thickness increases further and again changes are conspicuous in the stratum functionalis. The glands (**Gl**) assume a corkscrew shape, and thus they have a sinuous appearance in a section (Fig. 3). During the secretory stage the cells accumulate glycogen and the endometrium is ready for implantation. Note, however, that the basal layer is less changed.

The epithelium and supporting connective tissue stroma (secretory stage) are shown at higher magnification in Figure 4. Note the columnar epithelium (**Ep**) and the highly cellular connective tissue (**CT**). The surface epithelium (not shown) is also columnar, except that in some patches it is ciliated. The stromal cells are capable of transforming into decidual cells. They require the sequential action of estrogen and progesterone in order to develop this potential. The actual stimulus for the transformation is the implanting blastocyst. (Artificial stimuli can also induce the transformation.)

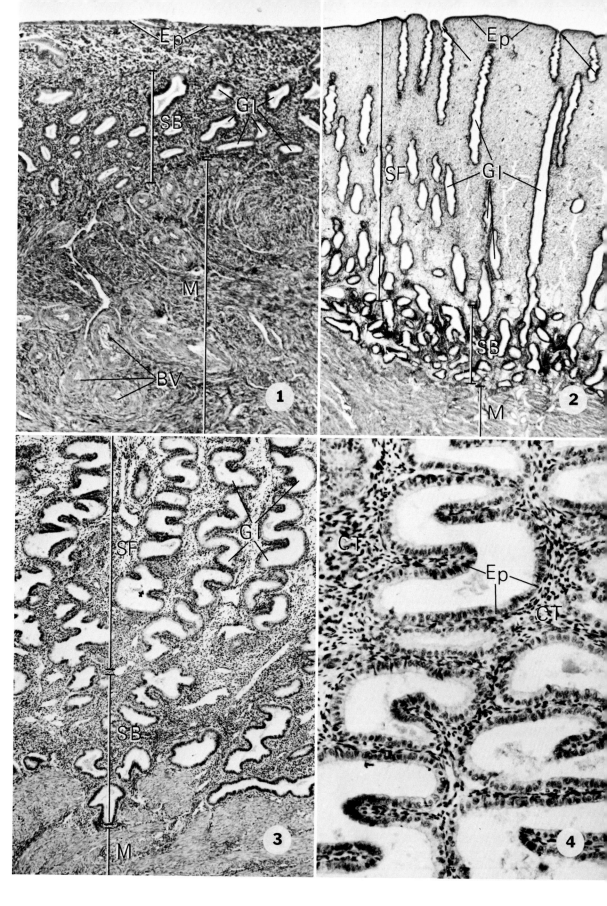

PLATE 14-5

Plate 14-6. THE CERVIX

The *cervix* is the narrow or constricted portion of the uterus. It projects into the anterior wall of the vagina. A canal traverses the cervix and provides for communication between the vaginal canal and the uterine cavity. In its general features, the structure of the cervix resembles the remainder of the uterus in that it consists of a mucosa (endometrium) and a myometrium. There are, however, some differences in the mucosa.

A section through the cervix is shown in Figure 1. The plane of section passes through the long axis of the *cervical canal;* the lumen of the cervical canal (**CC**) is on the right and the *vaginal canal* (**VC**) is above.

The mucosa (**Muc**) of the cervix differs according to the cavity it faces. The three small **rectangles** in Figure 1 delineate representative areas of the mucosa which are shown at higher magnification in Figures 2, 3, and 4. Each figure illustrates the essential features of the epithelium in the different portions of the cervix. The portion which projects into the vagina, referred to as the *portio vaginalis,* is surfaced by stratified squamous epithelium (Fig. 2). The epithelial–connective tissue junction presents an even contour (in contrast to the irregular profile seen in the vagina). In other respects the epithelium has the same general features as the vaginal epithelium. Another similarity is that the epithelial surface of the portio vaginalis undergoes cyclical changes similar to those of the vagina in response to ovarian hormones (see page 234). The mucosa of the portio vaginalis, like that of the vagina, is devoid of glands.

The portion of the cervical mucosa which faces the cervical canal is surfaced by columnar epithelium (Fig. 4). An abrupt change from stratified squamous epithelium to columnar epithelium occurs at the ostium of the uterus, i.e., where the portio vaginalis meets the cervical canal (Fig. 3). A large number of round cells, most of which are lymphocytes, are present in the connective tissue. This is not an uncommon occurrence. Glands extend from the surface of the cervical canal into the underlying connective tissue. The cervical glands differ from those in the uterus proper in that they branch (**arrows**, Fig. 1). One of the glands seen in Figure 1 has become markedly dilated. [It is not uncommon

for cervical glands to develop into cysts (**Cy**) owing to obstruction in the duct. Such cysts are referred to as *Nabothian cysts.*] The endometrium of the cervix does not undergo the cyclical loss of tissue that is characteristic of the body and fundus of the uterus. However, the amount and character of its mucous secretion varies at different times of the uterine cycle.

The myometrium forms the major thickness of the cervix. It consists of interweaving bundles of smooth muscle cells situated in a more extensive, continuous network of fibrous connective tissue.

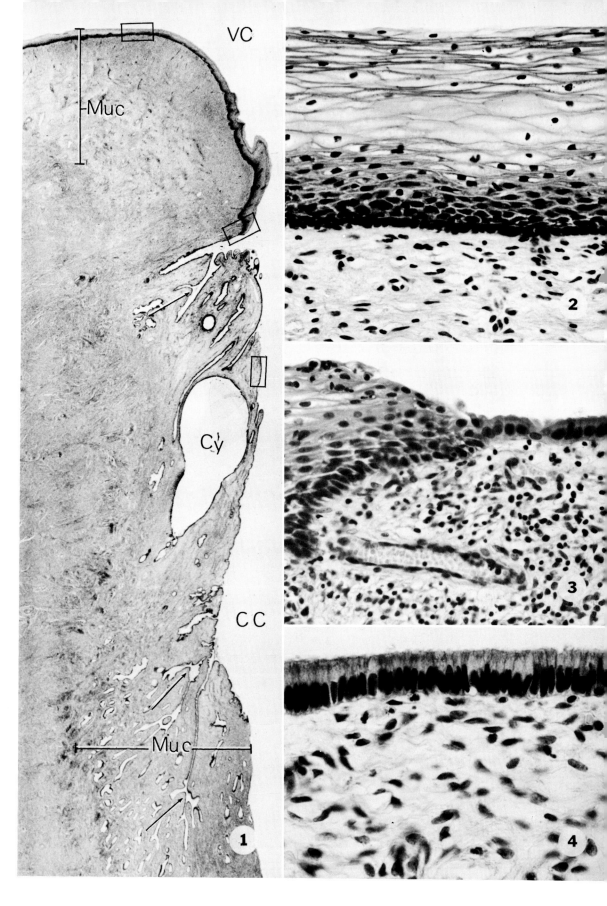

VC

Muc

Cy

CC

Muc

1

2

3

4

PLATE 14-6

Plate 14-7. VAGINA

The vagina is a fibromuscular tube which forms the opening of the female reproductive tract to the exterior. The wall of the vagina (Fig. 1) consists of three layers: a mucous membrane, a muscular layer, and an outer adventitia. The mucous membrane, in turn, consists of stratified squamous epithelium (**Ep**) and an underlying connective tissue (**CT**). The boundary between the two is readily identified, owing to the more intense staining of the deep portion of the epithelium. Connective tissue papillae project into the under surface of the epithelium, giving the epithelial-connective tissue junction an uneven appearance. The papillae (**arrows**) may be cut obliquely or in cross section, and appear as connective tissue islands within the epithelium.

The muscular layer (**Mus**) of the vaginal wall is made up of smooth muscle, except at the opening of the tube (ostium) where a ring of striated muscle (bulbocavernosus) is present. The smooth muscle is arranged in two ill-defined layers. The outer one being somewhat longitudinal. The area marked by the **circle** in the upper left of Figure 1 is shown at higher magnification in the **inset** to illustrate the smooth muscle cells. They are organized as small interlacing bundles surrounded by connective tissue.

The **rectangle** in Figure 1 marks an area of vaginal epithelium and connective tissue which is examined at higher magnification in Figure 2. The epithelium is characteristically thick. Although keratohyaline granules may be present in the superficial cells, keratinization (in the human) does not occur. In this connection, nuclei can be observed throughout the entire thickness of the vaginal epithelium.

One of the features of vaginal epithelium which aids in its identification is that, except for the deepest layers, the cells have an empty appearance. This is due, in part, to the fact that the cells accumulate glycogen as they migrate toward the surface, and in the preparation of routine H & E sections, the glycogen is lost.

Vaginal epithelium is influenced by ovarian hormones and undergoes cyclical changes which correspond to the ovarian cycle. In rodents, these changes are manifest by marked

KEY

BV, blood vessels
CT, connective tissue
Ep, epithelium
L, leucocytes
Mus, muscular layer
arrows, connective tissue papillae

Fig. 1 (human), x 40, (inset), x 250; Fig. 2 (human), x 180.

alterations in the cells. In the human, however, the epithelial changes are less pronounced, but nevertheless evident. For example, the amount of glycogen increases under the influence of estrogen; moreover, the desquamation, which the epithelium continuously undergoes, increases under the influence of progesterone.

The connective tissue immediately under the vaginal epithelium contains large numbers of cells, many of which are lymphocytes and granulocyte neutrophils (**L**). The lymphocytes are characterized by their deep-staining, round nuclei. The number of leucocytes fluctuates during the ovarian cycle. The cells invade the epithelium around the time of menstruation and they appear along with the epithelial cells in vaginal smears. The connective tissue includes large amounts of elastic material in addition to collagen fibers; however, this is not evident in H & E sections. The connective tissue also characteristically contains a large number of blood vessels (**BV**).

The histological identification of the vagina should take into account the following points: 1) the epithelium does not keratinize and, except for the deepest layers, the cells appear to be empty in routine H & E sections; 2) the mucous membrane contains neither glands nor a muscularis mucosae; 3) the muscle is chiefly smooth and not well ordered. (In contrast, the muscle of the oral cavity, pharynx, and upper part of the esophagus is striated; in its more distal portion, where the esophagus contains smooth muscle, it can be easily distinguished from the vagina by the presence of a muscularis mucosae.)

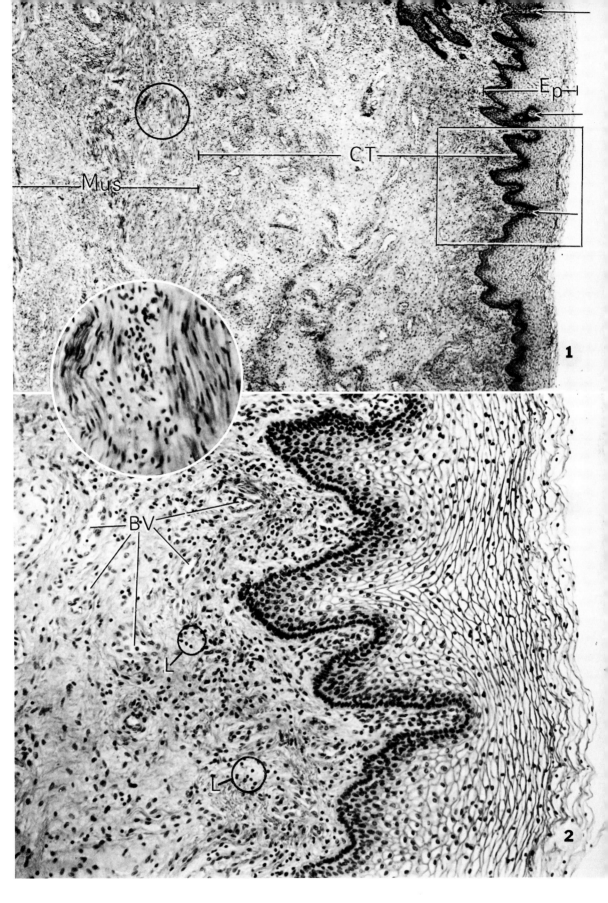

Mus

CT

Ep

BV

L

L

1

2

PLATE 14-7

Plate 14-8. MAMMARY GLAND, INACTIVE

The *mammary glands* are branched tubulo-alveolar glands which develop from the epidermis and come to lie in the subcutaneous tissue (superficial fascia). They begin to develop at puberty in the female, but do not reach a full functional state until after pregnancy. The glands also develop more or less slightly in the male at puberty. However, the development is limited and the glands usually remain in a stabilized state.

Figure 1 is a section through an inactive gland. The parenchyma is sparse and consists mainly of duct elements. Four longitudinally cut ducts (**D**) are shown in the center of the field. A small lumen can be seen in each. A resting lobule is to the right of the ducts and is shown at higher magnification in Figure 2.

The epithelial elements of the *resting mammary gland* are contained in a loose, cellular connective tissue [**CT(L)**] which is readily distinguished from the more dense connective tissue [**CT(D)**] beyond the area of the lobule. Note the greater number of cells in the loose connective tissue in contrast to the lesser number in the dense connective tissue. Note also that the dense connective tissue contains fibers which appear thicker. Loose irregular connective tissue also surrounds the duct elements, but it is not as clearly delineated from the dense connective tissue as it is in the lobules. Variable amounts of adipose tissue (**AT**) are found in the dense connective tissue.

The epithelial cells (**Ep**) within the resting lobule (Fig. 2) are regarded as being chiefly duct elements. It is generally considered that alveoli are not present, however, their precursors are represented as cellular thickenings of the duct wall. The epithelium of the resting lobule is cuboidal and in addition, myoepithelial cells are present. Some of the nuclei at the periphery of the epithelium belong to myoepithelial cells.

During pregnancy the glands begin to proliferate. This can be thought of as a dual process in which ducts proliferate and alveoli spring from the ducts. Figure 3 shows a lobule and its ducts in an early state of proliferation. The *proliferating gland* shows many epithelial sprouts from the enlarged duct (**arrows**). In contrast, the resting duct (Fig. 1) shows smooth contours without any conspicuous

KEY

AT, adipose tissue
CT(D), dense connective tissue
CT(L), loose connective tissue
D, duct
Ep, epithelium
arrows, epithelial sprouts

Fig. 1 (human), x 65; Fig. 2 (human), x 160; Fig. 3 (human), x 65.

branching or evidence of proliferation. In the proliferating gland, the loose connective tissue appears less prominent.

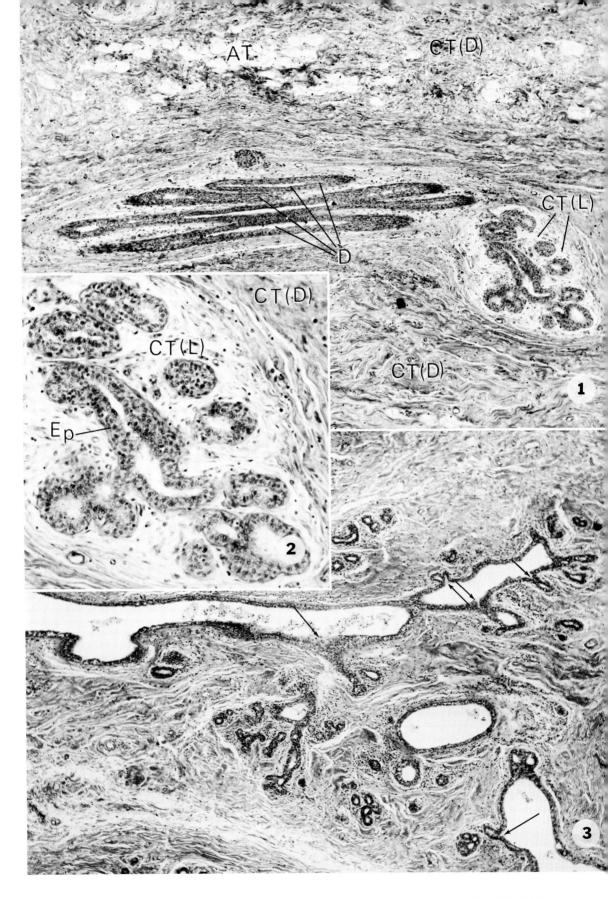

PLATE 14-8

Plate 14-9. Mammary Gland, Proliferative

Whereas the development of the duct elements in the mammary gland is well marked during the early proliferative period, the development of the alveolar elements becomes conspicuous at a later time. Figure 1 shows several lobules (L) at a later stage of proliferation than is shown in the preceding plate. Distinct alveoli (A) can now be recognized. These are all joined to a duct (D), although the connections are usually not seen in a two-dimensional section. Lobules are separated by dense connective tissue septa (S), and some ducts can be recognized as being in an interlobular location. Although alveolar development is well under way (Fig. 1), some regions of the gland are still in a relatively early stage of proliferation. For example, the inset (Fig. 1) shows where epithelial sprouting is occurring along the length of a duct (arrowheads).

A higher magnification of one of the proliferating lobules is provided in Figure 2. Numerous alveoli (A) are evident. The alveoli consist of a single layer of cuboidal epithelium as well as *myoepithelial cells.* A small amount of precipitate is located in the lumen of some of the alveoli. This represents the early secretory activity of the cells.

The duct (D) through which the alveoli will discharge their product is shown on the left, almost like a stalk. It can be recognized because of its location and its elongated profile. Some of the flattened nuclei that are at the epithelial–connective tissue junction of the duct belong to myoepithelial cells.

The connective tissue (CT) surrounding the alveoli is loose, and contains delicate collagenous fibers and large numbers of round cells (arrows). The identity of these cells is difficult to establish at this magnification, though most are probably lymphocytes.

KEY

A, alveoli
CT, connective tissue
D, duct
L, lobule
S, septa
arrowheads, epithelial sprouts
arrows, round connective tissue cells

Fig. 1 (human), x 65, (inset), x 160; Fig. 2 (human), x 160.

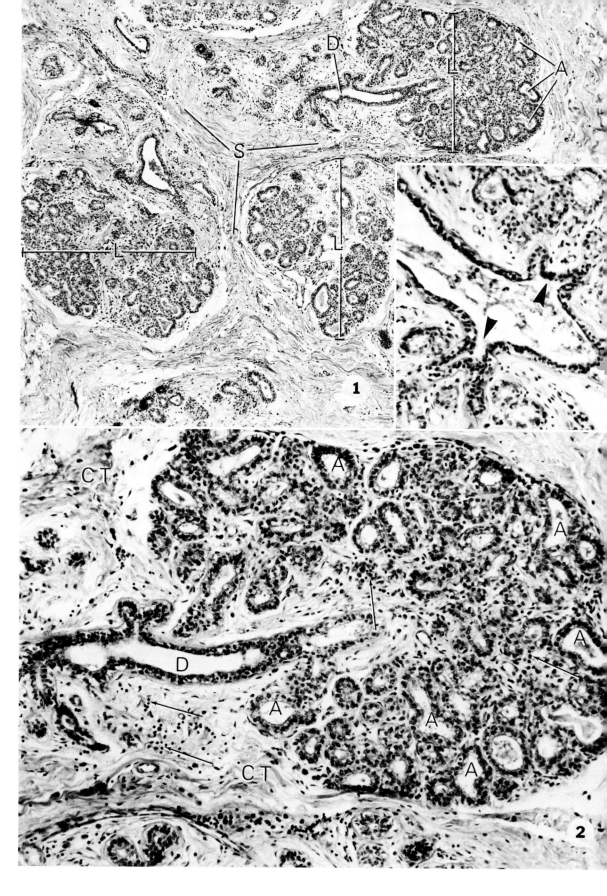

PLATE 14-9

Plate 14-10. Mammary Gland, Lactating

The *lactating mammary gland* is characterized by the presence of large numbers of alveoli (Fig. 1). Many of these appear as oval or spherical profiles and in this respect, on cursory examination, the gland is easy to confuse with the thyroid gland. However, all of the alveoli in the mammary gland are joined to a duct and often the place where several alveoli open into a central channel can be seen. These connections represent branchings of a terminal duct system. The presence of connected alveoli (**asterisks**) enable one to identify the lactating mammary gland and distinguish it from thyroid tissue even if the duct elements are not conspicuous. Sections of mammary glands usually include duct elements, but the small ducts are difficult to identify since they resemble the alveoli.

A large duct (**D**), easily recognized by its size, is in the upper left of the figure. A number of connective tissue septa (**S**) separate the alveoli of neighboring lobules. Large blood vessels (**BV**) are within the connective tissue septa.

Figure 2 shows several alveoli at higher magnification. The alveoli of lactating mammary glands are made up of cuboidal epithelium and myoepithelial cells. Frequently, some precipitated product can be seen within the lumen of the alveolus. Only a small amount of connective tissue separates the neighboring alveoli. Capillaries (**Cap**) can be seen in this connective tissue.

Figure 3 is a special preparation showing some of the lipid that is present in the mammary secretion. The lipid appears as the black spheres of various size within the alveolar lumen as well as within most of the cells. In its production the lipid first appears as small droplets within the cells. These droplets become larger and ultimately they are discharged into the alveolar lumen.

The lymphatic vessels of the mammary glands, which are important clinically, are not usually evident in histological sections.

KEY

BV, blood vessels
Cap, capillaries
D, duct
S, septa
asterisks, branchings of terminal duct system

Fig. 1 (human), x 160; Figs. 2 and 3 (human), x 640.

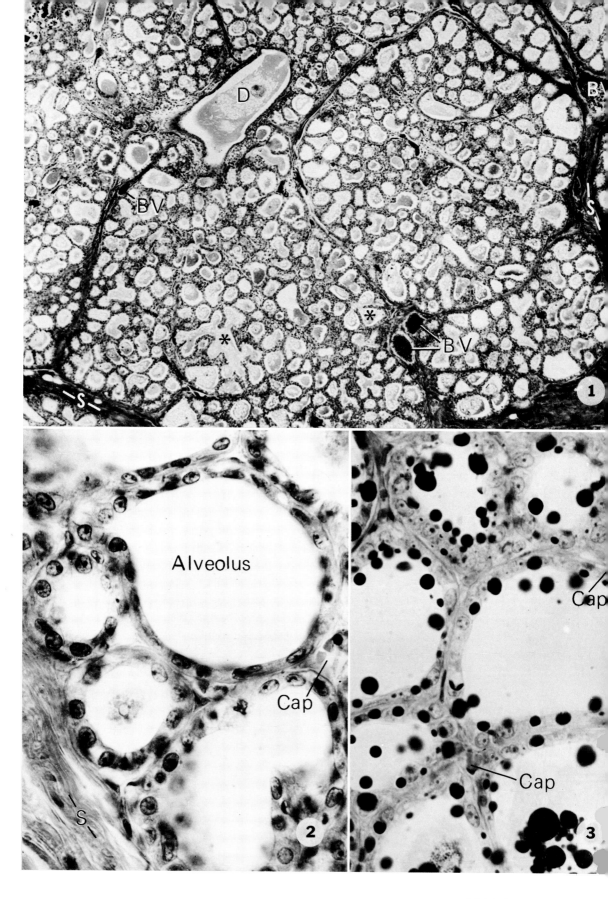

PLATE 14-10

Plate 14-11. PLACENTA I

The *placenta* is a discoid-shaped organ which serves for the exchange of materials between the fetal and maternal circulations during pregnancy. It develops primarily from embryonic tissue; however, it also has a component derived from the uterus, namely, the *stratum basalis*. The development of the placenta is complex and requires descriptions and illustrations beyond the scope of this book. The reader can find this information in a standard embryology text.

One side of the placenta is embedded in the uterine wall; the other side faces the amniotic cavity which contains the fetus. After birth, the placenta separates from the wall of the uterus and is discharged along with the contiguous membranes of the amniotic cavity.

A section extending from the amniotic surface into the substance of the placenta is shown in Figure 1. This includes the *amnion* (**A**), the *chorionic plate* (**CP**), and the *chorionic villi* (**CV**). The amnion consists of a layer of simple cuboidal epithelium (**Ep**) and an underlying layer of connective tissue (**CT**) (**inset**). The connective tissue of the amnion is continuous with the connective tissue of the chorionic plate as a result of their fusion at an earlier time. The plane of fusion, however, is not evident in H & E sections; the separation (**asterisk**) in parts of Figure 1 in the vicinity of the fusion is an artefact.

The chorionic plate is a thick connective tissue mass which contains the ramifications of the umbilical arteries and vein. These vessels (**BVp**) do not have the distinct organizational features characteristic of arteries and veins; rather, they resemble the vessels of the umbilical cord. While their identification as blood vessels is relatively simple, it is difficult to distinguish which vessels are branches of an umbilical artery and which are tributaries of the vein.°

The main substance of the placenta consists of *chorionic villi* of different sizes (see page 244). These emerge from the chorionic

KEY

A, amnion
BVp, blood vessel in chorionic plate
BVv, blood vessel in chorionic villi
CP, chorionic plate
CV, chorionic villi
CT, connective tissue
DC, decidual cells
Ep, epithelium
SB, stratum basalis
asterisk, see text

Fig. 1 (human), x 16, (inset), x 370; Fig. 2 (human), x 70, (inset), x 370.

plate as large stem villi which branch into increasingly smaller villi. Branches of the umbilical arteries and vein (**BVv**) enter the stem villi and ramify through the branching villous network. Some villi extend from the chorionic plate to the maternal side of the placenta and make contact with the maternal tissue; these are called *anchoring villi*. Other villi, the *free villi*, simply arborize within the substance of the placenta without anchoring onto the maternal side.

The maternal side of the placenta is shown in Figure 2. The *stratum* basalis (**SB**) is on the right side of the illustration. This is the part of the uterus to which the chorionic villi anchor. Along with the usual connective tissue elements, the stratum basalis contains specialized cells called *decidual cells* (**DC**). The same cells are shown at higher magnification in the **inset**. Decidual cells are usually found in clusters; moreover, their cytoplasmic limits can be readily discerned, thus imparting an epitheloid appearance. Because of these features they are easily identified.

Septa from the stratum basalis extend into the portion of the placenta which contains the chorionic villi. These do not contain the branches of the umbilical vessels and, on this basis, they can frequently be distinguished from stem villi or their branches.

° The umbilical cord contains two arteries which carry blood to the placenta and a vein which returns blood to the fetus. The umbilical arteries have thick muscular walls. These are arranged as two layers, an inner longitudinal and an outer circular. Elastic membranes are poorly developed in

these vessels and, indeed, may be absent. The umbilical vein is similar to the arteries, also having a thick muscular wall arranged as inner longitudinal and outer circular layers. Near its connection to the fetus, the umbilical cord may contain remnants of the allantois and yolk sac.

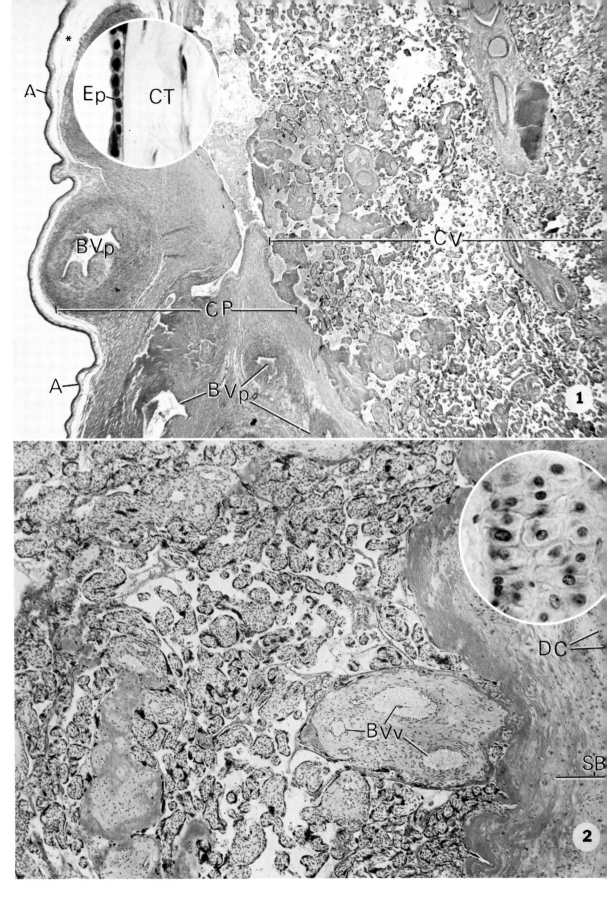

PLATE 14-11

Plate 14-12. PLACENTA II

Chorionic villi consist of a connective tissue core and a two-layered cellular covering. The outermost cellular layer is the *syncytial trophoblast*; immediately under this is another layer of cells referred to as *cytotrophoblasts*. The latter are numerous in the early placenta; however, relatively few are present in the term placenta.

A section through the substance of a term placenta is illustrated in Figure 1. This shows chorionic villi (**CV**) of different size, and the surrounding intervillous space (**IS**). The connective tissue of the villi contains branches and tributaries of the umbilical arteries and vein (**BV**). The smallest villi contain only capillaries; larger villi contain correspondingly larger blood vessels. The intervillous space contains maternal blood. This blood may drain from the specimen prior to its preparation and therefore not be seen in the section.

The nuclei of the syncytial trophoblast may be more or less evenly distributed, giving this layer an appearance in H & E sections similar to that of cuboidal epithelium. There are, however, sites where the nuclei are gathered in clusters (**arrowheads**), as well as regions of syncytium relatively free of nuclei (**arrows**). These stretches of syncytium may be so attenuated as to give the impression that the villous surface is devoid of a cover. It is thought that the nuclear clusters and the vicinal cytoplasm may separate from the villus and enter the maternal blood pool.

The syncytial trophoblast contains microvilli which project into the intervillous space. These may appear as a striated border in paraffin sections (**oval inset**); however, they are not always adequately preserved and may not be evident.

Most of the cells within the core of the villus are typical connective tissue fibrocytes and fibroblasts. The nuclei of these cells stain well with hematoxylin; but the cytoplasm cannot be distinguished from the delicate intercellular fibrous material. Other cells have a recognizable amount of cytoplasm about the nucleus. These are considered to be phagocytic and are named *Hofbauer cells.* The Hofbauer cells (**HC**) shown in Figure 1 do not contain any distinctive cytoplasmic inclusions; however, the

KEY

BV, blood vessels
CV, chorionic villi
Cy, cytotrophoblasts
HC, Hofbauer cells
IS, intervillous space
arrowheads, clusters of syncytial trophoblast nuclei
arrows, attenuated syncytial cytoplasm

Fig. 1 (human), 280, (insets), x 300 and x 640; Fig. 2 (human), x 280.

Hofbauer cell shown in the circle inset has become filled with rounded vesicular bodies; moreover, the cell itself now appears rounded.

A midterm placenta is shown in Figure 2. This has a much larger number of cytotrophoblasts than the term placenta. The cytotrophoblasts (**Cy**) form an almost complete layer of cells immediately deep to the syncytial trophoblast. Cytotrophoblasts are the source of syncytial trophoblasts. Cell division occurs in the cytotrophoblast layer (note mitotic figure in **circle inset**). The newly formed cells become incorporated into the syncytial layer.

The syncytial trophoblast covers not only the surface of the chorionic villi, but also extends from the anchoring villi onto the surface of the stratum basalis and onto the placental septa. As a consequence, the entire compartment in which maternal blood is contained is walled by syncytial trophoblast.

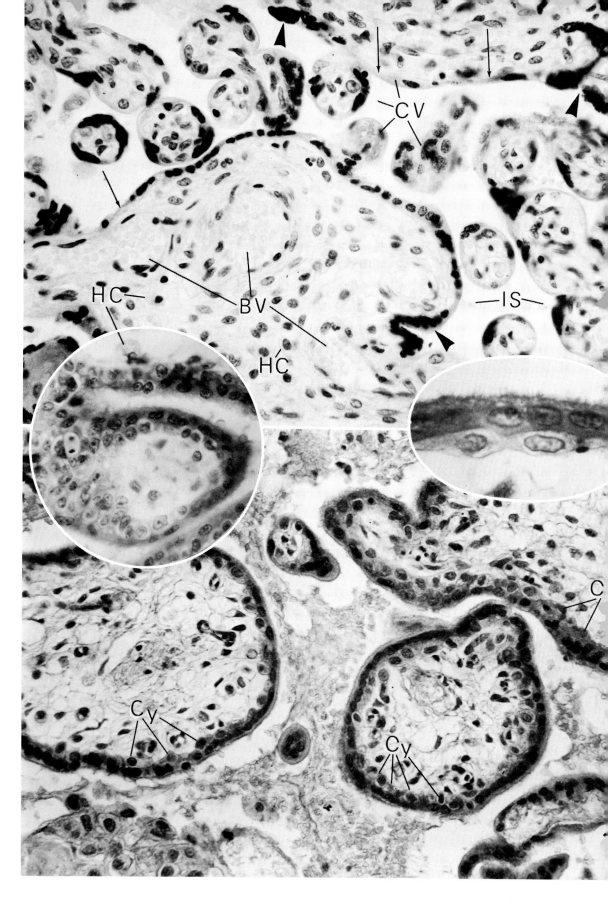

PLATE 14-12

15 ENDOCRINE SYSTEM

THE ENDOCRINE SYSTEM consists of the following glands: the *thyroid, para-thyroids, pituitary, adrenals,* and *parts of the testes* (Plate 13-2), *ovaries* (Plates 14-2 and 14-3) and *pancreas* (Plate 10-20). The *pineal gland* (Plate 15-7) is included with the endocrine system, although its function is not clearly understood. Although hormones are produced by the placenta and the gastrointestinal mucosa, these structures are not primarily thought of as endocrine glands. This applies also to the kidney and liver which produce circulating regulatory substances.

Whereas exocrine glands secrete their products onto a surface either directly or via a duct, the products of endocrine glands, the *hormones,* pass into neighboring blood vessels and by means of the blood vessels the hormones reach their site of action. Endocrine glands are also called *ductless glands* or *glands of internal secretion.*

The various endocrine glands differ in their manner of development and in the nature of their product. They display a variety of structural forms which makes it difficult to generalize about them. For example, the parathyroid, adenohypophysis (part of the pituitary gland), adrenal glands, and the islets of Langerhans (in the pancreas) are arranged as cords of cells that are richly supplied with blood vessels. The thyroid gland is also richly supplied with blood vessels, but it has an additional provision, in the form of follicles, for storing its product. The ovaries have a distinctive feature in that transient endocrine-producing structures appear during different parts of the ovarian cycle. The hormone-producing cells of the testes are arranged as small, isolated islands of cells. The neurohypophysis (part of the pituitary gland) bears some resemblance to nerve tissue. It is, in fact, not a hormone-producing structure, but rather a hormone-storing and hormone-releasing structure.

The structural feature which is most common to the endocrine glands is that the cells have an epithelial arrangement, but they do not possess a free surface. Rather they are closely opposed to blood vessels. But even here, the neurohypophysis is an exception to the generalization in that it does not develop the characteristics of epithelial tissue.

247

Plate 15-1. THYROID GLAND

The *thyroid gland* is located in the neck in close relation to the upper part of the trachea and the lower part of the larynx. It consists of two lateral lobes that are joined by a narrow isthmus. The functional unit of the thyroid gland is the *follicle*, which consists of a single layer of cuboidal or low columnar epithelium surrounding a colloid-filled space. A rich capillary network is present in the connective tissue that separates the follicles. The connective tissue also contains lymphatic capillaries. The posterior aspect of the thyroid gland is in relation to the parathyroid glands, which are frequently imbedded in the thyroid tissue.

A histological section of the thyroid gland is shown in Figure 1. The follicles (**F**) vary somewhat in size and shape, and they appear closely packed. The homogeneous mass in the center of each follicle is the *colloid* (**C**). The thyroid cells (*principal cells*) appear to form a ring around the colloid. Although the individual cells are difficult to distinguish at this magnification, the nuclei of the cells serve as an indication of their location and arrangement.

Large groups of cells (**X**) are present between some of the follicles. Where the nuclei are of the same size and staining characteristics, one can conclude that the section went through the wall of the follicle in a tangential manner without including the lumen. Connective tissue (**CT**) and small blood vessels can be recognized between the follicles. At the bottom of the field is a portion of a parathyroid (**P**) gland which was removed with the thyroid specimen.

Thyroid follicles are shown at higher magnification in Figure 2. In this specimen, the thyroid cells are cuboidal, but they may be more flattened (when they are in a less active state) or columnar (when they are in a more active state). In some follicles, there are vacuolar spaces at the periphery of the colloid (**arrowheads**). These spaces, from which colloid was lost, are regarded as artefacts; however, they reflect differences in the state of the colloid. Examination of Figure 2 (and Fig. 1) reveals that adjacent follicles are extremely close and separated by a small amount of connective tissue (**CT**). As already mentioned, a rich capillary network is present

KEY

C, colloid
CT, connective tissue
F, follicles
P, parathyroid gland
X, tangential section of follicular epithelium
arrowheads, vacuolar spaces in colloid
arrows, connective tissue or vascular nuclei

Fig. 1 (monkey), x 190; Fig. 2 (monkey), x 480.

in this connective tissue. The elongated nuclei (**arrows**) between the follicles belong to connective tissue cells or to the capillary (and lymphatic) endothelium. The blood capillaries are not conspicuous in this specimen. Lymphatic capillaries are always difficult to identify in paraffin sections except in certain tissues (e.g., villi of small intestine).

The role of the thyroid gland in the production of thyroid hormone is well known. Thyroid hormone is produced by the principal cells. A second cell type, present in relatively small numbers, also occurs in the thyroid follicle. These cells are referred to as "C" cells, ultimobranchial cells, or most often as parafollicular cells. They have also been referred to as light cells because of their appearance in the light microscope. It should be noted, however, that not every cell whose cytoplasm has a "light" appearance, or stains poorly, is a parafollicular cell since an occasional principal cell may be pale staining. Positive identification requires the application of special techniques (e.g., silver), or examination with the electron microscope. Parafollicular cells are in the same epithelial layer as the principal cells, but they do not reach the lumen of the follicle. These cells are also found in the perifollicular connective tissue. Parafollicular cells produce thyrocalcitonin, a hormone which lowers the calcium level of the blood.

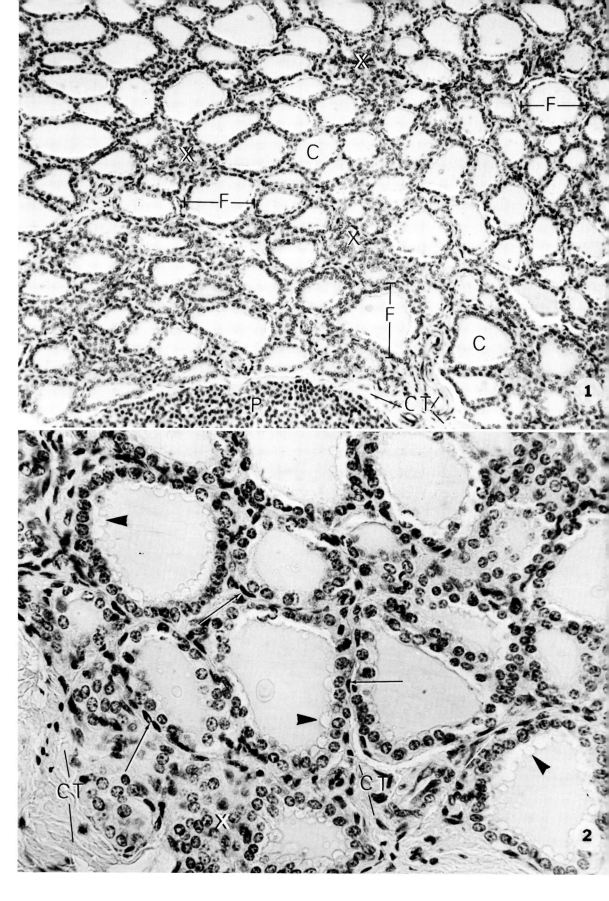

PLATE 15-1

Plate 15-2. PARATHYROID GLAND

The parathyroid glands are usually four in number. Each is surrounded by a capsule (**Cap**). Connective tissue trabeculae extend from the capsule into the substance of the gland, and, as seen in Figure 1, associated with the trabeculae are the larger blood vessels (**BV**) and, occasionally, fat cells (**FC**). The parenchyma of the parathyroid glands appears as cords or sheets of cells, separated by capillaries and delicate connective tissue septa.

Two parenchymal cell types can be distinguished in routine H & E sections: *chief cells (principal cells)* and *oxyphil cells* (**rectangle,** Fig. 1). These are shown at higher magnification in Figure 2. The **curved broken line** indicates the boundary between the oxyphil cells (**OC**) and the chief cells (**CC**). The chief cells are more numerous. They contain a spherical nucleus surrounded by a small amount of cytoplasm. The boundaries between the cells are evident in some places. Oxyphil cells are larger than chief cells, but have a slightly smaller and more intensely staining nucleus. Their cytoplasm stains with eosin and the boundaries between the cells are well marked. They are arranged in small or large groups that are scattered about in a much larger field of chief cells. Even with low magnification it is often possible to identify clusters of oxyphil cells, because a unit area contains fewer nuclei than a comparable unit area of chief cells. This point is clearly evident in the region of the rectangle of Figure 1. Oxyphil cells are not found in some species. In man they are said to appear during the first decade of life and increase somewhat in number in older individuals.

In addition to the chief and oxyphil cells which are easy to identify, there are other cells intermediate between these two, more difficult to identify. The significance of these intermediate cell types is not clear at present. Some variation in cell characteristics (as seen with the light microscope) may be due to artefacts of tissue preparation. Other variations are thought to represent the presence of transitional cells. Recent observations with the electron microscope verify the presence of cells which appear to be transitional between chief and oxyphil cells. This finding tends to support the concept that chief and

KEY

BV, blood vessels
Cap, capsule
CC, chief cells
FC, fat cells
OC, oxyphil cells
arrows, nuclei of fibroblasts or endothelial cells

Fig. 1 (human), x 160; Fig. 2 (human), x 640.

oxyphil cells represent two functional variations of the same cell.

The delicate connective tissue septa in the parathyroids are not conspicuous in H & E preparation. However, the elongated nuclei (**arrows,** Fig. 2) that can be seen between the parenchymal cells belong either to connective tissue cells or capillary endothelium.

The parathyroid glands elaborate a hormone that influences calcium and bone metabolism. Injection of parathyroid hormone into laboratory animals results in the release of calcium from bone by the action of osteocytes (osteocytic osteolysis) and osteoclasts (osteoclasia). Removal of parathyroid glands results in a rapid drop in blood calcium levels.

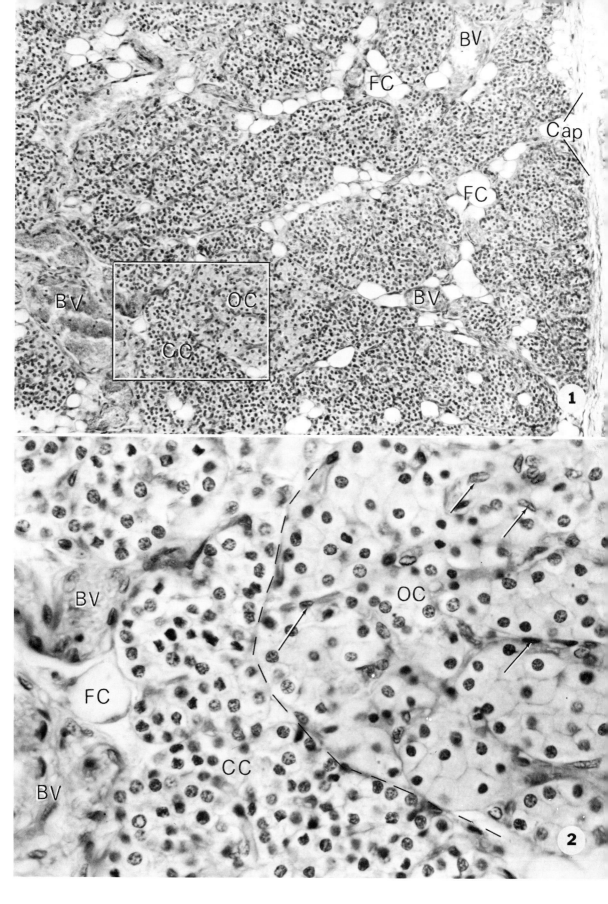

PLATE 15-2

Plate 15-3. Pituitary Gland I

The *pituitary gland,* or *hypophysis cerebri,* is located in a small bony fossa in the floor of the cranial cavity. It is connected by a stalk to the base of the brain. Although it is joined to the brain, only part of the pituitary gland develops from neural ectoderm; this is referred to as the *neurohypophysis.* The larger part of the pituitary gland develops from the oral ectoderm; this part is called the *adenohypophysis.* The adenohypophysis develops as a diverticulum of the buccal epithelium, called *Rathke's pouch.* In the fully developed gland, the lumen of Rathke's pouch may be retained as a vestigial cleft.

Both the adenohypophysis and neurohypophysis are further subdivided as follows:

Adenohypophysis
    a) pars distalis (anterior lobe)
    b) pars tuberalis
    c) pars intermedia

Neurohypophysis   (posterior lobe)

    a) pars nervosa
    b) infundibulum (infundibular stem and median eminence of tuber cinereum).

These parts are shown in a sagittal section of the pituitary gland in the accompanying figure. The neurohypophysis is marked by the **broken lines.** The pars nervosa is the expanded portion which is continuous with the infundibulum (**I**). The pars tuberalis (**PT**) is located around the infundibular stem. The pars intermedia (**PI**) is between the pars distalis and the pars nervosa. It borders a small cleft (**C**) which constitutes the remains of the lumen of Rathke's pouch. The pars distalis is the largest part of the pituitary gland. It contains a variety of cell types, some of which are more numerous in one region, some in another. This accounts for the difference in staining (light and dark areas) that is to be seen throughout the pars distalis.

The parts of the pituitary gland can be identified largely on the basis of their location and relation to each other. For example, the pars nervosa can be identified readily if it is continuous with a stem or stalk of essentially the same kind of material. The pars intermedia is in an intermediate location, and in relation to the vestigial cleft; however, the cleft may not

KEY

C, vestigial cleft of Rathke's pouch
I, infundibulum
PI, pars intermedia
PT, pars tuberalis

Fig. (monkey), x 40.

be evident and the pars intermedia may be more extensive (in this specimen it continues along the surface of the gland).

Upon considering the cell types at higher magnification (Plate 15-4), one comes to realize that these also serve as a major indication as to the part of the gland that is being examined.

The blood supply to the pars distalis of the pituitary gland is unique and requires special mention in that it is supplied by two sets of vessels. The capillaries of the pars distalis receive blood from arteries in the usual manner, but they also receive blood via a hypophyseal portal system. The latter originates as capillaries in the infundibulum. They then drain into a venous network which flow to the pars distalis where they empty into a second capillary network. This system serves as a route whereby releasing factors (hormones) from the hypothalamus are conveyed to the pars distalis. There is reported to be a specific releasing factor for each of the anterior pituitary hormones. The releasing factors cause the release, or discharge, of the specific pituitary hormones and in this way the hypothalamus regulates the secretory activity of the pars distalis.

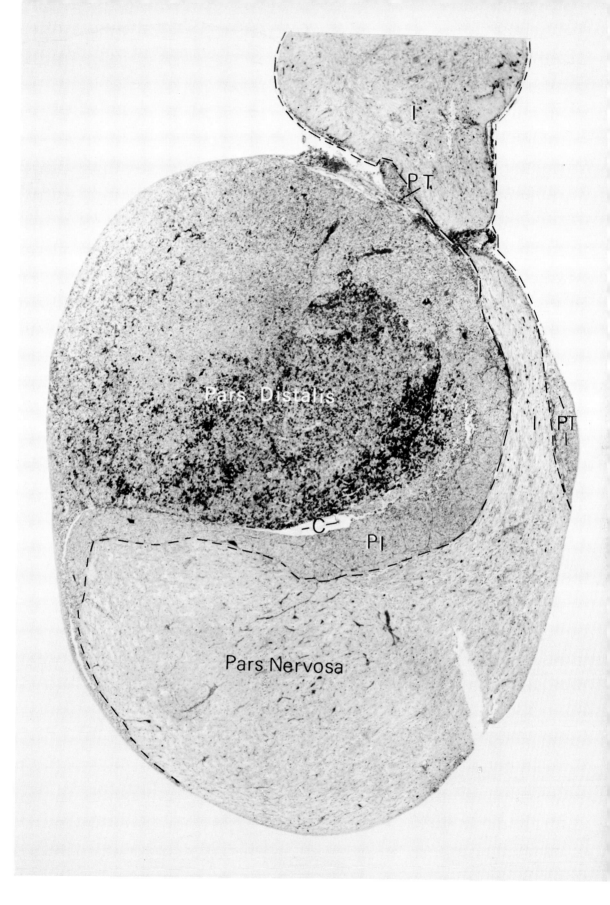

PLATE 15-3

Plate 15-4. Pituitary Gland II

The *pars distalis* contains two main cell types, *chromophobes* and *chromophils*. Chromophobes stain poorly; chromophils stain well. Chromophils are further subdivided into *acidophils* and *basophils*. Basophils stain with basic dyes or hematoxylin, whereas the cytoplasm of the acidophil stains with acid dyes such as eosin. Also, the cytoplasm of basophils stains with the PAS reaction due to the glycoprotein in the secretory granules.

A region of the pars distalis which shows a large number of basophils is illustrated in Figure 1. The field also contains acidophils, chromophobes, and stromal elements. The basophils (**B**) can be distinguished from acidophils (**A**) because the basophils are slightly larger and the cytoplasm of the acidophils stains with eosin. Both of these cell types can be distinguished from the chromophobes (**C**), which contain only a small amount of poorly staining cytoplasm. The parenchymal components of the pars distalis are arranged as cords of cells. These are separated by a delicate connective tissue stroma which contain capillaries. The elongated nuclei (**arrows**) belong to either cells of the connective tissue stroma or to the endothelial cells.

A region of pars distalis predominating in acidophils is shown in Figure 2. Eosinophilic cytoplasm can be seen in each cell. In contrast, the nuclei of chromophobes. (**C**) are surrounded by a small amount of poorly staining cytoplasm. Acidophils can be further subdivided into two groups on the basis of special cytochemical and ultrastructural features. One group, called somatotropes, produces the growth hormone (somatotropic hormone, **STH**); the other group of acidophils, called mammotropes or luteotropes, produce the lactogenic hormone (luteotropic hormone, **LTH**). Two groups of basophils can also be distinguished with the electron microscope and/or with special cytochemical procedures. One group produces the thyroid stimulating hormone (**TSH**); the other produces the gonadotropic hormones (**FSH** and **LH**). Chromophobes are also a heterogenous group of cells. Many are considered to be depleted acidophils or basophils, however, one group of chromophobes is considered to produce the hormone ACTH.

KEY

A, acidophils
B, basophils
BV, blood vessel
C, chromophobes
HB, Herring bodies
PI, pars intermedia
PN, pars nervosa
V, vesicles
arrows, nuclei of stromal or vascular cells

Figs. 1 and 2 (cat), x 640; Figs. 3–5 (cat), x 400.

The *pars tuberalis* (Fig. 3) surrounds the infundibular stem. It consists of small acidophil and basophil cells. Frequently, these are arranged as small vesicles (**V**) that contain colloid. Its function is not known.

The *pars intermedia* (**PI**) varies in size in different mammals (Fig. 4). It is relatively small in the human. It consists of cords of cells which resemble basophils, except that they are smaller. They sometimes form colloid-filled vesicles. Cells from the pars intermedia are occasionally seen in the pars nervosa (**PN**). The function of the pars intermedia in man is not clear. Studies with frogs indicate that a hormone from the intermedia, called the melanocyte stimulating hormone (**MSH**) brings about a darkening of the skin.

The *neurohypophysis* (Fig. 5) contains cells called *pituicytes* and nonmyelinated nerve fibers from the supraoptic and paraventricular nuclei of the hypothalamus. The pituicytes are comparable to neuroglial cells of the central nervous system. The nuclei of the cells are round or oval; the cytoplasm extends from the nuclear region of the cell as long processes. In H & E preparations, the cytoplasm of the pituicytes cannot be distinguished from the nonmyelinated nerve fibers. The hormones of the neurohypophysis, oxytocin and the antidiuretic hormone, ADH (also called vasopressin because of its action on vascular smooth muscle), are formed in the hypothalamic nuclei, pass via the fibers of the hypo-*thalamo-hypophyseal* tract to the neurohypophysis where they are stored in the expanded terminal portions of the nerve fibers. In histological sections, the stored neurosecretory material appears as the *Herring bodies* (**HB**).

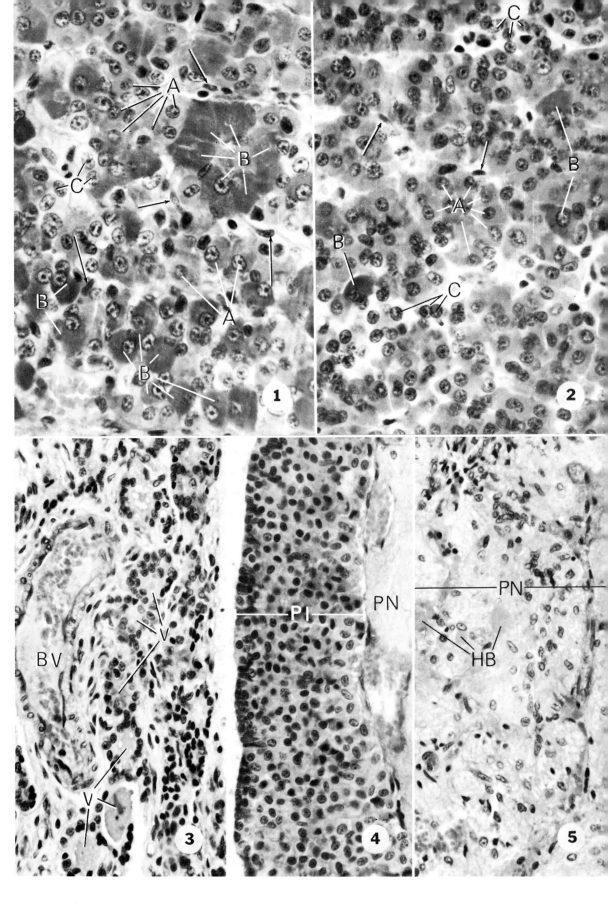

PLATE 15-4

Plate 15-5. ADRENAL GLAND I

There are two adrenal glands, one situated at the upper pole of each kidney. An adrenal gland is a composite of two distinct structural and functional components, the cortex and the medulla. The cortex develops from mesoderm, the medulla from ectoderm.

A section through the entire thickness of an adrenal gland is shown in Figure 1. Several histological features are readily evident in this low-power micrograph. The outer part of the gland, the *cortex*, has a distinctly different appearance from the inner portion, the *medulla*. Several large blood vessels (**BV**) are in the medulla. These are veins which drain both the cortex and medulla. A capsule (**Cap**) surrounds the gland and from it, delicate trabeculae extend into the substance of the gland.

The cortex is divided into three parts according to the type and arrangement of cells. These are designated as the *zona glomerulosa* (**ZG**), the *zona fasciculata* (**ZF**), and the *zona reticularis* (**ZR**).

The zona glomerulosa is located at the outer part of the cortex, immediately under the capsule (Figs. 1 and 2). The parenchyma of this zone consists of small cells which appear as arching cords or as oval groups. The nuclei of the parenchymal cells are spherical, and the cells possess a small amount of lightly staining cytoplasm. Because of the small amount of cytoplasm, the nuclei in this zone appear relatively crowded. Between the cords of cells are elongated nuclei (**arrows**, Figs. 2 and 3) which belong either to cells of the delicate connective tissue stroma or to the capillary endothelium.

The zona fasciculata consists of radially oriented cords of cells, usually two cells in width. It can be divided into two parts, an outer and an inner, based on the appearance of the cells in routine H & E preparations. The outer part of the zona fasciculata (**ZF**) is shown in Figure 3 and in the lower part of Figure 2. The nuclei of these cells are about the same size as those of the zona glomerulosa; however, there is more cytoplasm and the nuclei are more distant from one another than those of the zona glomerulosa. Occasionally, binucleate cells (**asterisks**) are seen in the zona fasciculata. These may be difficult to recognize because the cell boundaries are not

KEY

BV, blood vessels
Cap, capsule
ZF, zona fasciculata
ZG, zona glomerulosa
ZR, zona reticularis
arrows, nuclei of endothelial cells, or of connective tissue cells
asterisks, binucleate cells

Fig. 1 (monkey), x 30; Figs. 2 and 3 (monkey), x 400.

always conspicuous. The cells of the outer part of the zona fasciculata contain a considerably greater amount of lipid than the cells in the other parts of the cortex. During the preparation of routine H & E specimens, the lipid is lost, and as a consequence, the cytoplasm has a noticeably empty or spongy appearance.

The zones of the adrenal cortex are not only morphologically distinct, but the zones also reflect a functional specialization. The zona glomerulosa secretes the mineralocorticoids (aldosterone and deoxycorticosterone). On the other hand, the zona fasciculata secretes the glucocorticoids (cortisol, cortisone and corticosterone), and the zona reticularis is active in the production of adrenal androgens. The zona fasciculata has also been found to secrete adrenal androgens. There is yet another functional distinction in that the inner two zones of the adrenal cortex are regulated by ACTH whereas the zona glomerulosa is not.

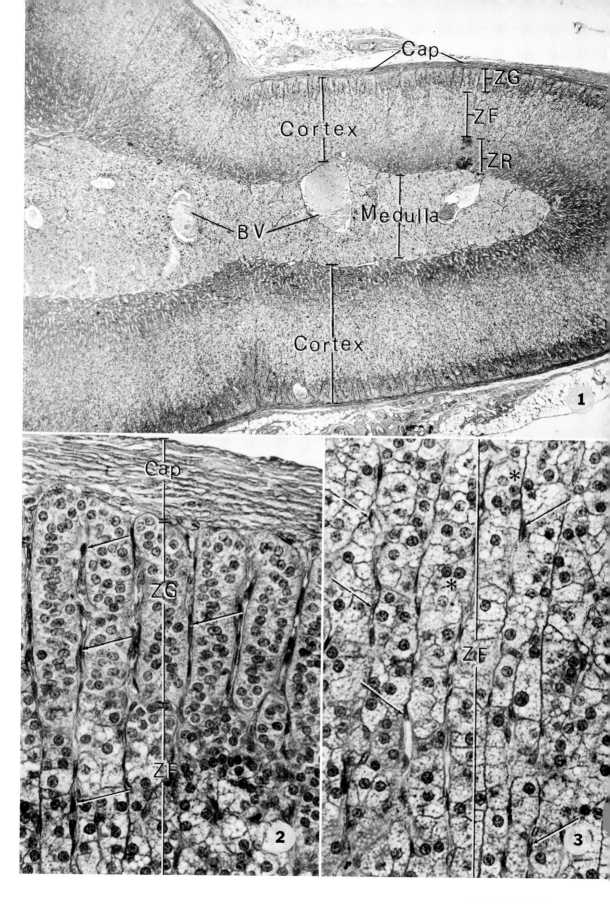

PLATE 15-5

Plate 15-6. ADRENAL GLAND II

The junction between the outer and inner parts of the *zona fasciculata* is shown in Figure 1. The outer part of the zona fasciculata, as described in the previous plate, consists of cells whose cytoplasm has a spongy appearance [**ZF(S)**]. This constitutes the bulk of the fascicular zone. The inner part of the zona fasciculata consists of smaller cells [**ZF(C)**]. The cytoplasm of these cells appears more compact than that of the cells in the outer part. As previously mentioned, the spongy appearance is due to the loss of lipid that occurs during the preparation of the tissue. Throughout the entire zona fasciculata the cells are arranged as cords, and between the cords one can see the elongated nuclei (**arrows**) that belong either to cells of the delicate connective tissue stroma or to endothelial cells.

The *zona reticularis* (**ZR**) is shown in Figure 2. This is the deepest part of the cortex, immediately adjacent to the medulla. It consists of interconnecting, irregular cords of relatively small cells. The cords are narrower than those of the other parts of the cortex; in many places they are only one cell wide. Between the cords of cells are the capillaries which in this zone are usually dilated. As in the other parts of the gland, the spherical nuclei belong to the parenchymal cells, the elongated nuclei (**arrows**) belong to the endothelial cells or to cells of the connective tissue stroma.

The cells which make up the human fetal adrenal gland display ultrastructural features which indicate that they are active in steroid synthesis. Functionally, the fetal adrenal cooperates with the placenta in the production of estrogens and other steroids. For example, neither the fetal adrenal nor the placenta contain all the necessary enzymes for estrogen synthesis, but together they do. As such, they constitute a "fetal-placental unit" which produces estrogen.

In mammals, the adrenal *medulla* (**M**) is in the center of the gland, surrounded by the cortex. It consists of large cells (Fig. 3) which are organized in ovoid groups or as short, interconnecting cords. The cytoplasm of neighboring cells may stain with different intensity. These cells color when treated with chromate reagents, and for this reason they are some-

KEY

M, adrenal medulla
ZF(C), zona fasciculata, compact cells
ZF(S), zona fasciculata, spongy cells
ZR, zona reticularis
arrows, nuclei of endothelial cells, or of connective tissue cells

Figs. 1–3 (monkey), x 400.

times called *chromaffin cells.* Elongated nuclei (**arrows**) of vascular or connective tissue cells can be seen in the delicate stroma which separates the groups of parenchymal cells. *Ganglion cells* are occasionally seen in sections of the adrenal medulla.

The cells of the adrenal medulla develop from the same source as the postganglionic cells of the sympathetic nervous system. They are directly innervated by preganglionic cells of the sympathetic system and may be regarded as modified postganglionic cells that are specialized to secrete. These cells produce epinephrine and norepinephrine.

The adrenal medulla receives its blood supply via two routes. It is supplied by arterioles which pass through the cortex, and it is supplied by capillaries that continue from the cortex. This means that some of the blood reaching the medulla contains cortical secretion.

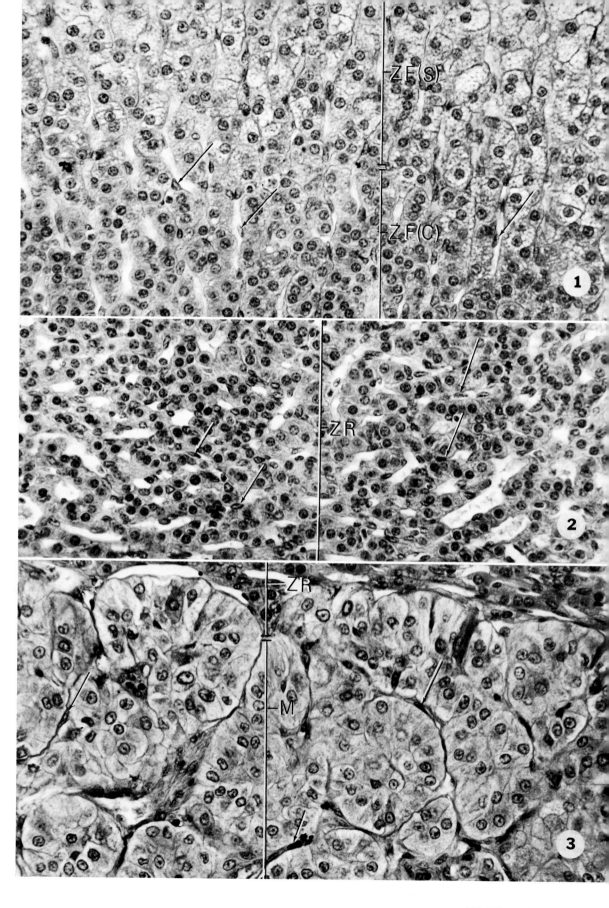

PLATE 15-6

Plate 15-7. PINEAL GLAND

The *pineal gland, (pineal body, epiphysis cerebri)* is located in the brain above the superior colliculi. It develops from neuroectoderm, but in the adult it bears little resemblance to nerve tissue.

The pineal gland is surrounded by a capsule (**Cap**), except at its stalk. The capsule is formed by the *pia mater*. Trabeculae extend from the capsule into the substance of the gland and divide it into lobules (Fig. 1). The lobules (**L**) appear as the indistinct groups of cells surrounded by connective tissue (**CT**). The adult pineal body contains calcareous deposits (**BS**) which are regularly found in histological sections. They are called *brain sand* or *corpora amylacea*. When viewed with higher magnification they can be seen to possess a lamellated structure.

Two cell types have been described within the pineal gland: parenchymal cells and glial cells. The full extent of these cells cannot be appreciated without the application of special methods. These would show that the glial cells and the parenchymal cells have processes and that the processes of the parenchymal cells are expanded at their periphery. The parenchymal cells are more numerous. In an H & E preparation, the nuclei of the parenchymal cells are pale staining and somewhat vesicular. The nuclei of the glial cells, on the other hand, are smaller and stain more intensely. In Figure 2, two nuclear types can be seen. The more numerous nuclei are the larger ones; they stain less intensely and are somewhat vesiculated; they belong to parenchymal cells (**PC**). The less numerous nuclei are the smaller ones; they stain more intensely and belong to glial cells (**GC**).

Although the physiology of the pineal gland is not well understood, the secretions of the gland evidently have an antigonadal effect. For example, hypogenitalism has been reported in pineal tumors which consist chiefly of parenchymal cells, whereas, sexual precocity is associated with nonparenchymal tumors (presumably in these the parenchymal cells have been destroyed). In addition, numerous experiments with laboratory animals indicate that the pineal gland has a neuroendocrine function whereby the pineal gland serves as an intermediary which relates endocrine function (particularly gonadal func-

KEY

BS, brain sand
Cap, capsule
CT, connective tissue
GC, nuclei of glial cells
L, lobules
PC, nuclei of parenchymal cells

Fig. 1 (human), x 80; Fig. 2 (human), x 185.

tion) to cycles of light and dark. The external photic stimuli reach the pineal gland via optical pathways which connect with the superior cervical ganglion. In turn, the superior cervical ganglion sends postganglionic nerve fibers to the pineal gland. The extent to which these findings with laboratory animals apply to man is not yet clear.

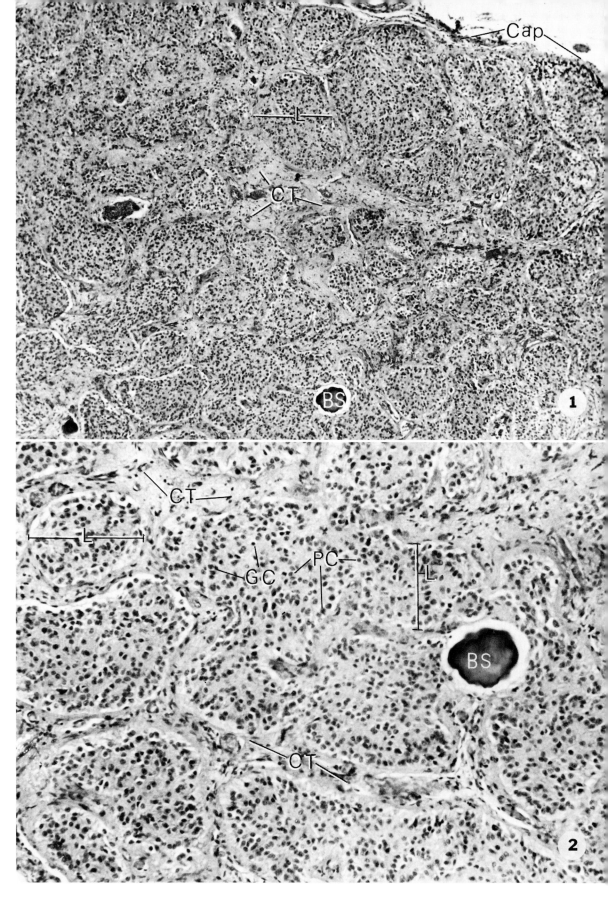

PLATE 15-7

16 THE ORGAN OF SPECIAL SENSE

Plate 16-1. THE EYE I

A section through the eyeball is shown in Plate 16-1. The micrograph illustrates most of the structural features of the eye at low magnification and provides orientation for the micrographs which follow.

The wall of the eyeball consists of three layers: the retina, the uvea, and an outer fibrous layer. Innermost is the *retina* (**R**) which is comprised of several layers of cells. Among these are *receptor cells* (rods and cones), *neurons* (e.g., bipolar and ganglion cells), *supporting cells*, and a *pigmented epithelium* (Plate 16-2). The receptor components of the retina are situated in the posterior three-fifths of the eyeball. At the anterior boundary of the receptor layer, the ora serrata (**OS**), the retina becomes reduced in thickness and nonreceptor components of the retina continue forward to cover the posterior, or inner, surface of the ciliary body (**CB**) and the iris (**I**). This anterior nonreceptor extension of the inner layer is highly pigmented, and the pigment (melanin) is evident as the black inner border of these structures.

The *uvea*, the middle layer of the eyeball, consists of the *choroid*, the *ciliary body*, and the *iris*. The choroid is a vascular layer; it is relatively thin and difficult to distinguish in the accompanying figure, except by location. On this basis, it is identified (**Ch**) as being just external to the pigmented layer of the retina. The choroid is also highly pigmented; the choroidal pigment is evident as a discrete layer in several parts of the section.

Anterior to the ora serrata, the uvea is thickened; here, it is called the ciliary body (**CB**). This contains the ciliary muscle (Plate 16-3) which brings about adjustments of the lens for the focusing of light. The ciliary body also contains processes, to which the zonular fibers are attached. These fibers function as suspensory ligaments of the lens. The iris (**I**) is the most anterior component of the uvea and contains a central opening, the pupil.

The outermost layer of the eyeball, the fibrous layer, consists of the *sclera* (**S**) and the *cornea* (**C**). Both of these contain collagenous fibers as their main structural element; however, the cornea is transparent and the sclera is opaque. The extrinsic muscles of the eye insert into the sclera and affect movements of the eyeball. These are not included

KEY

AC, anterior chamber
C, cornea
CB, ciliary body
Ch, choroid
I, iris
L, lens
ON, optic nerve
OS, ora serrata
PC, posterior chamber
R, retina
S, sclera

Fig. (human), x 7.

in the preparation except for a small piece of a muscle insertion (**arrow**) in the upper left of the illustration. Posteriorly, the sclera is pierced by the emerging optic nerve (**ON**).

The *lens* (**L**) will be considered on page 270. Just posterior to the lens is the large cavity of the eye, the *vitreal cavity*, which is filled with a thick jellylike material, the *vitreous humor* or *body*. Anterior to the lens, are two additional chambers of the eye, the anterior (**AC**) and posterior chambers (**PC**), separated by the iris.

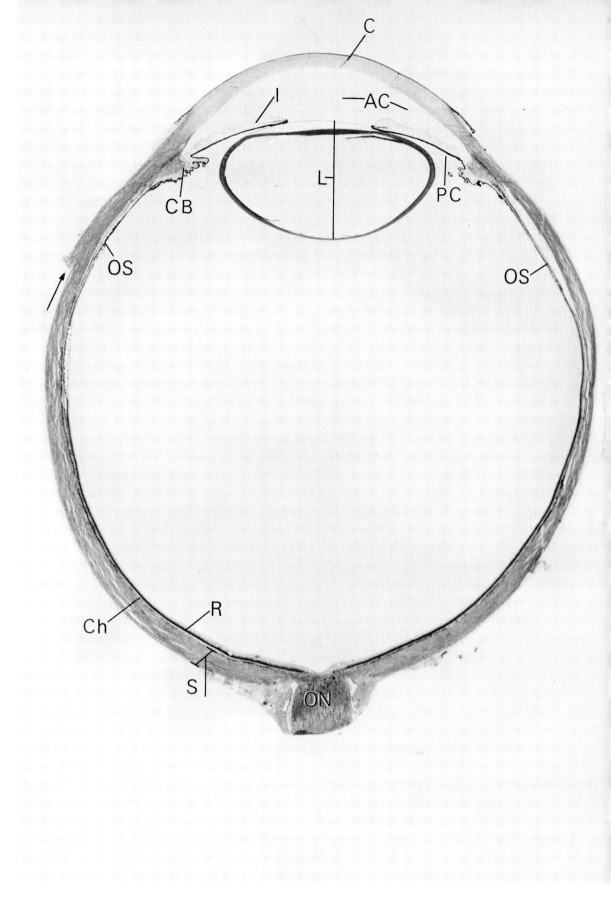

PLATE 16-1

Plate 16-2. THE EYE II

The site where the optic nerve leaves the eyeball is called the *optic disc* (**OD**). It is characteristically marked by a depression, evident in Figure 1. Receptor cells are not present at the optic disc and since it is not sensitive to light stimulation, it is sometimes referred to as the *blind spot*.

The fibers which give rise to the optic nerve originate in the retina, more specifically, in the ganglion cell layer (see below). They traverse the sclera through a number of openings (**arrows**, Fig. 1) to form the optic nerve. The region of the sclera which contains these openings is called the lamina cribrosa (**LC**). The optic nerve contains a central artery and vein (not shown in Figure 1) which also traverse the lamina cribrosa. Branches of these vessels (**BV**) supply the inner portion of the retina.

The optic nerve and retina are, in effect, a projection of the central nervous system, and the fibrous cover of the optic nerve is an extension of the meninges of the brain. As a consequence, pressure within the cranial cavity, transmitted along this channel, can be detected by examination of the optic disc.

On the basis of structural features which are readily evident in histological sections, the retina is divided into ten layers as listed below and labeled in Figure 2.

1. Pigment epithelium (**PEp**)
2. Layer of rods and cones (**R & C**)
3. External limiting membrane (**ELM**)
4. Outer nuclear layer (nuclei of rod and cone cells) (**ONL**)
5. Outer plexiform layer (**OPL**)
6. Inner nuclear layer (nuclei of bipolar, horizontal, amacrine, and Müller's cells) (**INL**)
7. Inner plexiform layer (**IPL**)
8. Layer of ganglion cells (**GC**)
9. Nerve fiber layer (**NFL**)
10. Internal limiting membrane (**ILM**)

The Müller's cells are supporting cells comparable to neuroglia. Processes of Müller's cells ramify virtually through the entire thickness of the retina. The inner limiting membrane is the basal lamina of the Müller's cells; the outer limiting membrane is not actually a membrane, rather it represents

junctional complexes between the processes of Müller's cells and photoreceptor cells (rods and cones).

Aside from the pigment epithelium and the Müller's cells, the other cells of the retina are neural elements arranged sequentially in three layers: 1) the rods and cones; 2) an intermediate neuronal layer (bipolar, horizontal and amacrine cells); and 3) ganglion cells. Nerve impulses originating in the rods and cones are transmitted to the intermediate layer and then to the ganglion cells. Synaptic connections occur in the inner and outer plexiform layers, resulting in some degree of neuronal integration. Finally, the ganglion cells send their axons to the brain as components of the optic nerve.

Figure 2 also shows the innermost layer of the choroid (**Ch**). This is a cell-free membrane, the *lamina vitrea* (**LV**), also called Bruch's membrane. Electron micrographs reveal that it corresponds to the basement membrane of the pigment epithelium. Immediately external to the lamina vitrea is the capillary layer of the choroid (lamina choriocapillaris). These vessels supply the outer part of the retina.

The posterior portion of the retina (see Fig. 3) contains a small depression called the *fovea centralis* (**FC**). This part of the retina contains only cone cells. The depression of the fovea is due to a spreading apart of the inner layers of the retina, leaving the cone elements relatively uncovered. The fovea centralis is associated with acute vision. As one moves from the fovea toward the ora serrata, the number of cone cells decreases and the number of rod cells increases.

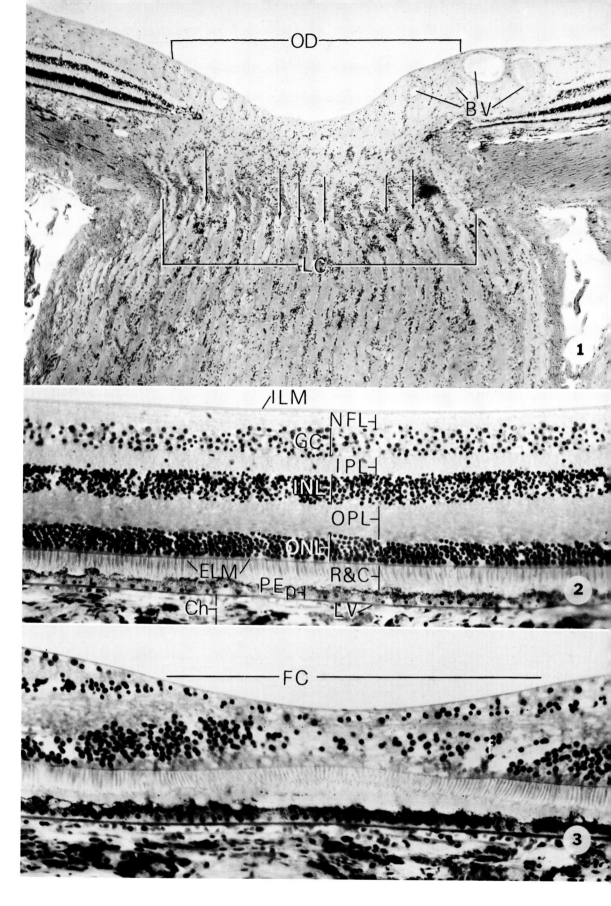

PLATE 16-2

Plate 16-3. The Eye III

A portion of the anterior of the eye is shown in Figure 1. Included in the illustration are parts of the cornea (**C**), sclera (**S**), iris (**I**), ciliary body (**CB**), anterior chamber (**AC**), posterior chamber (**PC**), lens (**L**), and zonular fibers (**ZF**). The zonular fibers function as a suspensory ligament of the lens.

The cornea is considered in detail in Plate 16-4. However, the relationship of the cornea to the *sclera* is illustrated to advantage in Figure 1. The junction between the two (**arrows**) is marked by a change in staining, the substance of the cornea appearing lighter than that of the sclera. The corneal epithelium (**CEp**) is continuous with the epithelium (**CjEp**) that covers the sclera. (The junction between these is marked by the small circle in Figure 1 and shown at higher magnification in the inset.) However, the latter is separated from the dense fibrous component of the sclera by a loose vascular connective tissue. Together, this connective tissue and its covering epithelium constitute the conjunctiva (**Cj**). The epithelial-connective tissue junction of the conjunctiva is irregular; in contrast, the undersurface of the corneal epithelium presents an even profile.

Just lateral to the junction of the cornea and sclera is a canal, seen in cross section, the *canal of Schlemm* (**CS**, Fig. 2). This canal takes a circular route about the perimeter of the cornea. It communicates with the anterior chamber through a loose trabecular meshwork of tissue called the spaces of Fontana. These spaces can only be seen adequately in ideal preparations and they are not evident in Figures 1 or 2. The canal of Schlemm also communicates with episcleral veins. By means of its communications, the canal of Schlemm provides a route for the fluid in the anterior and posterior chambers to reach the blood stream. The canal may form more than one channel as it encircles the cornea.

Immediately internal to the anterior margin of the sclera (**S**) is the *ciliary body* (**CB**, Fig. 2). The inner surface of this forms radially arranged, ridge-shaped elevations, the ciliary processes (**CP**), to which the zonular fibers (**ZF**) are anchored. From the outside in, the components of the ciliary body are: the ciliary muscle (**CM**), the connective tissue (vascular) layer (**VL**), the lamina vitrea (**LV**), and the

KEY

AC, anterior chamber
C, cornea
CAV, circular artery and vein
CB, ciliary body
CEp, corneal epithelium
CiEp, ciliary epithelium
Cj, conjunctiva
CjEp, conjunctival epithelium
CM, ciliary muscle
CP, ciliary processes
CS, canal of Schlemm
I, iris
L, lens
LV, lamina vitrea
nP, non-pigmented layer of the ciliary epithelium
P, pigmented layer of the ciliary epithelium
PC, posterior chamber
S, sclera
VL, vascular layer (of ciliary body)
ZF, zonular fibers
arrows, junction between cornea and sclera

Fig. 1 (human), x 30, (inset), x 300; Fig. 2 (human), x 65, (inset), x 570.

ciliary epithelium (**CiEp**). The ciliary epithelium consists of two layers (**inset**), the pigmented layer (**P**) and the non-pigmented layer (**nP**). The ciliary epithelium plays a role in the formation of the aqueous humor. The lamina vitrea is a continuation of the same layer of the choroid; it is the basement membrane of the pigmented ciliary epithelial cells.

The ciliary muscle is arranged in three patterns. The outer layer is immediately deep to the sclera. These are the meridionally arranged *fibers of Brücke*. The outermost of these continues more posteriorly into the choroid and is referred to as the tensor muscle of the choroid. The middle layer is the radial group. It radiates from the region of the sclero-corneal junction into the ciliary body. The innermost layer of muscle cells is circularly arranged. These are seen in cross section. The circular artery and vein (**CAV**) for the iris, also cut in cross section, are just anterior to the circular group of muscle cells.

The iris and lens are considered on page 270. The **rectangles** in Figure 1 mark those areas of the lens which are shown in Plate 16-4, (Fig. 3 and its inset).

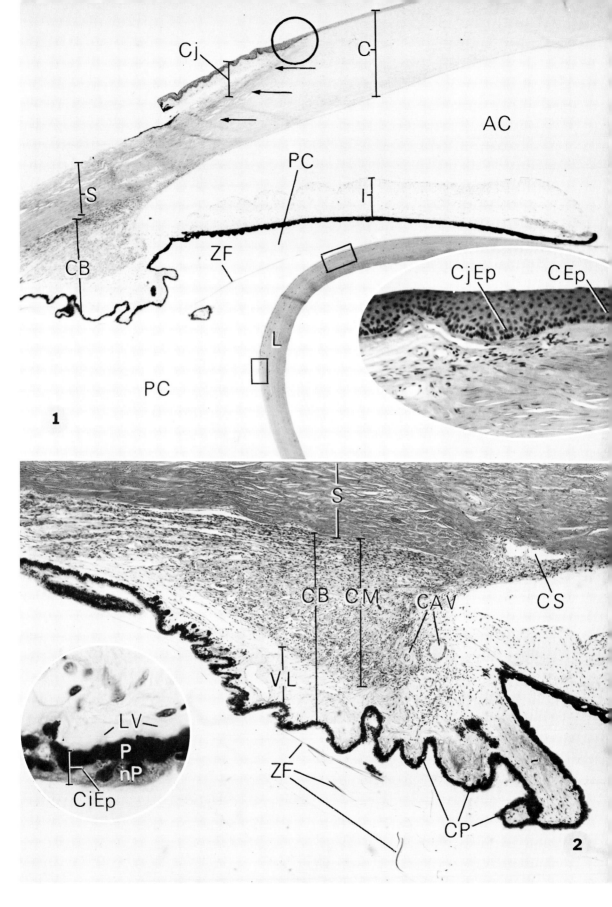

1

Cj   C   AC

S

CB   PC   ZF   PC   I

L   PC

CjEp   CEp

S

CB   CM   CAV   CS

VL

LV
P
nP
CiEp

ZF   CP

2

PLATE 16-3

Plate 16-4. THE EYE IV

The *cornea* is the transparent portion of the eye, anterior to the iris. It consists of five layers, three of which are cellular. The layers are: the *epithelium; Bowman's membrane,* which is acellular; the *substantia propria* (corneal stroma); *Descemet's membrane,* also acellular; and the *endothelium.* The full thickness of the cornea is illustrated in Figure 1, and the two surfaces, at higher magnification, in the insets.

The epithelium (**Ep**) is stratified squamous, about five cells in thickness. The basal cells exhibit a columnar or polyhedral shape, but they become progressively flattened as they migrate toward the surface. They do not keratinize and, accordingly, each cell contains a nucleus. The cells are joined by desmosomes which appear as "intercellular bridges" (**arrows**) in light micrographs (**inset**).

The undersurface of the corneal epithelium presents a smooth profile. It rests on a homogeneous-appearing substance called *Bowman's membrane* (**BwM**). The *substantia propria* (**SP**) forms most of the thickness of the cornea. It consists of regularly arranged sheets, or lamellae, of collagenous fibers and fibroblasts. The collagenous fibers within each lamella are parallel to each other, but at right angles to the fibers of adjacent lamellae. This orientation contributes to the transparency of the cornea. Indeed, opaqueness due to scarring of the cornea (e.g., after a wound), is accompanied by a failure to reestablish the normal orientation. The substantia propria is separated from the corneal endothelium by *Descemet's membrane* (**DM**). Like Bowman's membrane, this appears homogeneous with the light microscope. The *endothelium* (**En**) consists of a single layer of cuboidal cells whose lateral cell margins are sometimes evident (**arrowhead, inset**). The cornea is devoid of blood vessels. During inflammation, white cells migrate into the cornea from the vessels in the sclera. Even in noninflammatory states, lymphocytes are occasionally seen in the cornea. The corneal epithelium is richly supplied with nerve endings; however, these are not evident in H & E sections.

The pupillary margin of the iris is shown at higher magnification in Figure 2. The major portion of the iris consists of connective tissue (**CT**) which contains pigment cells (**PC**) to a

KEY

BwM, Bowman's membrane
CT, connective tissue
DM, Descemet's membrane
En, corneal endothelium
Ep, corneal epithelium
LCap, lens capsule
LF, lens "fibers"
PC, pigment cells
PE, pigmented epithelium
PMyE, pigmented myoepithelial cells
SM(C), circular smooth muscle
SP, substantia propria
ZF, zonular fibers
arrowhead, lateral margin of endothelial cells
arrows, intercellular bridges

Fig. 1 (human), x 135, (inset), x 600; Fig. 2 (human), x 250; Fig. 3 (human), x 800, (inset), x 250.

varying degree (only in the albino are these absent). The posterior surface of the iris consists of two layers of pigmented epithelial cells. The cells in the anterior of these two layers contain myofilaments. This anterior layer of pigmented epithelium is actually myoepithelium (**PMyE**) and it makes up the radial, or dilator, muscle fibers of the iris. The myoid character of these cells is largely obscured by the pigment. In addition, the iris contains smooth muscle cells arranged circularly around the pupil. These are cross sectioned in Figure 2 [**SM(C)**]. These circularly arranged muscle cells make up the pupillary constrictor of the iris.

The lens consists entirely of epithelial cells (Fig. 3) surrounded by a homogeneous capsule (**L Cap**) to which the zonular fibers (**ZF**) are joined. On the anterior surface of the lens the cells have a cuboidal shape. However, at the lateral margin the cells are extremely elongated (**inset**) and their cytoplasm extends toward the center of the lens. These elongated columns of epithelial cytoplasm are also referred to as lens fibers (**LF**). New cells are produced at the margin of the lens and displace the older cells toward the center. Upon aging, the older cells (fibers) lose their nucleus.

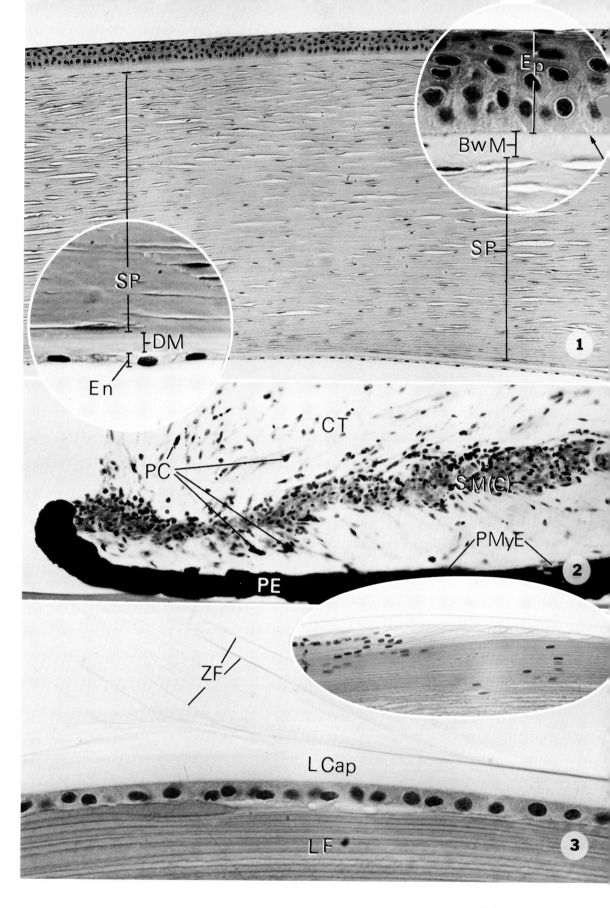

En

SP

DM

Ep

BwM

SP

1

CT

PC

SM(C)

PMyE

PE

2

ZF

L Cap

LF

3

PLATE 16-4

Plate 16-5. THE EAR

The inner ear consists of a number of chambers and canals in the temporal bone, which contain a network of membranous channels. These are referred to respectively as the *bony labyrinth* and *membranous labyrinth*. In places, the membranous labyrinth forms the lining of the bony labyrinth; in other places there is a separation of the two. Within the space lined by the membranous labyrinth is a watery fluid, called *endolymph*. External to the membranous labyrinth, i.e., between the membranous and bony labyrinths, is additional fluid, called *perilymph*.

The bony labyrinth is divided into three parts: the *cochlea, semicircular canals,* and the *vestibule.* The cochlea and semicircular canals each contain membranous counterparts of the same shape; however, the membranous components of the vestibule are more complex in their form, being comprised of ducts and two chambers, the *utricle* and *saccule.* The cochlea contains the receptors for hearing, the *organ of Corti;* the semicircular canals contain the receptors for movement; and the saccule and utricle contain receptors for position.

A section through the inner ear is shown in Figure 1. Bone surrounds the entire inner ear cavity. Because of its labyrinthine character, in sections, the inner ear appears as a number of separate chambers and ducts. These, however, are all interconnected (except that the perilymphatic and endolymphatic spaces remain separate). The largest chamber is the vestibule (**V**). The upper, right side of this chamber (**arrow**) leads into the cochlea (**C**). Just below the arrow which marks the entry into the cochlea is the oval ligament (**OL**) surrounding the base of the stapes (**S**). Both have been cut obliquely and are not seen in their entirety. The facial nerve (**FN**) is in an osseous tunnel to the right of the oval ligament. The communication of the vestibule with one of the semicircular canals is marked by the **arrowhead**. On the left are cross sections through components of the duct system (**DS**) of the membranous labyrinth.

The cochlea is a spiral structure having the general shape of a cone. The specimen illustrated in Figure 1 makes 3½ turns (in man, there are 2½ turns). The section goes through the central axis of the cochlea. This consists

KEY

C, cochlea
CN, cochlea nerve
CT, connective tissue
Cu, cupula
DS, duct system (of membranous labyrinth)
Ep, epithelium
FN, facial nerve
HC, hair cell
M, modiolus
OL, oval ligament
S, stapes
SC, sustentacular cell
SG, spiral ganglia
V, vestibule
arrows (**curved**), entry to cochlea
arrowhead, entry to semicircular canal

Fig. 1 (guinea pig), x 20; Fig. 2 (guinea pig), x 225.

of a bony stem called the modiolus (**M**). It contains the beginning of the cochlear nerve (**CN**) and the spiral ganglia (**SG**). Because of the plane of section, the spiral arrangement of the cochlear tunnel, the tunnel is cut crosswise in seven places (note, 3½ turns).

The **rectangle** in Figure 1 is shown at higher magnification in Figure 2. It illustrates a receptor for movement, the *crista ampullaris,* one of which is present in each of the semicircular canals. The epithelial (**Ep**) surface of the crista consists of two cell types, sustentacular (*supporting*) cells and hair (*receptor*) cells. (Two types of hair cells are distinguished with the electron microscope.) It is difficult to identify these cells on the basis of specific characteristics; however, they can be distinguished on the basis of location, the hair cells (**HC**) being situated in a more superficial location than the sustentacular cells (**SC**). A gelatinous mass, the cupula (**Cu**), surmounts the epithelium of the crista ampullaris. Each receptor cell sends a hairlike projection deep into the substance of the cupula.

The epithelium rests on a loose, cellular, connective tissue (**CT**) which also contains the nerve fibers associated with the receptor cells. The nerve fibers are difficult to identify, since they are not organized as a discrete bundle.

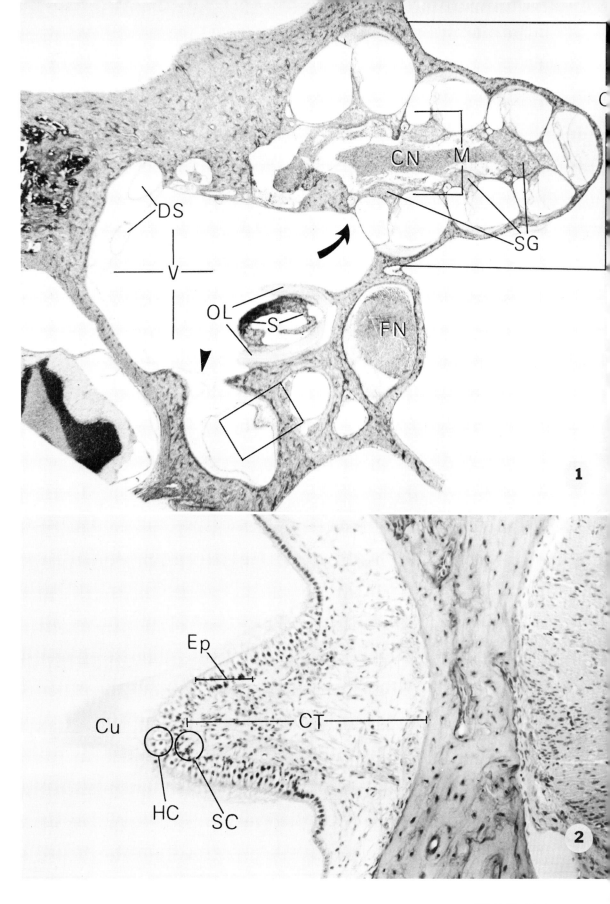

1

2

PLATE 16-5

Plate 16-6. ORGAN OF CORTI

A section through one of the turns of the cochlea is shown in Figure 1. The most important functional component of the cochlea is the organ of Corti. It is enclosed by the rectangle and is examined at higher magnification in Figure 2. Other structures included in Figure 1 are as follows. The *spiral ligament* (**SL**) is a thickening of the periostium on the outer part of the tunnel. Two membranes, the *basilar membrane* (**BM**) and the *vestibular membrane* (**VM**), join with the spiral ligament and divide the cochlear tunnel into three parallel canals, namely the *scala vestibuli* (**SV**), the *scala tympani* (**ST**), and the *cochlear duct* (**CD**). Both the scala vestibuli and scala tympani are perilymphatic spaces; these communicate at the apex of the cochlea. The cochlear duct, on the other hand, is the space of the membranous labyrinth and is filled with endolymph. It is thought that the endolymph is formed by the portion of the spiral ligament which faces the cochlear duct, the *stria vascularis* (**StV**). This is highly vascularized and contains specialized cells considered to perform the above mentioned function.

A shelf of bone, the *osseous spiral lamina* (**OSL**), extends from the modiolus to the basilar membrane. Branches of the cochlear nerve (**CN**) travel along the spiral lamina to the modiolus where the main trunk of the nerve is formed. [The components of the cochlear nerve are bipolar neurons whose cell bodies constitute the spiral ganglia (**SG**)]. The spiral lamina supports an elevation of cells, the limbus spiralis (**LS**). The surface of the limbus is comprised of columnar cells.

The components of the organ of Corti are as follows (Fig. 2), beginning at the limbus spiralis (**LS**): inner border cells (**IBC**); inner phalangeal and hair cells (**IP & HC**); inner pillar cells (**IPC**); (the sequence continues, repeating itself in reverse) outer pillar cells (**OPC**); outer phalangeal and hair cells (**OP & HC**); and outer border cells (**CH**) (cells of Hensen). Hair cells are receptor cells; the other cells are collectively referred to as supporting cells. The outer hair and phalangeal cells can be distinguished in Figure 2 by their location and because their nuclei are well aligned. Since the hair cells rest on the phalangeal cells, it can be concluded that the upper three nuclei belong to outer hair cells,

KEY

BM, basilar membrane
CB, cells of Boettcher
CC, cells of Claudius
CD, cochlea duct
CH, cells of Hensen
CN, cochlear nerve
IBC, inner border cells
IP & HC, inner phalangeal and hair cells
IPC, inner pillar cells
IST, internal spiral tunnel
IT, inner tunnel
LS, limbus spiralis
OP & HC, outer phalangeal and hair cells
OPC, outer pillar cells
OSL, osseous spiral lamina
OT, outer tunnel
RM, reticular membrane
SG, spiral ganglia
SL, spiral ligament
ST, scala tympani
StV, stria vascularis
SV, scala vestibuli
TM, tectorial membrane
VM, vestibular membrane

Fig. 1 (guinea pig), x 65, (inset), x 380; Fig. 2 (guinea pig), x 380.

the lower three to outer phalangeal cells.

The supporting cells extend from the basilar membrane (this is not evident in Figure 2 but can be seen in the **inset**) to the surface of the organ of Corti where they form a reticular membrane (**RM**). The free surface of the receptor cells fit into openings in the reticular membrane and the "hairs" of these cells project toward, and make contact with, the tectorial membrane (**TM**). The latter is a cuticular extension from the columnar cells of the limbus spiralis. In ideal preparations, nerve fibers can be traced from the hair cells to the cochlear nerve.

In their course from the basilar membrane to the reticular membrane, groups of supporting cells are separated from other groups by spaces which form spiral tunnels. These tunnels are named the *inner tunnel* (**IT**), the *outer tunnel* (**OT**), and the *internal spiral tunnel* (**IST**). Beyond the supporting cells are two additional groups of cells, the cells of Claudius (**CC**) and the cells of Boettcher (**CB**).

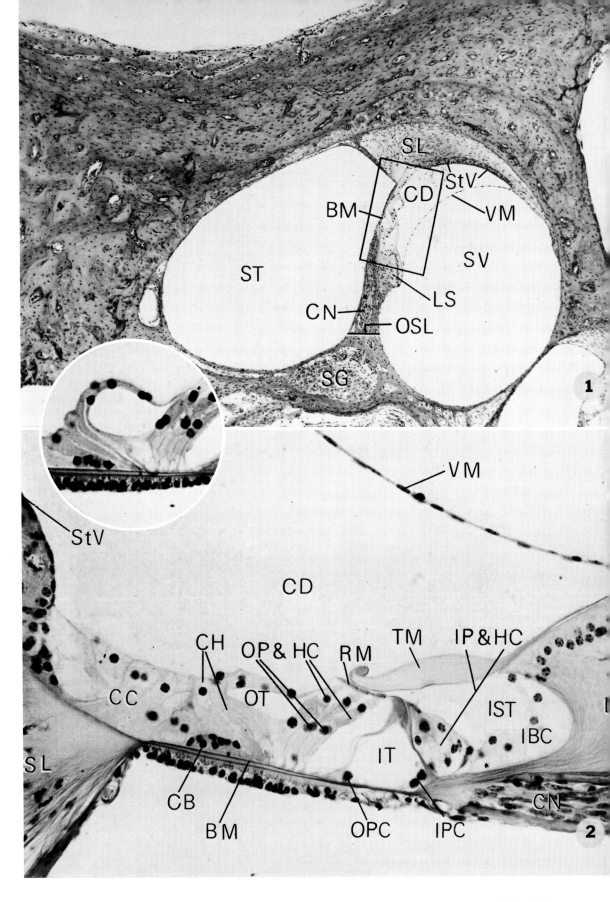

PLATE 16-6

INDEX

A Band, 78, 80
Absorptive cells, 8–12, 166, 168, 174
Acini, mucous salivary, 150, 152
    serous salivary, 150, 152
Actin filaments, 69, 72, 80
Adipose tissue, 18
Adrenal gland, 256–289
Agranulocytes, 62, 64
Alimentary canal, organization, 142
Alveolar duct, 194
Alveolar sac, 194
Alveoli, lung, 185, 194
    serous, pancreas, 182
Ameloblasts, 154
Amnion, 242
Antidiuretic hormone, ADH, 254
Aorta, 112
    nerva vasorum, 112
    tunica adventitia, 112
    tunica intima, 112
    tunica media, 112
    vasa vasorum, 112
Appendix, 172
Argentaffine cells, large intestine, 172
    small intestine, 166
    stomach, 160
Arrector pili muscle, 136, 138
Arterioles, 108, 116
Artery(ies), 108
    arcuate, 197
    conducting, 112
    elastic, 30
    hepatic, 134, 176, 178
    interlobular, 197

internal elastic membrane, 144
    muscular, 114
    tunica adventitia, 114
    tunica intima, 114
    tunica media, 114
    umbilical, 242
Astrocytes, 89
Atretic follicles, ovary, 222, 224
Auerbach's plexus, 170
Axon, 88–106
Axon terminal, 94
Azurophilic granules, 64

Basal bodies, ciliated epithelium, 8, 190, 192
Basal cells, 8
Basal lamina, 3, 14, 100, 118
Basal membrane, 3
Basement lamina, 14
Basement membrane, 3
    relationship to epithelium, 3
    trachea, 190
Basilar membrane, 274
Basket cells, 104
Basophiles, 62, 66
Betz cells, cerebrum, 102
Bile canaliculi, 178
Billroth's cords, 130, 132
Binucleate cells, liver, 178
    transitional epithelium, 10
    urinary bladder, 206
Bladder, gall, 180
    urinary, 206
Blood, agranulocytes, 62, 64
    basophiles, 62, 64

Blood (*Continued*)
eosinophiles, 62, 64
erythrocytes, 62, 64
granulocytes, 62, 66
leucocytes, 62, 64
lymphocytes, 62, 64
monocytes, 62, 64
neutrophiles, 62, 64
platelets, 62
thrombocytes, 62
Blood-testis barrier, 208
Bone, 32, 52, 54
canaliculi, 32, 46
cancellous, 28, 32
capillaries, electron microscopy, 48
cement line, electron microscopy, 48
compact, 32
cortical, electron microscopy, 48
decalcified sections, 33
epiphyseal plate (disc), 42, 50, 52
formation, endochondral, 50, 52
intramembranous, 54
ground sections, 33, 46
Haversian canal, 33, 46
Haversian systems, 33, 46
interstitial lamellae, electron microscopy, 48
lacunae, 32, 42, 46
lamellae, 46
lamellar, 32
marrow, 42, 52
marrow cells, 52
matrix, 52
medullary cavity, 50
non-lamellar, 32
osteoblasts, 50, 52, 54
osteoclasts, 54
osteocytes, 42, 52, 54
osteoid, 52, 54
osteons, 32, 46
perichondral, 50
periosteal, 50
preosteoblasts, electron microscopy, 48
primary spongy, 33
remodeling of, 50, 54
resorption, 54
spicules, 42, 52, 54
spongy, 33, 42
trabeculae, 42
Volkmanns canals, 46
woven compact, 42
Bony labyrinth, 272
Bowman's capsule, 196, 209
Bowman's glands, 186

Bowman's membrane, 270
Brain sand, 260
Bridges, intercellular, 140, 146
Bronchiole, 192
respiratory, 192, 194
terminal, 192
Bronchus, 190, 192
Bruch's membrane, 266
Brunner's glands, 166
Brush border, 4, 200

C Cell, pancreas, 182
C Cell, thyroid, 248
Calyx, renal, 196, 202
Canal, cervical, 232
portal, 176
semicircular, 272
Canaliculi, bile, 178
bone, 56
Capillaries, peritubular, 200
sinusoidal, liver, 176
Capsule, Bowman's, 192
Cardiac muscle (*see* Muscle), 82, 84, 86
Cardiovascular system, 108–119
arterioles, 108, 116
elastic tissue, 108, 112
endothelium, 108, 116
organization of, 108
valves, 108, 109
Cartilage, 32–42, 50, 52
appositional growth, 34
articular, 42
calcified, 50, 52
cells, 32, 33, 42, 44, 52
elastic, 32
electron microscopy, 36, 38
erosion of, 50
fibrocartilage, 44
ground substance, 32
hyaline, 32, 40, 42
hypertrophic, 50, 52
interstitial growth, 34
lacunae, 32, 34, 42, 44, 52
matrix, 32, 34, 36, 40, 44, 52
extraterritorial, 34
territorial, 34
proliferating, 52
reserve, 52
resorption of, 52
spicules, 52
Cavity, joint, 40
Cell(s), absorptive, 8, 10, 166, 168, 174
alpha (A), pancreas, 182
argentaffine, large intestine, 166

Cell(s) *(Continued)*
    small intestine, 170
    stomach, 160
  basal, 8
  basket, 104
  beta (B), pancreas, 182
  Betz, 102
  binucleate *(see* Binucleate cells)
  of Böettcher, 274
  C, pancreas, 182
  C, thyroid, 248
  centro-acinar, 182
  chief, stomach, 116, 158, 160
  of Claudius, 274
  connective tissue, 26
  D, pancreas, 182
  decidual, 230
  endothelial, 6, 118
  epithelial, 3–15
  epithelioid, 10
    testis, 212
    thymus, 134
  epithelio-reticular, 120, 134
  ganglion, 90–97
  goblet, 8, 166, 168, 174
  Golgi type II, 104
  granule, 102, 104
  granulosa lutein, 226
  hair, of ear, 272, 274
  of Hensen, 274
  hepatic, 176
  Hofbauer, 244
  interstitial, of Leydig, 209, 212
  juxtaglomerular, 197
  Kupffer, 178
  Langerhans, 136
  of Leydig, 209, 212
  macrophages, 121, 126
  of Martinotti, 102
  mast, 17, 18
  Merkel, 136
  mucous, salivary, 150
  mucous neck, stomach, 160
  Müller's, 266
  myoepithelial, 68, 140, 236, 238
  neuroglial, 68, 102, 106
  Paneth, 170, 172
  parietal, stomach, 160
  perichondrial, 36, 38
  plasma, 18, 121, 168
  pneumocytes
    type I, type II, 194
  primordial spermatogenic, 212
  Purkinje, 104
  pyramidal, 102
  replacement of, 6
  reticular, 84, 120, 124
  satellite, 92, 94
  Schwann, 92, 94
  septal, 194
  serous, salivary, 150
  Sertoli, 210
  sustentacular, ear, 272
    olfactory mucosa, 186
    testis, 210
  theca lutein, 226
  ultimobranchial cells, 248
Cerebellum, basket cells, 104
  cortex, 104
  Golgi type II cells, 104
  granular layer, 104
  granule cells, 104
  molecular layer, 104
  plexiform layer, 104
  Purkinje cells, 104
Cerebrum, Betz cells, 102
  cells of Martinotti, 102
  cortex, 102
  granule cells, 102
  layers, 102
  neuroglial cells, 102
  neuropil, 102
  pyramidal cells, 102
Cervix, 232
Chondrocytes, 32, 34, 36, 38
Chorionic gonadotropin, 221
Chorionic plate, 242
Chorionic villi, 200, 242, 244
Choroid, 222, 264
Cilia, 6
  bronchiole, 148
  efferent ductules, 170
  respiratory system, 146, 148
  uterine tube, 184
Ciliary body, 220, 224
Circumvallate papillae, tongue, 144, 146
Cochlea, 228, 230
Cohnheim's fields, 50
Collagen, 11, 13
Collagenous fibers, 11, 13, 14
Collecting tubules, 153, 156, 158
Colloid, thyroid gland, 204
Colon, 128
Conjunctiva, 224
Connective tissue, 16–31
  cell types, 13, 16, 17
  classification, 16
  dense, 16

Connective tissue *(Continued)*
  elastic, 30
  electron microscopy, 22
  embryonic, 30
  fibers, 17
  loose, 16
  mucous, 19
  organization, 16
    loose and dense, 16
  regular, 18
  reticular, 18
  staining, fibers, 17
Convoluted tubules, renal, 196, 197, 200, 202
Cornea, 264, 268, 270
Corpora amylacea, 260
Corpuscle(s), Hassall's, 134
  Malpighian *(see* Renal)
  Meissner's, 138, 140
  Pacinian, 140
  renal (Malpighian), 156, 196, 198, 200
Corpus luteum, 226
Crista ampullaris, 272
Cross striations, muscle, 69, 76, 78, 80
Crypts, of Lieberkuhn, 164, 166, 168, 174
  tonsilar, 122
Cumulus oophorus, 224
Cupula, 272
Cytoplasmic densities, smooth muscle, 118
Cytotrophoblast, 244

Decemet's membrane, 182
Decidual cells, 242
Demilunes, 108, 150, 152
Dendrite, 84, 94
Dental lamina, 154
Dental papilla, 154
Dental sac, 154
Dental tubule, 154
Dentin, 154
Dentino-enamel junction, 154
Dermis, 136, 138, 140
Desmosome, 14
Digestive system, 142–183
  glands, 142–143
Disse's space, 178
Duct, alveolar, 194
  cochlear, 274
  hepatic, 176, 178
  mammary gland, 236–240
  pancreatic, 182
  salivary, 150, 152
Ductless glands, 247–261

Ductus deferens, 216
Duodenum, 120, 122, 164, 166

Ear, basilar membrane, 274
  bony labyrinth, 272
  cochlea, 272, 274
  cupula, 272
  membranous labyrinth, 272
  organ of Corti, 272, 274
  reticular membrane, 274
  semicircular canal, 272
  spiral ganglion, 272, 274
  stapes, 272
  stria vascularis, 274
  tectorial membrane, 274
  vestibular membrane, 274
  vestibule, 272
Efferent ductules, 214
Elastic artery, 80
Elastic cartilage, 28
Elastic fibers, 17, 38
Elastic tissue, 18
Electron microscopy, 2
  cartilage, 36
  columnar epithelium, 12
  connective cells, 24
  connective tissue, 22
  cortical bone, 48
  developing bone, 56, 58
  lymph node, 126, 128
  osteoclast, 60
  perineurium, 100
  skeletal muscle, 78, 80
  smooth muscle, 72, 74
  sympathetic ganglion, 92, 94
Enamel, 154
Enamel organ, 154
  inner enamel epithelium, 154
  outer enamel epithelium, 154
  stellate reticulum, 154
  stratum intermedium, 154
Endocardium, 110
Endocrine glands, 247–261
Endometrium, 230
Endomysium, 76, 78
Endoneurium, 98, 100
Endoplasmic reticulum, granular, 24, 38, 56, 58, 60, 72, 94, 100
Endothelium, 4, 6, 108–119
  replacement, 6
Eosinophiles, 62, 66
Ependyma, 89
Epicardium, 110
Epidermis, 96, 136, 138, 140

Epididymis, 214
  stereocilia, 214
Epineurium, 98–100
Epiphyseal plate (disc), 36, 42, 50, 52
Epithelial cells, functions, 4
Epitheloid cells, 10
  testis, 212
  thymus, 134
Epithelium, 4–15
  classification of, 4
  columnar, 8, 12
  cuboidal, 8
  general description, 3
  glandular, 10
  pseudostratified columnar, 8
    ciliated, 8
  replacement of, 6
  simple squamous, 6
  stratified squamous, 6
  surface modifications, 4
  transitional 10, 204, 206
Erythrocytes, 62, 64
Esophagus, 156–159
Estrogen, 221
Eye, choroid, 264, 266
  ciliary body, 220, 224, 264, 268
  conjunctiva, 224, 268
  cornea, 220, 224, 226, 264, 268, 270
  iris, 220, 224, 226, 264, 268, 270
  lens, 264, 268, 270
  optic nerve, 264, 266
  retina, 264, 266
  sclera, 264, 268

Fascia adherens, 84
Fat cells, 17, 18
Fenestrated membranes, 30
Fiber(s), collagenous, 17, 18, 20, 22
  connective tissue, 16
  elastic, 17, 30, 42
  mossy, 104
  muscle, 68
  nerve, 90, 96, 98
  Purkinje, heart, 86
  reticular, 17, 18
    lymph nodes, 124
    spleen, 132
Fibroblast, 17, 18, 22, 24, 72
Fibrocartilage, 32, 44
Fibrocyte, 17
Filaments
  actin, 69, 72
  myosin, 69, 72
Filiform papillae, 144

Follicle(s), antral, 222
  atretic, 224
  Graafian, 224
  primordial ovarian, 222
  secondary ovarian, 224
  thyroid gland, 248
  unilaminar, 222
Fungiform papillae, 144

Gall bladder, 180
Ganglia, 89
Ganglion, capsule cell, 96
  cell, 90, 96
    lung, 192
    pancreas, 182
    small intestine, 170
  dorsal root, 96
  satellite cell, 96
  spiral, 272, 274
  supporting cells, 96
  sympathetic, 90
Gap junction, 74, 84
Gastric pits, 158, 160, 162
Germinal centers, lymph node, 124, 126
  spleen, 130
  tonsil, 122
Germinal epithelium, ovary, 222
Glands, adrenal, 256, 258
  Bowman's, 186
  Brunner's, 166
  cervical, 232
  development of, 3
  ductless, 247
  endocrine, 247–261
  exocrine, 247
  holocrine, 140
  of internal secretion, 247
  mucous, soft palate, 148
  parathyroid, 250
  parotid, 152
  pineal, 260
  pituitary, 252–254
  prostate, 218
  salivary, 150, 152
  sebaceous, 138, 140
  sero-mucous, soft palate, 148
  serous, tongue, 146
  sublingual, 152
  submandibular, 150
  sweat, 138, 140
  thymus, 134
  thyroid, 248
  uterine, 230
  van Ebner's 146

Glomerulus, 197
Glucagon, 182
Glycogen, 36, 38, 80
Glycosaminoglycans, 16, 32
Goblet cells, 8
Golgi apparatus, 58
Graafian follicle, 224
Granule(s), azurophilic, 64
    keratohyaline, 138
    secretory, 152
    zymogen, 152
Granulocytes, 62, 66
Granulosa lutein cells, 226
Ground substance, 16, 17, 32
    cartilage, 32
    connective tissue, 16, 17
    staining, 16, 17

H Band, 78, 80
Hair follicle, 138, 140
Hassall's corpuscles, 134
Haversian canal, 33
    electron microscopy, 48
Haversian systems, 32, 33, 46
Heart, endocardium, 110
    epicardium, 110
    myocardium, 110
    Purkinje fibers, 69, 86, 110
    subendocardial layer, 110
    subendothelial layer, 110
Henle's loop, 196, 202
Herring bodies, 210
Histocytes, 17
Hofbauer cells, 244
Howship's lacuna, 54
Hydroxyapatite crystals, 56, 60
Hypodermis, 136
Hypophysis cerebri (*see* Pituitary gland)

I Band, 78, 80
Ileum, 164
Integument (*see* Skin)
Intercellular bridges, 140, 146
Internal elastic membrane, 114, 116, 118
Interstitial cells of Leydig, 209, 212
Intestine, large, 172, 174
    small, 164
Iris, 264, 268, 270
Islets of Langerhans, 182

Jejunum, 164
Joint, developing, 40
Joint cavity, 40
Junction, gap, 74

Junctional complex, 12

Keratin, 138
Keratohyaline granules, 138
Kidney, 196–203
    calyx, 202
    collecting tubules, 200, 202
    convoluted tubules, 198, 200, 202
    cortex, 198
    cortical labyrinth, 198, 200
    Henle's loop, 202
    medulla, 198
    medullary rays, 198
    peritubular capillaries, 200
    pyramid(s), 198, 202
    renal (Malpighian) corpuscles, 198
    sinus, 202
Kupffer cells, 178

Lacteal, 168, 170
Lacunae (*see* Bone; Cartilage)
Lamina, basal, 3
    basement, 14
    reticular, 3
Lamina propria, 18, 120
    appendix, 172
    duodenum, 166
    esophagus, 156, 158
    large intestine, 174
    stomach, 158, 160, 162
    trachea, 190
Larynx, 188
Lens, 264, 268, 270
Leucocytes, 62
Leuteotropes, 254
Leuteotropic hormone (LH), 254
Leydig cells, 209, 212
Ligament(s), 28
    developing, 40
Light microscopy, 1
Lipid, 36
Lipofuchsin, 90
Liver, 176–179
    bile canaliculi, 178
    central veins, 176
    hepatic cells, 176, 178
    hepatic ducts, 178
    Kupffer cells, 178
    lobules, 176
    sinusoids, 176, 178
Lobule, liver, 176
Lungs, 185, 190, 192
Lymph node(s), 122, 124
    capsule, 122

Lymph nodes(s) *(Continued)*
  cortex, 122, 124
  cortical sinus, 122, 124, 126
  germinal center, 122, 124
  hilus, 122
  medulla, 122, 124
  medullary cords, 122
  medullary sinuses, 122
  reticular cells, 124, 126, 128
  stroma, 124, 128
  trabeculum, 124
Lymph nodule(s), 120
  lymph node, 122, 124
  small intestine, 164
  stomach, 158
  tonsil, 122
Lymphatic capillaries, 109
Lymphatic organs, 120
Lymphatic tissue, 120
  dense, 120
  diffuse, 120
  distribution, 120
Lymphatic vessels, 116
Lymphocytes, 120, 126, 128
  circulating, 62, 64
Lysosomes, 74

M Band, 78, 80, 84
Macrophages, 17, 18, 74, 121, 126
Macula adherens, 84
Macula densa, 200
Malpighian corpuscles, kidney, 196
  spleen, 130
Mammary gland, 236–241
  inactive, 236
  lactating, 240
  proliferative, 238
Mammotropes, 254
Mast cell, 17, 18
Matrix *(see* Bone; Cartilage)
Meckel's cartilage, 54
Medullary cavity, 50
Medullary ray, 198
Meissner's corpuscles, 138, 140
Meissner's plexus, 170
Melanocyte stimulating hormone (MSH),
    254
Membrana granulosa, 227
Membrane, basal, 3
  basement, 3
  basilar, 274
  Bruch's, 266
  fenestrated, elastic, 30, 118
  reticular, 274

  synovial, 40
  tectorial, 274
  vestibular, 274
Membranous labyrinth, 272
Mesenchyme, 16, 19
Mesentery, 164
Mesothelium, 4, 6
  replacement of, 6
  small intestine, 170
Microglia, 89
Microvilli, 12
Mineralization front, 56, 60
Modiolus, 272
Monocytes, 62, 64
Mucopolysaccharide, 32
Mucosa, appendix, 172
  cervical, 232
  duodenum, 166
  esophagus, 156, 158
  gall bladder, 180
  large intestine, 172
  nasal, 148
  olfactory, 186
  oral, 148
  small intestine, 164
  stomach, 158, 160
  tongue, 144
  trachea, 190
  ureter, 204
  urinary bladder, 206
  vaginal, 234
Mucous, connective tissue, 16, 19
Muller's cells, 266
Muscle, 68–87
  arrector pilli, 138
  cardiac, 69, 82, 86, 110
    cross striations, 82, 84
    fibers, 82, 84
    intercalated discs, 69, 82, 84
    myofibrils, 82
  cross striations, 69, 76, 78, 80
  fibers, 68, 69, 76, 78, 80, 82, 84
  myofibrils, 69
  myofilaments, 68, 69, 78, 84
  sarcolemma, 68, 69, 76
  skeletal, 68, 76, 78, 80
  smooth, 68, 70, 72, 74
    distribution, 68 *(see also* Muscularis;
        Muscularis externa; Muscularis
        mucosae)
    organization, 68, 70, 74
  striated, 69, 76–86
    Cohnheim's fields, 76
    cross striations, 69, 76–80

Muscle *(Continued)*
    developing, 30
    endomysium, 76, 78
    fibers, 68, 69, 76–80
    myofibrils, 69, 76–80
    sarcostyles, 76
  visceral, 68, 69
Muscularis, gall bladder, 180
  ureter, 204
  urinary bladder, 206
Muscularis externa, appendix, 172
  duodenum, 166
  esophagus, 156
  large intestine, 172
  small intestine, 164, 170
  stomach, 160, 162
Muscularis mucosae, appendix, 172
  duodenum, 166
  esophagus, 156
  large intestine, 174
  stomach, 160, 162
Myelin, 89, 92, 96, 98, 100
Myocardium, 110
Myoepithelial cells, 68, 140
  pigmented, 268
Myofibrils, 69, 76–82
  Purkinje fibers, heart, 86
Myofibrocyte, 22, 24, 68
Myofilaments, 68, 69, 78, 80, 84, 100
Myometrium, 230
Myosin filaments, 68, 69, 72, 78

Nerva vasorum, aorta, 112
Nerve(s), 98, 100
  endoneurium, 98, 100
  epineurium, 98, 100
  fibers, 88–106
  neurilemma (Schwann cell), 89, 92–100
  perineurium, 92, 98, 100
  sheath of Schwann *(see* Neurilemma)
Nervous system, 88–106
  divisions, 88, 89
  neuroglia, 88, 89, 102, 106
  node of Ranvier, 89
  organization, 88, 89
  Schwann cell *(see* Neurilemma)
Neurilemma (Schwann cell), 89, 92–100
Neuroglia, 88, 89, 102, 106
Neuron(s), 88
  in adrenal gland, 258
  in alimentary canal, 142, 160, 170, 172
  in bronchus, 192
  types
    amacrine cells, 266
    basket cells, 104
    bipolar cells of retina, 266
    Cajal, horizontal cells of, 102
    dorsal root, 96
    ganglion cells of retina, 266
    Golgi, type II, 104
    granule cells, 102
    horizontal cells of retina, 266
    Müller's cells, 266
    polymorphic cells, 102
    Purkinje cells, 104
    pyramidal cells, 102
    stellate cells, 102
    sympathetic ganglia, 90, 92, 94
    ventral (anterior) horn cells, 106
Neutrophils, 62, 66
Nexus, 74
Nissl bodies, 94, 106
Nodules [*see* Lymph Nodule(s)]

Odontoblasts, 154
Olfactory mucosa, 186
  basal cells, 186
  glands, 186
  lymphatic vessels, 186
  receptor cells, 186
  sustentacular cells, 186
Oligodendrocytes, 88
Oocyte, 222
Optic nerve, 264, 266
Organ of Corti, 272, 274
Osteoblasts, 50–58
Osteoclasia, 250
Osteoclasts, 54, 60
Osteocytes, 42, 52–56
Osteocytic osteolysis, 50, 250
Osteoid, 52–60
Osteons, 32, 33
  electron microscopy, 48
Ovary, 222–226
  atretic follicles, 222–224
  corpus luteum, 226
  cortex, 222
  cumulus oophorus, 224
  follicle cells, 222
  germinal epithelium, 222
  granulosa lutein cells, 226
  medulla, 222
  oocyte, 222
  primordial follicles, 222
  theca lutein cells, 226
  tunica albuginea, 222
  unilaminar, 222
  zona pellucida, 224

Oviduct, 228
Oxytocin, 254

Pacinian corpuscles, 137, 140
Palatine tonsils, 124
Pancreas, 182
Paneth cells, 170, 172
Papillae, dermal, 138
  tongue, 144, 146
Parathyroid gland, 250
  chief cells, 250
  oxyphil cells, 250
Parietal cells, 160
Parotid gland, 152
Perichondrium, 34, 36, 42
Pericytes, 109
Perikaryon, 88
Perineurium, 92, 98, 100
Periosteum, 50, 56
Peyers patches, 142, 164
Pia mater, cerebellum, 104
  spinal cord, 106
Pituicytes, 254
Pituitary gland, 252–255
  blood supply, 252
  cell types, 254
  divisions, 252
Placenta, 242, 244
Plasma cells, 18, 121, 168
Platelets, 62
Plexus, Auerbach's, 170
  Meissner's, 170
Plicae circulares, 164
Pneumocytes types, I and II, 194
Polysaccharides, 16
  sulfated, 32
Portal canal, 176
Portal system, 178
Portal triad, 178
Portal vein, 176, 178
Predentin, 154
Preosteoblast, 56
Progesterone, 221
Prostate gland, 218
Prostatic concretions, 218
Proteoglycans, 32
Purkinje cells, 104
Purkinje fibers, 69, 86, 110
Pyramidal cells, 102
Pyramids, renal, 198, 202

Ranvier, node of, 89
Red blood cells see Erythrocytes)
Renal corpuscles (Malpighian), 198, 200

Renal sinus, 202
Renin, 197
Reproductive system, female, 218–241
  male, 209–219
Respiratory system, 185–195
Rete testes, 212
Reticular cells, lymph nodes, 120, 124, 126,
    128
Reticular fibers, 17, 128
  lymph nodes, 124
  spleen, 132
Reticular membrane, 274
Reticular tissue, 16, 18
Reticulum, sarcoplasmic, 80, 84
Retina, 264, 266
Ribosomes, 94
Romanowsky type stains, 63
Ruffled border, 60

Sac, alveolar, 194
Salivary glands, 150–153
  ducts, 150–152
  excretory, 150–152
  intercalary, 150–152
  striated, 150–152
Sarcolemma, 69, 76
Sarcomere, 78
Sarcoplasmic reticulum, 80, 84
Sarcostyles, 76
Satellite cell, 92, 94
Scala tympani, 274
Scala vestibuli, 274
Schwann cell, 89, 92, 94, 100
Sclera, 264, 268
Sebaceous glands, 138, 140
Semicircular canal, 272
Seminal vesicle, 216
Seminiferous tubules, 209, 210
Septal cell, 196
Serosa, appendix, 172
  large intestine, 172
  small intestine, 164, 170
  stomach, 160
  urinary bladder, 206
Serous glands, tongue, 146
Sertoli cells, 210
Sheath of Schwann, 89
Sinus, cortical, 124, 126
  renal, 202
  venous, spleen, 132
Sinusoids, 109
  liver, 134
Skeletal muscle, 68
Skeleton, fetal, 40

Skin, 136–141
  glands, 136–140
  organization of, 136
  receptors, 136, 140
  stratum corneum, 138
  stratum germinativum, 138
  stratum granulosum, 138
  stratum lucidum, 138
Smooth muscle, 68, 72, 74
  cytoplasmic densities, 100, 118
Soft palate, 148
Somatomammotropin, 221
Somatotropes, 254
Somatotropic hormone, 254
Space of Disse, 178
Sperm, 210
Spermatids, 210
Spermatocytes, primary, 210
  secondary, 210
Spermatogenesis, 210
Spermatogonia, 210
Spinal cord, anterior horn cells, 106
  neurological cells, 106
  neuropil, 106
  pia mater, 106
Spiral ganglia, 272, 274
Spleen, 130–132
  Billroth's cords, 130, 132
  capsule, 130, 132
  central artery, 130, 132
  circulation, 132
  germinal centers, 130
  red pulp, 130, 132
  reticular stroma, 132
  trabecula, 130, 132
  venous sinuses, 130, 132
  white pulp, 130, 132
Splenic nodules, 130
Spongy bone, 32, 33, 42
Stains,
  Romanowsky type, 63
  H & E, 1
Stapes, ear, 272
Stereocilia, 8
  ductus deferens, 216
  epididymis, 214
Stomach, 119, 158–162
  cardiac glands, 158–162
  fundic glands, 158–162
  glands, 158–162
  mamillated areas, 160
  pyloric glands, 158, 162
  pyloric region, 162
Straight tubules, 212

Stratum basalis, 230
Stratum corneum, 138
Stratum functionalis, 230
Stratum germinativum, 138
Stratum granulosum, 138
Stratum lucidum, 138
Stria vascularis, 274
Striated border, 8
  gall bladder, 180
  large intestine, 174
  osteoclasts, 54
  placenta, 244
  small intestine, 168
Striated muscle, visceral, 69
Striations, cross, 69, 76, 78, 82
Sublingual glands, 152
Submandibular glands, 150
Submucosa, appendix, 172
  duodenum, 166
  esophagus, 156
  large intestine, 172
  small intestine, 164
  stomach, 160, 162
  trachea, 190
Supporting tissue, 32–54
Surfactant, 194
Sustentacular cells, testis, 210
Sweat glands, 138, 140
Synapse, 88
Synapse, axodendritic, 94
  axosomatic, 94
Synaptic vesicles, 94
Syncytial trophoblast, 244

T tubule (system), 80
Taste buds, 144, 146
Tectorial membrane, 274
Tela subcutanea, 136
Tendon, 28
Terminal bars, 8
  web, 14
Testis, 210, 212
  interstitial cells, 212
  Leydig cells, 209, 212
  rete testis, 212
  seminiferous tubules, 210
  straight tubules, 212
  testosterone, 212
  undescended, 212
Theca externa, 224
  interna, 224
Theca lutein cells, 226
Thrombocytes, 62
Thymocytes, 134

Thymus, epitheloid (epithelio-reticular) cells, 134
  gland, 134
  gland cortex, 134
    involution, 134
    lobes, 134
    medulla, 134
Thyrocalcitonin, 248
Thyroid gland, 248
  colloid, 248
  follicles, 248
Thyroid stimulating hormone (TSH), 254
Tongue, 144–146
  filiform papillae, 144
  fungiform papillae, 144
  vallate papillae, 144
Tonofilaments, 84
Tonsil, 122
  crypts, 122
  epithelium, 122
  germinal center, 122
  lingual, 188
  lymph nodules, 122
  palatine, 122
Tooth, developing, 154
Tooth germ, 154
Trachea, 190
  basement membrane, 190
  glands, 190
  hyaline cartilage, 190
Triad, 80
Trophoblast, 244
Tube, uterine, 228
Tubules, convoluted, 198–202
  seminiferous, 209, 210
Tunica adventitia, 114
  aorta, 112
  arteriole, electron microscopy, 118
Tunica albuginea, ovary, 222
  testis, 210
Tunica intima, 114
  aorta, 112
  arteriole, electron microscopy, 118
Tunica media, 114
  aorta, 112
  arteriole, electron microscopy, 118

Umbilical arteries and vein, 242
Umbilical cord, 30, 242
Ureter(s), 204
  transitional epithelium, 204
Urinary bladder, 206
  transitional epithelium, 206

Urinary system, 196–206
Uterine tube, 228
  peg cells, 228
Uterus, 230
  decidual cells, 230
  endometrium, 230
  myometrium, 230
  stratum basalis, 230
  stratum functionalis, 230
Uvea, 264

Vagina, 234
Valves of Kerckring, 164
Valvulae conniventes, 164
Vasa vasorum, aorta, 112
Vasopressin, 254
Vein, 109
Vein(s), 114
  central, liver, 176
  hepatic, 176, 178
  portal, 176, 178
  umbilical, 242
Venous sinuses, spleen, 130
Venules, 109
Vesicle, seminal, 216
Vestibular membrane, 274
Vestibule, ear, 272
Villi, 168, 179
  absorptive cells, 168
  basement membrane, 168
  chorionic, 242, 244
  endothelial cells, 168
  goblet cells, 168
  lacteal, 168
  lamina propria, 168
  lymphocytes, 168
  smooth muscle cells, 168
  striated border, 168
Visceral striated muscle, 69
Vocal folds, 188
Volkmanns canals, 46
Von Ebner's glands, 146

White blood cells (*see* Leucocytes)
White matter, cerebrum, 102
  spinal cord, 106

Z line, 78, 80, 84
Zona fasciculata, adrenal gland, 256–258
Zona glomerulosa, adrenal gland, 256
Zona pellucida, 224
Zona reticularis, adrenal gland, 258
Zonula adherens, 14
Zonula occludens, 14

76 77 78 79 80 9 8 7 6 5 4 3 2 1